....
Aging and the Gastrointestinal Tract

Interdisciplinary Topics in Gerontology

Vol. 32

KARGER

Aging and the Gastrointestinal Tract

Volume Editors
Alberto Pilotto, San Giovanni Rotondo
Peter Malfertheiner, Magdeburg
Peter R. Holt, New York, N.Y.

20 figures and 20 tables, 2003

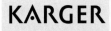

Basel · Freiburg · Paris · London · New York ·
Bangalore · Bangkok · Singapore · Tokyo · Sydney

· ·

Alberto Pilotto, MD

Geriatric Unit,
'Casa Sollievo della Sofferenza' Hospital,
IRCCS, San Giovanni Rotondo, Italy

Peter Malfertheiner, MD

Department of Gastroenterology,
Hepatology and Infectious Diseases,
Otto-von-Guericke
University of Magdeburg, Germany

Peter R. Holt, MD

St. Luke's Hospital Center, and
Institute for Cancer Prevention
New York, N.Y., USA

Library of Congress Cataloging-in-Publication Data

Aging and the gastrointestinal tract / volume editors, Alberto Pilotto, Peter Malfertheiner,
    Peter R. Holt.
        p. ; cm. – (Interdisciplinary topics in gerontology, ISSN 0074–1132 ; v. 32)
        Includes bibliographical references and index.
        ISBN 3–8055–7555–6 (hard cover : alk. paper)
            1. Geriatric gastroenterology. 2. Gastrointestinal system–Diseases–Age factors. I.
        Pilotto, A. II. Malfertheiner, P. (Peter), 1950– III. Holt, Peter R. IV. Series.
            [DNLM: 1. Gastrointestinal Diseases–Aged. 2. Aging–physiology. 3. Gastrointestinal
        System–Aged. WI 140 A267 2003]
        RC802.4.A34A35 2003
        618.97′633–dc21

                                                                                    2003040047

Bibliographic Indices. This publication is listed in bibliographic services.

Drug Dosage. The authors and the publisher have exerted every effort to ensure that drug selection and dosage set forth in this text are in accord with current recommendations and practice at the time of publication. However, in view of ongoing research, changes in government regulations, and the constant flow of information relating to drug therapy and drug reactions, the reader is urged to check the package insert for each drug for any change in indications and dosage and for added warnings and precautions. This is particularly important when the recommended agent is a new and/or infrequently employed drug.

© Copyright 2003 by S. Karger AG, P.O. Box, CH–4009 Basel (Switzerland)
www.karger.com
Printed in Switzerland on acid-free paper by Reinhardt Druck, Basel
ISSN 0074–1132
ISBN 3–8055–7555–6

Contents

Preface

With the dramatic increase in the aging population, the study and care of gastrointestinal disorders in the elderly have become priority topics for both clinicians and researchers.

Little attention was focused on the gastrointestinal tract of the elderly until very recently. In the last few years, however, the medical literature has provided more studies on the changes that occur in gastrointestinal physiology as a function of advanced age, as well as on gastrointestinal diseases associated with aging.

The aim of this book is to assemble in one place the results of the more recent studies in geriatric gastroenterology and to review both basic research and clinical aspects of this field. The book explores selected subjects of wide interest. The geriatric approach to gastrointestinal disorders includes the epidemiology of gastrointestinal disorders in the elderly and the effect of aging on the pharmacokinetics of gastrointestinal drugs, as well as a comprehensive clinical assessment of older patients with gastrointestinal disorders. A comprehensive multidimensional assessment is particularly important in managing older patients with chronic and disabling illnesses, such as gastrointestinal disorders, since these patients are likely to have multiple interacting problems that interfere with their daily function and complicate their treatment. For example, an older patient who presents with a common gastrointestinal problem such as peptic ulcer or chronic diarrhea typically has a multitude of other age-related disorders that can complicate diagnostic and therapeutic options. These clinical situations are particularly suited to a comprehensive geriatric assessment approach.

The effect of aging upon the physiology of the gastrointestinal tract is a crucial area for geriatric gastroenterology. Since the elderly patient may present with particularly unique variables, such as altered visceral function, which can impact profoundly on the presentation, diagnosis and treatment of disease, a deeper understanding of these variables is critical in order to provide optimal diagnostic modalities and design specific treatment care plans for elderly individuals. A section of the book is devoted to closely examining the structural and functional effects of aging on the physiology of the esophagus and stomach, small intestine and colon, liver and pancreas, focusing on distinctive features as they relate to pathophysiology as well as diagnostic and treatment modalities that are particularly relevant to the elderly population.

A significant component of this book is devoted to identifying the physician's clinical approach to the elderly with gastroenterological problems. Recent advances in diagnostic tools and treatments of elderly patients with dysphagia and gastroesophageal reflux disease, as well as with nonsteroidal antiinflammatory drug-related or *Helicobacter pylori*-associated gastroduodenal diseases, are reported in updated chapters. Moreover, the physician's approach to the management of disorders of the small intestine, colon, pancreas and liver is discussed, highlighting the specific aspects of such disorders in old age. Colon cancer, the scourge of the aged as a cause of gastrointestinal-related deaths in the older patient, is discussed in depth.

Diagnostic testing becomes very important in the elderly since clinical features such as history and physical signs are frequently most difficult to interpret in older individuals. There is no evidence that the risk of performing invasive diagnostic tests such as endoscopy of the upper or lower gastrointestinal tract is greater in the elderly than in the young. Clearly both the course and the therapy of a disease may be altered in an older individual. Indeed, very frequently, clinical manifestations and the response to therapy may appear to differ because the older patient has several concomitant disorders that may distort the classic features of the primary gastrointestinal disease. Due to these multidimensional aspects of the elderly subject, the process of geriatric assessment often requires the involvement of a multidisciplinary team with experienced specialists as well as primary care physicians and/or community health workers focused on identifying functional problems and disabilities of older persons.

We hope that this book will be useful for general physicians, specialists in geriatrics and gastroenterology and all health care providers who are involved in planning the care and management of elderly people with gastrointestinal disorders.

Alberto Pilotto
Peter R. Holt
Peter Malfertheiner

Pilotto A, Malfertheiner P, Holt PR (eds): Aging and the Gastrointestinal Tract.
Interdiscipl Top Gerontol. Basel, Karger, 2003, vol 32, pp 1–11

······················

Epidemiology of Gastrointestinal Disorders in the Elderly

Carla Destro, Stefania Maggi, Gaetano Crepaldi

Aging Section, Institute of Neuroscience, National Research Council, Padua, Italy

Introduction

With the marked increase in the population aged 65 years and over, the study and care of gastrointestinal disorders should be a high priority for both clinicians and researchers.

Over the years, geriatricians and gastroenterologists have speculated that the functioning of the gastrointestinal tract may decline with aging. It was thought that the efficiency of digestion and absorption declines with aging. Once this hypothesis was rigorously tested, however, it was found not to be true [1].

Gastrointestinal diseases are frequent in older patients and their presentation, complications and treatment may be different from those in younger patients. Oesophagus-stomach and colon-rectum disorders have higher prevalence rates than small intestine, liver and pancreas disorders, although few studies have been carried out in the general population [2].

The aim of this review is to summarize recent data and the current thinking of clinicians and researchers on the epidemiology of gastrointestinal disorders in the elderly.

Disorders of the Upper Gastrointestinal Tract

The two most significant oral diseases in older people are root caries and periodontal disease. The World Health Organization has a global oral data bank that includes epidemiological studies from 1986 to 1996 on non-institutionalized

European adults aged 65–74 years. Results revealed that 12.8–69.6% of subjects were edentulous, the mean number of teeth ranged from 15.1 to 3.8 and the decayed, missing and filled teeth index ranged from 22.2 to 30.2. This wide range in scores suggests that oral health policies need to be developed and implemented, taking into consideration geographical and socio-economic differences in populations.

Dysphagia, i.e. the inability to swallow or difficulty in swallowing solid and/or liquid meals, increases with advancing years. European surveys suggested that up to 10% of people over 50 years of age experience some difficulty with swallowing [3], and a study of people in long-term care found that the prevalence of under-nutrition was close to 50% and was significantly associated with eating and swallowing problems [4]. The causes of dysphagia in older people are mostly associated with cerebrovascular and neurological diseases, including Parkinson's disease, motor neuronal disease, myasthenia gravis and Alzheimer's disease.

Dyspepsia, i.e. the presence of episodic or persistent pain or discomfort localized to the epigastrium or upper abdomen [5], is a very common syndrome. In the United States, about 25% of people report recurrent epigastric discomfort that occurs at least once a year. At least 10% of these persons seek medical care. Dyspepsia is the primary complaint of approximately 5% of all patients who visit their family physician [6]. An American survey of a randomly selected community sample of 1,120 people aged from 34 to 64 years identified a prevalence of upper abdominal pain within the preceding year of 25.8%; a subgroup of reflux-like dyspepsia was identified in 9.4%. One third of dyspeptics also had irritable bowel symptoms [7]. Community surveys in the United Kingdom [8] show that over one third of people reported dyspepsia within the previous 6 months, with the frequency appearing to fall with age (24% of women and 15% of men aged over 80). About half of the people with dyspepsia reported both heartburn and upper abdominal pain. Only one in four had consulted their general practitioner, with consultation rates increasing with age.

Gastroesophageal reflux disease (GERD) appears to be more common in the elderly than in younger persons, possible because of a reduction in the intra-abdominal length of the lower oesophageal sphincter and an increased incidence of hiatus hernia. The prevalence and incidence of GERD are not accurately known. Estimates vary depending upon whether studies have examined reported symptoms or used investigational methods. Study has been hampered by a lack of methodologically rigorous studies using validated survey instruments in truly random community samples, as well as the lack of a gold-standard disease definition. GERD defined as heartburn is extremely common; 44% of adult Americans surveyed by the Gallup Organization experienced it monthly. Recent work based on an age- and sex-stratified random sample of 2,200 residents of

Olmsted County, Minnesota, USA, aged 25–74 years incorporated a valid and reliable self-report questionnaire. The overall age- and sex-adjusted prevalence of any episode of heartburn in the preceding year was 42.4% [95% confidence interval (CI) 39.8–45.1%]. The proportion with frequent (weekly) heartburn was 17.8% (95% CI 15.8–19.9%). The prevalence of yearly and weekly acid regurgitation was 45% (95% CI 42.3–47.7%) and 6.3% (95% CI 5.0–7.6%), respectively. The overall prevalence of GERD (defined as either heartburn or acid regurgitation) in the preceding year was 58.7% (95% CI 56.1–61.3%), and for weekly episodes, it was 19.8% (95% CI 17.7–21.9%). There were no overall significant differences with respect to age or sex for GERD, although heartburn was inversely associated with age [9].

Given that the prevalence of hiatus hernia and oesophageal dysfunction increases with age [10], GERD may be thought to be more common in older people. A population-based random sample of 600 non-institutionalized Finnish subjects aged 65 years or over suggested an overall prevalence of at least monthly GERD (heartburn or regurgitation) of 53.5% in men and 66.2% in women [11].

Severe oesophagitis is much more common in patients beyond the age of 65 than in young people. The magnitude of the symptoms does not correlate well with the severity of mucosal disease, and so, very severe oesophagitis may be associated with a relative paucity of symptoms. Manifestations of GERD are thus more likely to be late-stage complications such as bleeding from a haemorrhagic oesophagitis, dysphagia from a peptic structure or adenocarcinoma associated with Barrett's oesophagus. GERD-induced chest pain may mimic, or occur concomitantly with, cardiac disease.

Oesophageal carcinoma is a problem of advancing years, as most patients are over 65 years of age. Cancers of the middle and lower third of the oesophagus are most common. There is considerable geographic variation in this disease, suggesting that environmental factors are important. The highest annual incidence rates, exceeding 100 per 100,000, are reported in Iran, China and parts of Russia, whereas in Western Europe and among white Americans, rates are under 10 per 100,000. Several important risk factors for squamous cell carcinoma are recognized, including smoking, alcohol, chronic thermal injury, achalasia, nitrosamines, the Plummer-Vinson syndrome and diet. An estimated 0.2–2.0% of patients with Barrett's oesophagus eventually develop oesophageal adenocarcinoma. Because the prevalence of Barrett's oesophagus is higher in patients with GERD than without GERD, a possible causal relationship between GERD and oesophageal adenocarcinoma is suggested [12].

Drugs and the oesophagus is an important topic in older people since approximately half of adverse drug reactions affecting the oesophagus occur in patients aged over 65. Drugs damage the oesophagus either directly by local contact, i.e. aspirin, non-steroidal anti-inflammatory drugs (NSAIDs), corticosteroids, alendronate, potassium and ferrous salts, or as a result of a reduction of the lower oesophageal sphincter pressure, i.e. dopaminergics, nitrates, theophylline, benzodiazepines and tricyclic antidepressants.

Recent studies have demonstrated that acid and peptic gastric secretion do not decline with age [13, 14]. In contrast, evidence indicates that aging is associated with a lower capacity of the gastric mucosae to resist damage, even in healthy persons. Indeed, many factors involved in cytoprotection, such as mucosal blood flow and gastric mucosal prostaglandin, glutathione, bicarbonate and mucus secretion, decline with age. These changes may account for the impaired barrier function of the gastric mucosa and the increased risk of peptic ulcer disease in the elderly, particularly in association with the use of NSAIDs. Aging is associated with a modest slowing of gastric emptying, which may predispose subjects to anorexia and weight loss by prolonging gastric distension and increasing meal-induced fullness and satiety.

Non-erosive gastritis is a histological entity that is common in the general population and is associated with advanced age. It is now accepted that *Helicobacter pylori* infection is the cause of approximately 80% of cases of non-erosive gastritis, which may progress to peptic ulcer disease. Gastritis is present in almost all patients with duodenal ulcer and nearly 80% of patients with gastric ulcer [15].

During the last 3 decades, the incidence of peptic ulcer and, concomitantly, its associated complications and mortality, has increased in the elderly. Complications occur in about 50% of patients aged over 70 years. The high mortality rate (up to 30%) may relate to the presence of co-morbidity [16].

H. pylori infection in patients with peptic ulcer aged over 65 years has been reported to range from 58 to 78%. However, in one study of elderly patients hospitalized for ulcer disease, the rate of diagnostic screening for *H. pylori* was less than 60%, and only 50–73% of patients who had a positive *H. pylori* test were treated with antibiotics [17].

Recent studies have shown that NSAID gastropathy and its life-threatening complications occur primarily in elderly patients [18]. Although increased NSAID use by elderly people is an obvious risk factor, epidemiological data suggest that aging itself is an independent risk factor for the development of NSAID gastropathy and its complications [19]. Patients who have had peptic ulcers or ulcer complications in the past are more likely to develop NSAID gastropathy. Other risk factors for upper gastrointestinal lesions are high dosages of NSAIDs and the concomitant use of more than one NSAID or corticosteroids, aspirin and warfarin [20]. In particular, an *H. pylori*-positive patient receiving aspirin or NSAID treatment should be carefully asked about any upper abdominal complaints she/he might have [21, 22].

Complications occur in about 50% of elderly patients with peptic ulcers. The most common complication is bleeding, which occurs in about 10–15% of ulcer patients of all ages, yet most frequently in elderly patients. About 10–20% of patients with bleeding ulcers do not have preceding symptoms. The mortality rate in elderly patients with bleeding ulcers is estimated to be 29–60%. Perforation occurs in about 5–10% of ulcer patients and is more frequent in duodenal ulcers. The risk is increased by the use of NSAIDs. Although most elderly patients with perforated ulcers report abdominal discomfort, about 16% have minimal pain [23].

Acute upper gastrointestinal haemorrhage constitutes a significant fraction of acute general medical admissions and an increasing proportion of these patients are elderly. Age is an independent risk factor for gastrointestinal bleeding, with the annual incidence of haematemesis or melaena in patients over 75 being 10 times that of those aged less than 44. The reasons for this are not clear, but almost certainly comprise a complex mix of risk factors, including the use of NSAIDs and the presence of significant co-morbidity resulting in a previous hospital admission [24].

The rate of benign gastric tumours increases with age. Hyperplastic polyps account for 75–90% of such growths and typically are small, solitary lesions that are not considered pre-malignant. They rarely produce symptoms and thus may be found incidentally during an evaluation of the upper gastrointestinal tract. In contrast, adenomatous polyps are true neoplasms and account for 10–25% of benign gastric tumours, which probably reflects their heterogeneity in size, age and histology.

Gastric cancer (primarily adenocarcinoma) is the second most common cancer worldwide. Its incidence has been declining in the United States, but it still causes approximately 6 deaths per 100,000, or 14,000 deaths annually [25]. Its incidence also increases with advancing age. Gastric cancer presents most frequently in the sixth decade of life, and men are affected twice as often as women. Implicated aetiological factors include habitual ingestion of smoked foods, foods with high salt contents, increased uses of nitrites, various vitamin deficiencies, carcinogens such as aflatoxin and the development of atrophic gastritis with achlorhydria.

Liver Disorders

Several studies suggest that a significant proportion of patients with alcoholic liver disease not only present in old age but also are more likely to have severe disease at the time of diagnosis. In a British study, 28% of patients were diagnosed for the first time when over 60 years of age [26]. In France, a large retrospective study found that 20% of patients were over the age of 70 years. In the United States, one study among white males showed that the seventh decade was the peak for presentation with cirrhosis. Prognosis is related to age. In one study, mortality among those less than 60 years old at presentation was 5% at 1 year and 24% at 3 years, whereas mortality among those presenting at over 70 years of age was 75% at 1 year and 90% at 3 years [27].

Adverse drug reactions are reported to occur more frequently in older than in younger people. Drug consumption rises with age, and it is therefore possible that much of the increased incidence of adverse drug reactions in later life is secondary to high drug consumption and polypharmacy. Primary biliary cirrhosis is found above all in middle-aged and older women. The average age at presentation is 55–60 years, but about 25% of patients present with this disease when over 65 years of age [28]. Its prevalence rate in women over 50 was found to be 1 in 1,500 in parts of Europe. In developed countries, primary hepatocarcinoma is predominantly a disease of older people, with more than 50% of patients being over 60 years of age and more than 40% over 70 years of age at presentation. It is usually associated with cirrhosis, regardless of the underlying cause, and it is probable that the length of time for which an individual has had cirrhosis is an important determinant factor [28].

Pancreatic Disorders

Pancreatic disease is a common cause of morbidity and mortality in older persons. Acute gallstones, pancreatitis and pancreatic cancer are responsible for the great majority of pancreatic disease. As the numbers of elderly continue to increase, pancreatic disease will become even more common. Acute pancreatitis is responsible for 5–7% of cases of acute abdominal pain in older persons. The most important causes are ethanol consumption, gallstones and obesity. Drugs are another important cause of pancreatitis in elderly patients, among whom multiple-drug use is common. The mechanism of drug-induced pancreatitis is not well understood, as the association is often weak and rechallenge is usually contraindicated. Cardiovascular disease, common in older persons, may cause ischaemic injury to the pancreas. Pancreatic carcinoma can present as acute pancreatitis at any age, and it is the cause in 1–3% of cases of the latter condition. Despite this low frequency, there is a relatively high risk of pancreatic cancer in the elderly.

Alcohol is the most common cause of chronic pancreatitis and is responsible for 70–80% of cases. As alcohol consumption varies widely among nations, the incidence of chronic pancreatitis is also highly variable. Idiopathic causes of chronic pancreatitis are the second most common aetiology (20%).

Others include hypertriglyceridaemia, hyperparathyroidism, drug therapy, biliary stones, hereditary pancreatitis and obstruction or disruption of the main pancreatic duct. The aging process itself seems to be a risk factor for chronic pancreatitis in developed countries [29].

Carcinoma of the pancreas is the fifth leading cause of cancer death in the industrialized world. Age is a major risk factor, with three quarters of all pancreatic cancers occurring in patients over the age of 60. Other risk factors for pancreatic cancer include diabetes, cigarette smoking and chronic pancreatitis. Ninety percent of pancreatic tumours arise from the exocrine pancreas, while islet cell tumours, neuroendocrine tumours, sarcomas and primary lymphoma of the pancreas are rare. Ductal pancreatic adenocarcinomas, which are responsible for more than 90% of exocrine pancreatic tumours, are typically a disease of the elderly patient [29].

Gallbladder Disorders

Gallstones are three times more common in women than in men and are more prevalent with increasing age. One in 5 women and 1 in 10 men above the age of 55 have gallstones. The prevalence of cholelithiasis increases with age, and by 70 years, around 30% of women and 19% of men have gallstones [30]. Most are asymptomatic, but some subjects will develop biliary pain and complications. An epidemiologic study carried out in Italian subjects over 60 years of age demonstrated that gallstones were present in 13.9% of the participants, while 12.8% had had a cholecystectomy; the overall prevalence of gallstone disease was 26.7% [31]. Risk factors for the development of cholesterol gallstones include female gender, pregnancy, the use of contraceptives, obesity and rapid weight loss.

Carcinoma of the gallbladder is a disease of old age, with the majority of patients being 70 years of age or over at presentation. Although this carcinoma is usually associated with gallstones, it is not clear whether the relationship is significant. The neoplasm is four times more common in women than in men [32].

Lower Gastrointestinal Tract

Aging has minor effects on the structure of the small intestine, with some alteration in villus architecture and a reduction in the neuronal content of the mesenteric plexus. Aging does not result in major changes in small intestine motility, transit, permeability or absorption.

Bleeding from the small intestine is an important cause of morbidity and mortality in older persons, particularly caused by NSAID use and angiodysplasia.

Constipation is more common in elderly persons than in middle-aged persons. In the United States, the prevalence of constipation in people aged over 60 years of age ranges from 4 to 50%. The wide range in prevalence data is in part attributable to how constipation is defined in a given study. The most widely accepted definition is the passage of less than two bowel movements per week. Constipation is a symptom that can arise as a result of dietary factors, functional abnormalities, perceptual factors, neuromuscular disease, metabolic disease, obstructing lesions or iatrogenic causes. Constipation is one of the most common gastrointestinal complaints in the elderly, with up to 60% of elderly outpatients reporting laxative use. The overall prevalence of self-reported constipation is 24–37%, with women reporting constipation more often than men. In the institutionalized elderly, up to 50% self-report constipation and up to 74% use laxatives daily [33].

In the elderly, the risk of diarrhoea increases due to diminished physiological reserves, the burden of acute or chronic multisystem illness, under-nutrition, general debility and cognitive impairment. Diarrhoea is also relevant in the elderly as it is an important cause of morbidity and mortality. Older patients may not admit having chronic diarrhoea, particularly if they are also incontinent. Institutionalised elderly are particularly prone to gastrointestinal infections, but the manifestations may not be overt [34].

Faecal incontinence affects quality of life and causes caregiver strain. Among older people in the United Kingdom who live at home, the prevalence of faecal incontinence is estimated to be between 2 and 6%, while the prevalence among people who live in nursing homes is estimated to be between 4 and 30%. Sufferers are often reluctant to seek help because of embarrassment and a perceived lack of effective treatment. Consequently, underestimation of its prevalence is well recognized. Co-morbidities, such as stroke, dementia and limited physical ability, can contribute to an increased risk of faecal incontinence. Other aetiological factors include anorectal pathology, sphincter or pelvic floor damage, inflammatory bowel syndrome, irritable bowel syndrome, neurological diseases, faecal impaction with overflow, poor toilet facilities or inadequate care. Faecal incontinence occurs more frequently among women, and it is associated with symptoms of anxiety, depression and disability [35].

The risk of developing diverticula of the colon increases with age [36]. In Western countries, diverticular disease occurs in about 50% of persons greater than 65 years of age and in about 65% of those greater than 80 years of age. Diarrhoea can be a consequence of diverticulitis when acute or chronic inflammation due to a mechanical obstruction within the diverticula occurs [37]. Diverticulosis is the most common cause of massive lower gastrointestinal bleeding in older persons [38]. Diverticular haemorrhage accounts for up to 25% of all complications in patients with diverticulosis. Overall, 3–5% of patients with diverticulosis will develop significant gastrointestinal bleeding, 70% of which occurs in the right colon and involves a single non-inflamed diverticulum. The presence of diverticular haemorrhage and diverticulitis are nearly mutually exclusive, with fewer than 5% having both processes simultaneously. The most common complication of diverticulosis is diverticulitis, which occurs in 10–20% of patients. It results from inflammation and increases the risk of subsequent perforation of a colonic diverticulum. Mild forms of diverticulitis usually present with gradually increasing symptoms from the lower left quadrant of the abdomen, whereas acute complicated disease is characterized by a dramatic onset of abdominal pain, followed by fever within a few hours [39].

Ischaemic colitis occurs almost exclusively in the elderly, as a result of the increased prevalence of atherosclerosis. When patients with iatrogenic causes, including surgical procedures and drugs, are excluded, more than 90% of patients are over 60 years of age. In the gastrointestinal tract, the colon is the part most frequently injured by ischaemia. This occurs in association with other pathologies characteristic in the elderly, including polycythaemia, diabetes mellitus, arteritis and digitalis preparations. Patients usually present with cramping, abdominal pain, faecal urgency and/or haematochezia.

Irritable bowel syndrome refers to a heterogeneous group of disorders in which the patient complains of abdominal pain and unstable bowel habits. Overall, 10–15% of the population of the United States has symptoms compatible with the diagnosis of irritable bowel syndrome, although only a minority seek medical attention [37].

Cancer of the colon or rectum is the most common malignancy of the gastrointestinal tract in older persons. It varies widely in frequency in different parts of the world, occurring much more commonly in North America, north-western Europe and New Zealand than in South America, south-western Asia, equatorial Africa and India. Colorectal cancer mortality is 44% higher for men than for women. The incidence rises sharply after the age of 50, with two thirds of all patients being over 50. The mean age at diagnosis is 62 years. Multiple epidemiologic studies have shown that rates of colorectal cancer are highest in countries with diets high in fat and calories but low in fibre. Up to half of colorectal cancer cases may be related to diet. Estimates suggest that 15–25% of colorectal cancer cases may be related to high fat intake and that 25–35% may be related to low intake of fruits and vegetables. An estimated 32% of colorectal cancer cases may be related to physical inactivity [25]. The importance of dietary factors has been shown in studies of immigrants. Japanese subjects who had immigrated to the United States acquired a higher incidence of colorectal cancer with each subsequent generation, with the incidence in the third generation similar to that of native-born Americans [40].

References

1   Bharucha AE, Camilleri M: Functional abdominal pain in the elderly. Gastroenterol Clin North Am 2001;30:517–529.
2   Russell RM: The aging process as a modifier of metabolism. Am J Clin Nutr 2000;72 (2 suppl):529S–532S.
3   Lindgren S, Janzon L: Prevalence of swallowing complaints and clinical findings among 50–79-year old men and women in an urban population. Dysphagia 1991;6:187–192.
4   Keller H: Malnutrition in institutionalized elderly: How and why? J Am Geriatr Soc 1993;41: 1212–1218.
5   Drossman DA, Funch-Jensen P, Janssens J: Identification of subgroups of functional bowel disorders. Gastroenterol Intern 1990;3:159–172.
6   Talley NJ, Phillips SF, Melton LJ 3rd, Wiltgen C, Zinsmeister AR: A patient questionnaire to identify bowel disease. Ann Intern Med 1989;111:671–674.
7   Talley NJ, Zinsmeister AR, Schleck CD, Melton LJ 3rd: Dyspepsia and dyspepsia subgroups: A population-based study. Gastroenterology 1992;102:1259–1268.
8   Jones R, Lydeard S: Prevalence of symptoms of dyspepsia in the community. BMJ 1989;298: 30–32.
9   Locke GR 3rd, Talley NJ, Fett SL, Zinsmeister AR, Melton LJ 3rd: Prevalence and clinical spectrum of gastroesophageal reflux: A population-based study in Olmsted Country, Minnesota. Gastroenterology 1997;112:1488–1456.
10 Cameron AJ: Barrett's esophagus: Prevalence and size of hiatal hernia. Am J Gastroenterol 1999; 94:2054–2059.
11 Raiha IJ, Hietanen E, Sourander LB: Symptoms of gastroesophageal reflux in elderly people. Age Ageing 1991;20:365–370.
12 Blot WJ, Devesa SS, Fraumeni JF Jr: Continuing climb in rates of esophageal adenocarcinoma: An update. JAMA 1993;270:1320–1324.
13 Pilotto A, Vianello F, Di Mario F, Plebani M, Farinati F, Azzini CF: Effect of age on gastric acid, pepsin, pepsinogen group A and gastrin secretion in peptic ulcer patients. Gerontology 1994; 40:253–259.
14 Guslandi M, Pellegrini A, Sorghi M: Gastric mucosal defences in the elderly. Gerontology 1999; 45:206–208.
15 Peek RM, Blaser MJ: Pathophysiology of *Helicobacter pylori*-induced gastritis and peptic ulcer disease. Am J Med 1996;102:200–207.
16 Seinela L, Ahvenainen J: Peptic ulcer in the very old patients. Gerontology 2000;46:271–275.
17 Pilotto A: *Helicobacter pylori*-associated peptic ulcer disease in older patients. Current management strategies. Drugs Aging 2001;18:487–494.
18 Singh G, Ramey DR, Morfeld D, Shi H, Hatoum HT, Fries JF: Gastrointestinal tract complications of nonsteroidal anti-inflammatory drug treatment in rheumatoid arthritis. A prospective observational cohort study. Arch Intern Med 1996;156:1530–1536.
19 Garcia Rodriguez LA, Cattaruzzi C, Troncon MG, Agostinis L: Risk of hospitalization for upper gastrointestinal tract bleeding associated with ketorolac, other nonsteroidal antiinflammatory drugs, calcium antagonists and other antihypertensive drugs. Arch Intern Med 1998;158:33–39.
20 Wolfe MM, Lichtenstein DR, Singh G: Gastrointestinal toxicity of non-steroidal anti-inflammatory drugs. N Engl J Med 1999;340:1888–1899.
21 Pilotto A, Franceschi M, Leandro G, Di Mario F, Valerio G: The effect of *Helicobacter pylori* infection on NSAID-related gastroduodenal damage in the elderly. Eur J Gastroenterol Hepatol 1997;9:951–956.
22 Huang JQ, Sridhar S, Hunt RH: Role of *Helicobacter pylori* infection and non-steroidal anti-inflammatory drugs in peptic ulcer disease: A meta-analysis. Lancet 2002;359:14–22.

23 Skander MP, Ryan FP: Non-steroidal anti-inflammatory drugs and pain-free peptic ulceration in the elderly. BMJ 1988;297:833–834.

24 Pahor M, Guralnik JM, Salive ME, Chrischilles EA, Manto A, Wallace RB: Disability and severe gastrointestinal hemorrhage. A prospective study of community-dwelling older persons. J Am Geriatr Soc 1994;42:816–825.

25 Silverberg E, Boring CC, Sauives TS: Cancer statistics, 1990. CA Cancer J Clin 1990;40:9–26.

26 Potter JR, James OFW: Clinical features and prognosis of alcoholic liver disease in respect of advancing age. Gerontology 1987;33:380–387.

27 Garagliano CF, Lilienfeld AM, Mendelhof AI: Incidence rates of liver cirrhosis and related diseases in Baltimore and selected areas of the United States. J Chronic Dis 1979;32:543–554.

28 Almdal TP, Sorensen TIA: Incidence of parenchymal liver diseases in Denmark, 1981 to 1985: Analysis of hospitalization registry data. The Danish Association for the Study of the Liver. Hepatology 1991;13:650–655.

29 Gloor B, Ahmed Z, Uhl W, Buchler MW: Pancreatic disease in the elderly. Best Pract Res Clin Gastroenterol 2002;16:159–170.

30 Jorgensen T, Kay L, Schultz-Larsen K: The epidemiology of gallstones in a 70-year-old Danish population. Scand J Gastroenterol 1990;25:335–340.

31 Lirussi F, Nassuato G, Passera D, Toso S, Zalunardo B, Monica F, Virgilio C, Frasson F, Okolicsanyi L: Gallstone disease in an elderly population: The Silea study. Eur J Gastroenterol Hepatol 1999;11:485–491.

32 Diehl AK: Gallstone size and the risk of gallbladder cancer. JAMA 1983;250:2323–2326.

33 Schiller LR: Constipation and fecal incontinence in the elderly. Gastroenterol Clin North Am 2001;30:497–515.

34 Holt PR: Diarrhea and malabsorption in the elderly. Gastroenterol Clin North Am 2001;30:427–444.

35 Edwards NI, Jones D: The prevalence of faecal incontinence in older people living at home. Age Ageing 2001;30:503–507.

36 Farrell RJ, Farrell JJ, Morrin MM: Diverticular disease in the elderly. Gastroenterol Clin North Am 2001;30:475–496.

37 Camilleri M, Lee JS, Viramontes B, Bharucha AE, Tangalos EG: Insights into the pathophysiology and mechanisms of constipation, irritable bowel syndrome, and diverticulosis in older people. J Am Geriatr Soc 2000;48:1142–1150.

38 Longstreth GF: Epidemiology and outcome of patients hospitalized with acute lower gastrointestinal hemorrhage: A population-based study. Am J Gastroenterol 1997;92:419–424.

39 Larsson PA: Diverticulitis is increasing among the elderly. Significant cause of morbidity and mortality (in Swedish). Lakartidningen 1997;94:3837–3840, 3842.

40 Boland CR: Malignant tumors of the colon; in Yamada T, Alpers DH, Owyang C (eds): Textbook of Gastroenterology. Philadelphia, Lippincott, 1995, pp 1967–2026.

Carla Destro, CNR Aging Section, Institute of Neuroscience,
c/o Clinica Medica 1°, Via Giustiniani, 2, I–35128 Padova (Italy)
Tel. +39 049 8218898, Fax +39 049 8211818, E-Mail cdestro@unipd.it

Pilotto A, Malfertheiner P, Holt PR (eds): Aging and the Gastrointestinal Tract.
Interdiscipl Top Gerontol. Basel, Karger, 2003, vol 32, pp 12–27

....

Comprehensive Geriatric Assessment of Older Patients with Gastrointestinal Disorders

Laurence Z. Rubenstein[a], Lisa V. Rubenstein[b]

[a] Geriatric Research Education and Clinical Center and
[b] Health Services Research and Development Field Program, Sepulveda VA Medical
     Center, UCLA School of Medicine, Los Angeles, Calif., USA

Geriatric assessment is a multidimensional, usually interdisciplinary diagnostic process intended to determine a frail elderly person's medical, psychosocial and functional capabilities and problems with the objective of developing an overall plan for treatment and long-term follow-up [1]. It differs from the standard medical evaluation in its concentration on frail elderly people with their complex problems, its emphasis on functional status and quality of life and its frequent use of interdisciplinary teams and quantitative assessment scales. It is particularly important in dealing with older patients with chronic and disabling illnesses, such as gastrointestinal disorders, since such patients are likely to have multiple and interacting problems interfering with their daily function and complicating treatment, all of which can be better understood and addressed through a comprehensive assessment process. An older patient presenting with a common gastrointestinal problem such as constipation or intestinal obstruction typically has a multitude of other disease conditions and age-related disorders that complicate the diagnostic and therapeutic options and make the comprehensive assessment approach particularly valuable.

The process of geriatric assessment can range in intensity from a limited assessment by primary care physicians or community health workers focused on identifying an older person's functional problems and disabilities (screening assessment) to a more thorough evaluation of these problems usually coupled with initiation of a therapeutic plan by a physician or multidisciplinary team with geriatric training and experience (comprehensive geriatric assessment). This chapter will discuss both limited geriatric assessment, such as can be performed by a single practitioner in an office setting, and comprehensive geriatric assessment, usually requiring a specialized geriatric setting.

The ultimate goal of geriatric assessment is to improve quality of life, a concept that includes both health status as well as socio-environmental factors. Health status can be quantified both by measures of disease, such as signs, symptoms and laboratory tests, and by measures of functional status. Functional status signifies the individual's ability to participate fully in the physical, mental and social activities of daily life. The ability to function fully in these arenas is strongly affected by an individual's physiologic health, and can often be used as a measure of the seriousness of a patient's multiple diseases. A comprehensive geriatric assessment is useful in planning care for all these areas.

Brief History of Geriatric Assessment

The basic concepts of geriatric assessment have evolved over the past 70 years by combining elements of the traditional medical history and physical examination, the social worker assessment, functional evaluation and treatment methods derived from rehabilitation medicine and psychometric methods derived from the social sciences. By incorporating the perspectives of many disciplines, geriatricians have created a practical means of viewing the 'whole patient'.

The first published reports of geriatric assessment programs (GAPs) came from the British geriatrician Marjory Warren, who initiated the concept of specialized geriatric assessment units during the late 1930s while in charge of a large London infirmary. This infirmary was filled primarily with chronically ill, bedfast and largely neglected elderly patients who had not received a proper medical diagnosis or rehabilitation and who were thought to be in need of life-long institutionalization. Good nursing care kept the patients alive, but the lack of diagnostic assessment and rehabilitation kept them disabled. Through evaluation, mobilization and rehabilitation, Warren was able to get most of the long bedfast patients out of bed and often discharged home. As a result of her experiences, Warren advocated that every elderly patient receive comprehensive assessment and an attempt at rehabilitation before being admitted to a long-term care hospital or nursing home [2].

Since Warren's work, geriatric assessment has evolved. As geriatric care systems have developed worldwide, GAPs have usually been assigned central roles, generally as focal points for entry into the care systems [3]. Geared to differing local needs and populations, GAPs vary in intensity, structure and function. They can be located in very different settings, including acute hospital inpatient units and consultation teams, chronic and rehabilitation hospital units, outpatient and office-based programs and home visit outreach programs. Despite their diversity, they share many characteristics. Virtually all programs provide multidimensional assessment, utilizing specific measurement instruments to quantify functional, psychological and social parameters. Most use interdisciplinary teams to pool expertise and enthusiasm in working toward common goals. Additionally, most programs attempt to couple their assessments with intervention, such as rehabilitation, counseling or placement.

Today, geriatric assessment continues to evolve in response to increased pressures for cost containment, avoidance of institutional stays and consumer demands for better care. Geriatric assessment can help achieve improved quality of care and plan cost-effective care. This has generally meant more emphasis on noninstitutional programs and shorter hospital stays. Geriatric assessment teams are well positioned to deliver effective care for elderly persons with limited resources. Geriatricians have long emphasized the judicious use of technology, systematic preventive medical activities and less institutionalization and hospitalization.

Structure and Process of Geriatric Assessment

Geriatric assessment begins with the identification of deteriorations in health status or the presence of risk factors for deterioration. These deteriorations include both worsening of disease and worsening of functional status. If disease alone has worsened, without affecting function, the patient should be able to be cared for in the usual primary care or specialty settings. In addition, when functional status problems are mild and are not rapidly progressive, it is appropriate for a primary care practitioner to proceed with the assessment. However, because families and patients identify functional status problems early, and because internists and family practitioners are often unfamiliar with the concept of 'treating' functional status impairment as a problem in its own right, patients often self-refer to geriatric care settings for these functional status problems when such settings are available. Patients who have new severe or progressive deficits should ideally receive comprehensive interdisciplinary geriatric assessment. Examples of such patients often seen in gastroenterological practices are frail elderly outpatients being evaluated for anemia and occult bleeding or older hospitalized patients with heart failure or hip fracture who develop acute upper gastrointestinal hemorrhage.

An elderly patient presenting with a deterioration in health status of any kind, be it a gastrointestinal hemorrhage, worsening constipation or a new inability to perform errands, should be evaluated briefly to determine the full extent of functional disabilities. Many experts believe that frail elderly people, defined generally as people over the age of 75, or over the age of 65 with chronic disease, should also be screened for functional disability or risk factors at regular intervals, e.g. once a year, even when no known acute health insults have occurred [4–7]. When a new disability or high-risk state is detected through screening, a full geriatric assessment may also be appropriate in such patients.

A typical geriatric assessment begins with a functional status 'review of systems' that inventories the major domains of functioning. The major elements of this review of systems are captured in two commonly used functional status measures: basic activities of daily living and instrumental activities of daily living. Several reliable and valid versions of these measures have been developed [8–12], perhaps the most widely used being those by Katz et al. [13], Lawton and Brody [14] and Barthel [15, 16]. These scales are used by clinicians to detect whether the patient has problems performing activities that people must be able to accomplish to survive without help in the community. Basic activities of daily living include self-care activities such as eating, dressing, bathing, transferring and toileting. Patients unable to perform these activities will generally require 12- to 24-hour support by caregivers. Instrumental activities of daily living include heavier housework, going on errands, managing finances and telephoning, activities that are required if the individual is to remain independent in a house or apartment.

To interpret the results of impairments in basic and instrumental activities of daily living, physicians will usually need additional information about the patient's environment and social situation. For example, the amount and type of caregiver support available, the strength of the patient's social network and the level of social activities in which the patient participates will all influence the clinical approach taken in managing deficits detected. This information could be obtained by an experienced nurse or social worker. A screen for mobility and fall risk is also extremely helpful in quantifying function and disability, and several observational scales are available [17, 18]. An assessment of nutritional status and the risk of undernutrition is also important in understanding the extent of impairment and for planning care [19]. Likewise, a screening assessment of vision and hearing will often detect crucial deficits that need to be treated or compensated for.

Two other key pieces of information must always be gathered in the face of functional disability in an elderly person. These are a screen for mental status (cognitive) impairment and a screen for depression [8, 9, 12]. Of the several validated screening tests for cognitive function, the Folstein Mini-Mental State is one of the best because it efficiently tests the major aspects of cognitive functioning [20]. Of the various screening tests for geriatric depression, the Yesavage Geriatric Depression Scale [21] and the Zung Self-Rating Depression Scale [22] are in wide use, and even shorter screening versions are available without significant loss of accuracy [23].

Table 1. Measurable dimensions of geriatric assessment with examples of specific measures

Dimension	Basic context	Specific examples
Basic ADL [23, 24]	strengths and limitations in self-care, basic mobility and incontinence	Katz et al. [13] (ADL), Lawton Personal Self-Maintenance Scale [14] and Barthel Index [15]
IADL [24]	strengths and limitations in shopping, cooking, household activities and finances	Lawton and Brody [14] (IADL); Older Americans Resources and Services, IADL Section [28]
Social activities and supports [25]	strengths and limitations in social network and community activities	Lubben Social Network Scale [29]; Older Americans Resources and Services, Social Resources Section [28]
Mental health – affective [27]	the degree to which the person feels anxious, depressed or generally happy	Yesavage Geriatric Depression Scale [21, 23]; Zung Self-Rating Depression Scale [22]
Mental health – cognitive [16, 27]	the degree to which the person is alert, oriented and able to concentrate and perform complex mental tasks	Folstein Mini-Mental State [20]; Kahn Mental Status Questionnaire [30]
Mobility – gait and balance [9, 11]	quantitative scale of gait, balance and risk of falls	Tinetti Performance Oriented Mobility Assessment [17], 'Get up and go' test [18]
Nutritional adequacy [19]	current nutritional status and risk of malnutrition	Nutrition Screening Initiative Checklist [19], Mini-Nutritional Assessment [26]

ADL = Activities of daily living; IADL, = instrumental activities of daily living.

The major measurable dimensions of geriatric assessment, together with examples of commonly used health status screening scales, are listed in table 1 [7–37]. The instruments listed are short, have been carefully tested for reliability and validity and can be easily administered by virtually any staff person involved with the assessment process. Both observational instruments (e.g. physical examination) and self-report (completed by patient or proxy) are available. Components of them – such as watching a patient walk, turn around and sit down – are routine parts of the geriatric physical examination, but in the instrument they become part of a quantitative score. Many other kinds of assessment measures exist and can be useful in certain situations. For example, there are several disease-specific measures for stages and levels of dysfunction for patients with specific diseases such as arthritis [31], dementia [32] and parkinsonism [33]. There are also several brief global assessment instruments that attempt to quantify all dimensions of the assessment in a single form [34–37]. These latter instruments can be useful in community surveys and some research settings but are not detailed enough to be useful in most clinical settings. More comprehensive lists of available instruments can be found by consulting published reviews of health status assessment [7–11, 38].

A number of factors must be taken into account in deciding where an assessment should take place. Most geriatric assessments do not require the full range of technology nor the intense monitoring found in an inpatient setting. Yet hospitalization becomes unavoidable if no outpatient setting provides sufficient resources to accomplish the assessment fast enough. Mental and physical impairment often make it difficult for patients to comply with recommendations and to navigate multiple appointments in multiple locations. Functionally impaired elders must depend on families and friends, who risk losing their jobs because of chronic and relentless demands on time and energy in their roles as caregivers, and who may be elderly themselves. Each separate medical appointment or intervention has a high time cost for these caregivers. Patient fatigue during periods of increased illness may require the availability of a bed during the assessment process. These factors would favor an inpatient setting.

A specialized geriatric setting outside an acute hospital ward, such as a day hospital or subacute inpatient geriatric evaluation unit, will provide the easy availability of an interdisciplinary team with the time and expertise to provide needed services efficiently, an adequate level of monitoring and beds for patients unable to sit or stand for prolonged periods. Inpatient and day hospital assessment programs have the advantages of intensity, rapidity and ability to care for particularly frail or acutely ill patients. Outpatient programs are generally cheaper and avoid the necessity of an inpatient stay.

Assessment in the Office Practice Setting

A streamlined approach is preferable in the office setting because of time limitations. An important first step is setting priorities among problems for initial evaluation and treatment. The 'best' problem to work on first might be the problem that most bothers a patient or, alternatively, the problem upon which resolution of other problems depends (obstipation or depression often fall into this category).

The second step in performing a geriatric assessment is to understand the exact nature of the disability by performing a task or symptom analysis. In a nonspecialized setting, or when the disability is mild or clear-cut, this may involve only taking a careful history. When the disability is more severe, more detailed assessments by an interdisciplinary team may be necessary. For example, a patient may present with difficulty dressing. There are multiple tasks associated with a task such as dressing, any one of which might be the stumbling block (e.g. buying clothes, choosing appropriate clothes to put on, remembering to complete the task, buttoning, stretching to put on shirts or reaching downward to put on shoes). By identifying the exact areas of difficulty, further evaluation can be targeted toward solving the problem.

Once the history has revealed the nature of the disability, a systematic physical examination and ancillary laboratory tests are needed to clarify the cause of the problem. For example, difficulty dressing could be caused by mental status impairment, poor finger mobility or dysfunction of shoulders, back or hips. Evaluation by a physical or occupational therapist may be necessary to pinpoint the problem adequately, and evaluation by a social worker may be required to determine the extent of family dysfunction engendered by or contributing to the dependency. Radiologic and other laboratory testing may be necessary.

Each abnormality that could cause the patient difficulty in dressing suggests different treatments. By understanding the abnormalities that contribute most to the functional disability, the best treatment strategy can be undertaken. Often one disability leads to another; impaired gait may lead to depression or decreased social functioning, and immobility of any cause, even after the cause has been removed, can lead to secondary impairments in performance of daily activities due to deconditioning and loss of musculoskeletal flexibility.

Almost any acute or chronic disease can reduce functioning. Common but easily overlooked causes of dysfunction in elderly people include impaired cognition, impaired special senses (vision, hearing, balance), unstable gait and mobility, poor health habits (alcohol, smoking, lack of exercise), poor nutrition, polypharmacy, incontinence, psychosocial stress and depression. To identify causes contributing to the disability, the physician must thus look for worsening of the patient's chronic diseases, occurrence of a new acute disease or appearance of one of the common occult diseases listed above. The physician does this through a refocused history guided by the functional disabilities detected and their differential diagnoses, as well as a focused physical examination. The physical examination always includes, in addition to the usual evaluations of the heart, lungs, extremities and neurologic function, postural blood pressure, screening of vision and hearing and careful observation of the patient's gait. The Mini-Mental State Examination, already recommended as part of the initial functional status screen, may also determine what parts of the physical examination require particular attention as part of the evaluation of dementia or acute confusion. Finally, basic laboratory testing including a complete blood count and a blood chemistry panel, as well as tests indicated on the basis of specific findings from the history and physical examination, will generally be necessary.

Once the disability and its causes are understood, the best treatments or management strategies for it are often clear. When a reversible cause for the impairment is found, a simple treatment may eliminate or ameliorate the functional disability. When the disability is complex, the physician may need the support of a variety of community or hospital-based resources. In most cases, a strategy for long-term follow-up and, often, formal case management should be developed to ensure that needs and services are appropriately matched up and followed through.

Multidimensional Geriatric Assessment

If referral to a specialized geriatric setting has been chosen, the process of assessment will probably be similar to that described above, except that the greater intensity of resources and the special training of all members of the interdisciplinary team in dealing with geriatric patients and their problems will facilitate carrying out the proposed assessment and plan more quickly and in greater breadth and detail. In the usual geriatric assessment setting, key disciplines involved include, at a minimum, physicians, social workers, nurses and physical and occupational therapists, and optimally may include other disciplines such as dieticians, pharmacists, ethicists and home care specialists. Special geriatric expertise among the team members is crucial.

The interdisciplinary team conference, which takes place after most team members have completed their individual assessments, is critical. Most successful trials of geriatric assessment have included such a team conference. By bringing the perspectives of all disciplines together, the team conference generates new ideas, sets priorities, disseminates the full results of the assessment to all those involved in treating the patient and avoids duplication or incongruity. Development of fully effective teams requires commitment, skill and time as the interdisciplinary team evolves through the 'forming, storming and norming' phases to reach the fully developed 'performing' stage [39]. Involvement of the patient (and carer if appropriate) at some stage is important in maintaining the principle of choice [39, 40].

Effectiveness of GAPs

A large and still growing body of literature supports the effectiveness of GAPs in a variety of settings. Early descriptive studies indicated a number of benefits from GAPs such as improved diagnostic accuracy, reduced discharges to nursing homes, increased functional status and more appropriate prescribing of medication. Because they were noncontrolled studies, they were not able to distinguish the effects of the programs from simple improvement over time. Nor did these studies look at long-term outcomes. Nonetheless, many of these early studies provided promising results [41–45].

Improved diagnostic accuracy was the most widely described effect of geriatric assessment, most often indicated by uncovering substantial numbers of important problems. Frequencies of new diagnoses found ranged from almost one to more than four per patient. Factors contributing to the improvement of diagnosis in GAPs include the validity of the assessment itself (the capability of a structured search for 'geriatric problems' to find them), the extra measure of time and care taken in the evaluation of the patient (independent of the formal elements of 'the assessment') and a probable lack of diagnostic attention on the part of referring professionals.

Improved living location on discharge from the health care setting was demonstrated in several early studies, beginning with T.F. Williams' classic descriptive pre/post study of an outpatient assessment program in New York [46]. Of patients referred for nursing home placement in the county, the assessment program found that only 38% actually needed skilled nursing care, while 23% could return home and 39% were appropriate for board and care or other assisted living facilities. Numerous subsequent studies have shown similar improvements in living location [47–62]. Several studies that examined mental or physical functional status of patients before and after comprehensive geriatric assessment coupled with treatment and rehabilitation showed patient improvement on measures of function [47–51, 55, 59].

Beginning in the 1980s, controlled studies appeared that corroborated some of the earlier studies and documented additional benefits such as improved survival, reduced hospital and nursing home utilization and, in some cases, reduced costs [47–71]. These studies were by no means uniform in their results. Some showed a whole series of dramatic positive effects on function, survival, living location and costs, while others showed relatively few benefits, if any. However, the GAPs being studied were also very different from each other in terms of the process of care offered and patient populations accepted. At present, controlled trials of GAPs continue, and as results accumulate, we are able to understand which aspects contribute to their effectiveness and which do not.

One striking effect confirmed for many GAPs has been a positive impact on survival. Several controlled studies of different basic GAP models demonstrated significantly increased survival, reported in different ways and with varying periods of follow-up. Mortality was reduced for Sepulveda geriatric evaluation unit patients by 50% at 1 year, and the survival curves of the experimental and control groups still significantly favored the intervention group at 2 years [47, 63, 64]. Survival was improved by 21% at 1 year in a Scottish trial of geriatric rehabilitation consultation [59]. Two Canadian consultation trials demonstrated significantly improved 6-month survival [55, 56]. Two Danish community-based trials of in-home geriatric assessment and follow-up demonstrated a reduction in mortality [48, 61], and two Welsh studies of in-home GAPs showed beneficial survival effects among patients assessed at home and followed for 2 years [50, 51]. On the other hand, several other studies of geriatric assessment found no statistically significant survival benefits [52, 54, 58, 59].

Multiple studies followed patients longitudinally after the initial assessment and thus were able to examine the longer-term utilization and cost impacts of assessment and treatment. Some studies found an overall reduction in days in a nursing home [47, 59, 65, 66]. Hospital utilization was examined in several reports. For hospital-based GAPs, the length of hospitalization was obviously affected by the length of the assessment itself. Thus, some programs appear to prolong the initial length of stay [45, 67, 68], while others reduce the initial stay [53, 59–61, 69]. However, studies following patients for at least 1 year have usually shown a reduction in use of acute care hospital services, even in those programs with initially prolonged hospital stays [41, 48, 57].

Compensatory increases in the use of community-based services or home care agencies might be expected with declines in nursing home placements and use of other institutional services. These increases have been detected in several studies [48, 50, 55, 70], but not in others [47, 57, 62]. Although increased use of formal community services may not always be indicated, it usually is a desirable goal. The fact that several studies did not detect increases in the use of home and community services probably reflects the unavailability of community service or referral networks rather than the fact that such services were not needed more.

The effects of these programs on costs and utilization parameters have less commonly been examined comprehensively, due to methodological difficulties in gathering comprehensive utilization and cost data, as well as statistical limitations in comparing highly skewed distributions. The Sepulveda study found that total first-year direct health care costs had been reduced due to overall reductions in nursing home and rehospitalization days, despite significantly longer initial hospital stays in the geriatric unit [47]. These savings continued through 3 years of follow-up [63]. The program of Hendriksen et al. [48] reduced the costs of medical care, apparently through successful early case-finding and referral for preventive intervention. The outpatient GAP of Williams et al. [57] detected reductions in medical care costs due primarily to reductions in hospitalization. Although it would be reasonable to worry that prolonged survival of frail patients would lead to increased service use and charges, or, of perhaps greater concern, to worry about the quality of the prolonged life, these concerns may be without substance. Indeed, the Sepulveda study demonstrated that a GAP could not only improve survival but prolong high-function survival [47, 63], while at the same time reducing the use of institutional services and costs.

A 1993 meta-analysis attempted to resolve some of the discrepancies between study results, and to try to identify whether particular program elements were associated with particular benefits [72, 73]. This meta-analysis included published data from the 28 controlled trials completed at that date, involving nearly 10,000 patients, and was also able to include substantial amounts of unpublished data systematically retrieved from many of the studies. The meta-analysis identified five GAP types: hospital units (six studies), hospital consultation teams (eight studies), in-home assessment services (seven studies), outpatient assessment services (four studies) and 'hospital-home assessment services' (three studies), the latter of which performed in-home assessments on patients recently discharged from hospitals. The meta-analysis confirmed many of the major reported benefits for many of the individual program types. These statistically and clinically significant benefits included reduced risk of mortality (by 22% for hospital-based programs at 12 months, and by 14% for all programs combined at 12 months), improved likelihood of living at home (by 47% for hospital-based programs and by 26% for all programs combined at 12 months), reduced risk of hospital (re)admissions (by 12% for all programs at study end), greater chance of cognitive improvement (by 47% for all programs at study end) and greater chance of improvement of physical function for patients in hospital units (by 72% for hospital units).

Clearly, not all studies showed equivalent effects, and the meta-analysis was able to indicate a number of variables at both the program and patient levels that tended to distinguish trials with large effects from ones with more limited ones. When examined on the program level, hospital units and home visit assessment teams produced the most dramatic benefits, while no major significant benefits could be confirmed for office-based programs. Programs that provided hands-on clinical care and/or long-term follow-up were generally able to produce greater positive effects than purely consultative programs or ones that lacked follow-up. Another factor associated with greater demonstrated benefits, at least in hospital-based programs, was patient targeting; programs that selected patients who were at high risk for deterioration yet still had 'rehabilitation potential' generally had stronger results than less selective programs.

The meta-analysis confirmed the importance of targeting criteria in producing beneficial outcomes. In particular, when the use of explicit targeting criteria for patient selection was included as a covariate, increases in some program benefits were often found. For example, among the hospital-based GAP studies, positive effects on physical function and likelihood of living at home at 12 months were associated with studies that excluded patients who were relatively 'too healthy'. A similar effect on physical function was seen in the institutional studies that excluded persons with relatively poor prognoses. The reason for this effect of targeting on effect size no doubt lies in the ability of careful targeting to concentrate the intervention on patients who can benefit, without diluting the effect with persons too ill or too well to show a measurable improvement.

Studies performed since this meta-analysis have been largely corroborative. However, with principles of geriatric medicine becoming more diffused into standard care, particularly at places where controlled trials are being undertaken, differences between GAPs and control groups seem to be narrowing [74–80]. For cost reasons, growth of inpatient units has been slow, despite their proven effectiveness, while outpatient programs have increased, despite their less impressive effect size in controlled trials. However, some newer trials of outpatient programs have shown significant benefits in areas not found in earlier outpatient studies, such as functional status, psychological parameters and well-being, which may indicate improvement in the outpatient care models being tested [75–80].

A continuing challenge has been obtaining adequate financing to support the addition of geriatric assessment services to existing medical care. Despite the many proven benefits of GAPs, and their ability to reduce costs as documented in controlled trials, health care financers have often been reluctant to fund GAPs – presumably out of concern that the programs might be expanded too fast and that costs for extra diagnostic and therapeutic services might increase out of control. Many practitioners have found ways to 'unbundle' the comprehensive geriatric assessment process into component services and receive adequate support to fund the entire process. In this time of continuing fiscal restraint, geriatric practitioners must remain constantly creative in order to reach the goal of optimal patient care.

Conclusion

Published studies of comprehensive geriatric assessment have confirmed its efficacy in many settings. While there is no single optimal blueprint for geriatric assessment, the participation of a multidisciplinary team and the focus on functional status and quality of life as major clinical goals are common to all settings. Although the greatest benefits have been found in programs targeted at the frail subgroup of older persons, a strong case can be made for a continuum of GAPs and screening assessments performed periodically for all older persons and comprehensive assessment targeted at frail and high-risk patients. Clinicians interested in developing these services will do well to heed the experiences of the programs reviewed here in adapting the principles of geriatric assessment to local resources. Future research is still needed to determine the most effective and efficient methods for performing geriatric assessment and to develop strategies for best matching needs with services.

References

1   Rubenstein LZ, Rubenstein LV: Multidimensional geriatric assessment; in Tallis RC, Fillit HM (eds): Brocklehurst's Textbook of Geriatric Medicine, ed 6. London, Churchill Livingstone, 2002, chapter 26, pp 291–300.
2   Matthews DA: Dr. Marjory Warren and the origin of British geriatrics. J Am Geriatr Soc 1984;32: 253–258.
3   Brocklehurst JC: Geriatric Care in Advanced Societies. Lancaster, MTP, 1975.
4   The periodic health examination. Canadian Task Force on the Periodic Health Examination. Can Med Assoc J 1979;121:1193–1254.
5   Rubenstein LZ, Josephson KR, Nichol-Seamons M, Robbins AS: Comprehensive health screening of well elderly adults. J Gerontol 1986;41:343–352.
6   US Congress, Office of Technology Assessment: Preventive Health Services for Medicare Beneficiaries: Policy and Research Issues (OTA-H-416). Washington, US Government Printing Office, 1990.
7   Rubenstein LV: Using quality of life tests for patient diagnosis or screening; in Spilker B (ed): Quality of Life and Pharmacoeconomics in Clinical Trials, ed 2. Philadelphia, Lippincott-Raven, 1996.
8   Rubenstein LZ, Campbell LJ, Kane RL: Geriatric Assessment. Philadelphia, WB Saunders, 1987.
9   Rubenstein LZ, Wieland D, Bernabei R: Geriatric Assessment Technology: The State of the Art. Milan, Kurtis, 1995.
10 Kane RL, Kane RA: Assessing Older Persons. New York, Oxford University Press, 2000.
11 Osterweil D, Brummel-Smith K, Beck JC: Comprehensive Geriatric Assessment. New York, McGraw-Hill, 2000.
12 Gallo JJ, Fulmer T, Paveza GJ, Reichel W: Handbook of Geriatric Assessment, ed 3. Rockville, Aspen, 2000.
13 Katz S, Ford AB, Moskowitz RW, et al: Studies of illness in the aged. The index of ADL: A standardized measure of biological psychosocial function. J Am Med Assoc 1963;185:914–919.
14 Lawton MP, Brody EM: Assessment of older people: Self-maintaining and instrumental activities of daily living. Gerontologist 1969;9:179–186.
15 Mahoney FI, Barthel DW: Functional evaluation – the Barthel Index. Md State Med J 1965;14: 61–65.
16 Wade DT, Collin C: The Barthel ADL Index: A standard measure of physical disability. Int Disabil Stud 1988;10:64–67.
17 Tinetti ME: Performance oriented assessment of mobility problems in elderly patients. J Am Geriatr Soc 1986;34:119–126.
18 Mathias S, Nayak USL, Isaacs B: Balance in elderly patients: The 'get up and go' test. Arch Phys Med Rehabil 1986;67:387–389.

19   Vellas B, Guigoz Y: Nutritional assessment as part of the geriatric evaluation; in Rubenstein LZ, Wieland D, Bernabei R (eds): Geriatric Assessment Technology: The State of the Art. Milan, Kurtis, 1995, pp 179–194.

20   Folstein M, Folstein S, McHugh P: 'Mini-mental state'. A practical method for grading the cognitive state of patients for the clinician. J Psychiatr Res 1975;12:189–198.

21   Yesavage J, Brink T, Rose T, Lum O, Huang V, Adey M, Leirer VO: Development and validation of a geriatric depression screening scale: A preliminary report. J Psychiatr Res 1982–83;17:37–49.

22   Zung WWK: A self rating depression scale. Arch Gen Psychiatry 1965;12:63–70.

23   Hoyl MT, Alessi CA, Harker JO, Josephson KR, Pietruszka FM, Koelfgen M, Mervis JR, Fitten LJ, Rubenstein LZ: Development and testing of a five-item version of the Geriatric Depression Scale. J Am Geriatr Soc 1999;47:873–878.

24   Hedrick SC: Assessment of functional status: Activities of daily living; in Rubenstein LZ, Wieland D, Bernabei R (eds): Geriatric Assessment Technology: The State of the Art. Milan, Kurtis, 1995, pp 51–58.

25   Kane RA: Assessment of social function: Recommendations for comprehensive geriatric assessment; in Rubenstein LZ, Wieland D, Bernabei R (eds): Geriatric Assessment Technology: The State of the Art. Milan, Kurtis, 1995, pp 91–110.

26   Rubenstein LZ, Harker JO, Salva A, Guigoz Y, Vellas B: Screening for undernutrition in geriatric practice: Developing the short-form Mini-Nutritional Assessment (MNA-SF). J Gerontol A Biol Sci Med Sci 2001;56:M366–M372.

27   Gurland BH, Wilder D: Detection and assessment of cognitive impairment and depressed mood in older adults; in Rubenstein LZ, Wieland D, Bernabei R (eds): Geriatric Assessment Technology: The State of the Art. Milan, Kurtis, 1995, pp 111–134.

28   Duke University Center for the Study of Aging and Human Development: The OARS Methodology. Durham, Duke University Press, 1978.

29   Lubben JE: Assessing social networks among elderly populations. Fam Community Health 1988; 8:42–52.

30   Kahn R, Goldfarb A, Pollack M, et al: Brief objective measures of mental status in the aged. Am J Psychiatry 1960;117:326–328.

31   Chambers LW, MacDonald LA, Tugwell P, Buchanan WW, Kraag G: The McMaster Health Index Questionnaire as a measure of quality of life for patients with rheumatoid disease. J Rheumatol 1982;9:780–784.

32   Reisberg B, Ferris SH, De Leon MJ, Crook T: The Global Deterioration Scale for assessment of primary degenerative dementia. Am J Psychiatry 1982;139:1136–1139.

33   Hoehn MM, Yahr MD: Parkinsonism: Onset, progression, and mortality. Neurology 1967;17:427–442.

34   Stewart AL, Hays RD, Ware JE: The MOS short-form general health survey: Reliability and validity in a patient population. Med Care 1988;26:724–735.

35   Nelson E, Wasson J, Kirk J, Keller A, Clark D, Dietrich A, Stewart A, Zubkoff M: Assessment of function in routine clinical practice: Description of the COOP Chart method and preliminary findings. J Chronic Dis 1987;40(suppl 1):55S–69S.

36   Bergner M, Bobbit R, Carter WB: The sickness impact profile: Validation of a health status measure. Med Care 1981;19:787–805.

37   Jette AM, Davies AR, Cleary PD, Calkins DR, Rubenstein LV, Fink A, Kosecoff J, Young RT, Brook RH, Delbanco TL: The Functional Status Questionnaire: Reliability and validity when used in primary care. J Gen Intern Med 1986;1:143–149.

38   Van Swearingen JM, Brach JS: Making geriatric assessment work: Selecting useful measures. Phys Ther 2001;81:1233–1252.

39   Campbell LJ, Cole KD: Geriatric assessment teams. Clin Geriatr Med 1987;3:99–110.

40   Wieland D, Kramer BJ, Waite MS, Rubenstein LZ: The interdisciplinary team in geriatric care. Am Behav Sci 1996;39:655–664.

41   Williamson J, Stokoe IH, Gray S, et al: Old people at home: Their unreported needs. Lancet 1964;i:1117–1120.

42   Lowther CP, MacLeod RDM, Williamson J: Evaluation of early diagnostic services for the elderly. Br Med J 1970;i:275–277.

43 Brocklehurst JC, Carty MH, Leeming JT, Robinson JH: Medical screening of old people accepted for residential care. Lancet 1978;ii:141–143.

44 Applegate WB, Akins D, Vander Zwaag R, Thoni K, Baker MG: A geriatric rehabilitation and assessment unit in a community hospital. J Am Geriatr Soc 1983;31:206–210.

45 Rubenstein LZ, Josephson KR, Wieland GD, Pietruszka F, Tretton C, Strome S, Cole KD, Campbell LJ: Geriatric assessment on a subacute hospital ward. Clin Geriatr Med 1987;3: 131–143.

46 Williams TF, Hill JH, Fairbank ME, Knox KG: Appropriate placement of the chronically ill and aged: A successful approach by evaluation. JAMA 1973;266:1332–1335.

47 Rubenstein LZ, Josephson KR, Wieland GD, English PA, Sayre JA, Kane RL: Effectiveness of a geriatric evaluation unit. A randomized clinical trial. N Engl J Med 1984;311:1664–1670.

48 Hendriksen C, Lund E, Stromgard E: Consequences of assessment and intervention among elderly people: A three-year randomised controlled trial. Br Med J (Clin Res Ed) 1984;289:1522–1524.

49 Thomas DR, Brahan R, Haywood BP: Inpatient community-based geriatric assessment reduces subsequent mortality. J Am Geriatr Soc 1993;41:101–104.

50 Vetter NJ, Jones DA, Victor CR: Effect of health visitors working with elderly patients in general practice: A randomised controlled trial. Br Med J (Clin Res Ed) 1984;288:369–372.

51 Vetter NJ, Lewis PA, Ford D: Can health visitors prevent fractures in elderly people? BMJ 1992;304:888–890.

52 Winograd CH, Gerety M, Lai N: A negative trial of inpatient geriatric consultation: Lessons learned. Arch Intern Med 1993;153:2017–2023.

53 Collard AF, Bachman SS, Beatrice DF: Acute care delivery for the geriatric patient: An innovative approach. QRB Qual Rev Bull 1985;11:180–185.

54 Allen CM, Becker PM, McVey LJ, Saltz C, Feussner JR, Cohen HJ: A randomized, controlled clinical trial of a geriatric consultation team. Compliance with recommendations. JAMA 1986;255:2617–2621.

55 Hogan DB, Fox RA, Badley BWD, Mann OE: Effect of a geriatric consultation service on management of patients in an acute care hospital. Can Med Assoc J 1987;136:713–717.

56 Hogan DB, Fox RA: A prospective controlled trial of a geriatric consultation team in an acute care hospital. Age Ageing 1990;19:107–113.

57 Williams ME, Williams TF, Zimmer JG, Hall WJ, Podgorski CA: How does the team approach to outpatient geriatric evaluation compare with traditional care: A report of a randomized controlled trial. J Am Geriatr Soc 1987;35:1071–1078.

58 Gilchrist WJ, Newman RH, Hamblen DL, Williams BO: Prospective randomised study of an orthopaedic geriatric inpatient service. BMJ 1988;297:1116–1118.

59 Reid J, Kennie DC: Geriatric rehabilitative care after fractures of the proximal femur: One-year follow-up of a randomised clinical trial. BMJ 1989;299:25–26.

60 Pathy MSJ, Bayer A, Harding K, Dibble A: Randomised trial of case finding and surveillance of elderly people at home. Lancet 1992;340:890–893.

61 Hansen FR, Spedtsberg K, Schroll M: Geriatric follow-up by home visits after discharge from hospital: A randomized controlled trial. Age Ageing 1992;21:445–450.

62 Gayton D, Wood-Dauphinee S, de Lorimer M, Tousignant P, Hanley J: Trial of a geriatric consultation team in an acute care hospital. J Am Geriatr Soc 1987;35:726–736.

63 Rubenstein LZ, Josephson KR, Harker JO, Wieland D: The Sepulveda GEU Study revisited: Long-term outcomes, use of services, and costs. Aging (Milano) 1995;7:212–217.

64 Rubenstein LZ, Wieland D, Josephson KR, Rosbrook B, Sayre J, Kane RL: Improved survival for frail elderly inpatients on a geriatric evaluation unit (GEU): Who benefits? J Clin Epidemiol 1988;41:441–449.

65 Schuman JE, Beattie EJ, Steed DA, Gibson JE, Merry GM, Campbell WD, Kraus AS: The impact of a new geriatric program in a hospital for the chronically ill. Can Med Assoc J 1978;118: 639–645.

66 Lefton E, Bonstelle S, Frengley JD: Success with an inpatient geriatric unit: A controlled study. J Am Geriatr Soc 1983;31:149–155.

67 Berkman LF, Campion E, Swagerty E, Goldman M: Geriatric consultation teams: Alternative approach to social work discharge planning. J Gerontol Soc Work 1983;5:77–88.

68   Lichtenstein H, Winogard CH: Geriatric consultation: A functional approach. J Am Geriatr Soc 1984;32:356–361.

69   Burley LE, Currie CT, Smith RG, Williamson J: Contribution from geriatric medicine within acute medical wards. Br Med J 1979;ii:90–92.

70   Tulloch AH, Moore V: A randomized controlled trial of geriatric screening and surveillance in general practice. J R Coll Gen Pract 1979;29:733–742.

71   Rubenstein LZ, Wieland D, Bernabei R: Geriatric assessment technology: International research perspectives. Aging (Milano) 1995;7:157–158.

72   Stuck AE, Siu AL, Wieland GD, Adams J, Rubenstein LZ: Comprehensive geriatric assessment: A meta-analysis of controlled trials. Lancet 1993;342:1032–1036.

73   Stuck AE, Wieland D, Rubenstein LZ, et al: Comprehensive geriatric assessment: Meta-analysis of main effects and elements enhancing effectiveness; in Rubenstein LZ, Wieland D, Bernabei R (eds): Geriatric Assessment Technology: The State of the Art. Milan, Kurtis, 1995, pp 11–26.

74   Reuben DB, Borok GM, Wolde-Tsadik G, Ershoff DH, Fishman LK, Ambrosini VL, Liu Y, Rubenstein LZ, Beck JC: A randomized clinical trial of comprehensive geriatric assessment in the care of hospitalized patients. N Engl J Med 1995;332:1345–1350.

75   Burns R, Nichols LO, Martindale-Adams J, Graney MJ: Interdisciplinary geriatric primary care evaluation and management: Two-year outcomes. J Am Geriatr Soc 2000;48:8–13.

76   Stuck AE, Minder CE, Peter-Wuest I, Gillmann G, Egli C, Kesselring A, Leu RE, Beck JC: A randomized trial of in-home visits for disability prevention in community-dwelling older people at low and high risk for nursing home admission. Arch Intern Med 2000;160:977–986.

77   Boult C, Boult LB, Morishita L, Dowd B, Kane RL, Urdangarin CF: A randomized clinical trial of outpatient geriatric evaluation and management. J Am Geriatr Soc 2001;49:351–359.

78   Elkan R, Kendrick D, Dewey M, Hewitt M, Robinson J, Blair M, Williams D, Brummell K: Effectiveness of home based support for older people: Systematic review and meta-analysis. BMJ 2001;323:719–725.

79   Cohen HJ, Feussner JR, Weinberger M, Carnes M, Hamdy RC, Hsieh F, Phibbs C, Courtney D, Lyles KW, May C, McMurtry C, Pennypacker L, Smith DM, Ainslie N, Hornick T, Brodkin K, Lavori P: A controlled trial of inpatient and outpatient geriatric evaluation and management. N Engl J Med 2002;346:905–912.

80   Rubenstein LZ, Stuck AE: Preventive home visits for older people: Defining criteria for success. Age Ageing 2001;30:107–109.

Prof. Laurence Z. Rubenstein
Professor of Geriatric Medicine, UCLA School of Medicine,
Geriatric Research Education & Clinical Center (GRECC),
Sepulveda VA Medical Center, Los Angeles, CA 91343 (USA)
Tel. +1 818 895 9311, Fax +1 818 891 8181, E-Mail lzrubens@ucla.edu

Pilotto A, Malfertheiner P, Holt PR (eds): Aging and the Gastrointestinal Tract.
Interdiscipl Top Gerontol. Basel, Karger, 2003, vol 32, pp 28–39

....

Effect of Aging on the Pharmacokinetics of Gastrointestinal Drugs

Ulrich Klotz

Dr. Margarete Fischer-Bosch Institute of Clinical Pharmacology,
Stuttgart, Germany

Introduction

Recently, about 100 major medical journals devoted considerable space to a topic regarded as the most important global issue – aging [1]. Aging affects everything (e.g. ethics, economics, society, cells, physiological systems, clinical medicine), including pharmacokinetics (drug disposition) and pharmacodynamics. In most industrial countries, about 15% of the population is aged over 65 years, a number that is generally taken as the lower limit for defining the elderly. The subjects who are investigated in clinical trials are usually in good health (the fit elderly) and the 'real oldies' (>75 years) are very seldom included. In addition, the elderly population represents a continuum from 'fit' to 'frail' [2].

General Pharmacokinetic Considerations

Rational drug use in the elderly requires an understanding of age-dependent changes in the function and composition of the body. Advanced age, in conjunction with coexisting diseases and polypharmacy, will complicate the prescription of proper dosage regimens [3]. Several physiological changes occur with aging, which all have the potential to modify the pharmacokinetics of drugs, including those agents affecting the gastrointestinal tract (table 1).

Despite the observed physiological changes summarized in table 1, absorption of drugs usually remains unchanged in the aging patient with intact

Table 1. Physiological changes that occur with aging and have the potential to influence the pharmacokinetics of drugs [2, 3]

System	Changes
General	reduced total body mass reduced basal metabolic rate reduced proportion of body water increased proportion of body fat
Circulation	decreased cardiac output altered relative tissue perfusion decreased plasma protein binding (?)
Gastrointestinal tract	reduced gastric acid production reduced gastric emptying rate reduced gut motility reduced gut blood flow reduced absorption surface intestinal uptake/transport (?) intestinal metabolism (?)
Liver	reduced liver mass reduced liver blood flow reduced albumin synthesis hepatic and biliary uptake/transport (?)
Kidney	reduced GFR reduced tubular function
Lung	reduced vital capacity

intestinal mucosa. For several drugs, such as antibiotics, anticonvulsants, salicylates, benzodiazepines, phenylbutazone, metronidazole or bumetanide, an unchanged intestinal absorption in old age has been reported [4]. Some so-called high clearance drugs, drugs that undergo substantial presystemic elimination (e.g. labetalol, verapamil, nifedipine, molsidomine, lidocaine), can exhibit increased oral bioavailability in old age because of decreased intestinal and/or hepatic first-pass effects [4, 5]. However, no differences in oral bioavailability of other high clearance drugs, such as imipramine, amitriptyline, metoprolol, morphine or pethidine, have been noted [5]. Thus, it is difficult to make any generalizations or predictions.

Because of an increase in body fat and decrease in lean body mass and total body water with age (table 1), it can be anticipated that such age-dependent changes can result in alterations of drug distribution. For instance, hydrophilic compounds (e.g. ethanol, lithium, digoxin, acebutolol, cimetidine) have a reduced apparent volume of distribution (V) in the elderly, which will result in higher plasma concentrations, whereas lipophilic agents (e.g. diazepam, amitriptyline, tolbutamide) show the opposite effect, i.e. an increase of V in the elderly [4, 6, 7]. In this context, it should be remembered that the elimination half-life ($t_{1/2}$) of a drug is a hybrid constant which changes directly – according to the equation $t_{1/2} = 0.693 \times V/CL$ – with V, where CL is the total (systemic) clearance. In other words, an increase in V implies longer drug retention in the body.

Any changes in plasma protein binding due to decreases in plasma albumin levels or increased α_1-acid glycoprotein in old age are of minor extent and usually not clinically relevant [4, 6]. It appears that age- and disease-dependent changes in body weight and composition are more substantial and should not be overlooked.

An important pharmacokinetic change in the elderly is a decrease in renal drug elimination irrespective of whether the unchanged drug is cleared from the blood (body) by glomerular filtration and/or tubular secretion (table 1). Hence, an age-dependent decrease in CL and an increase in $t_{1/2}$ (see above equation) is to be expected. Consequently, doses of drugs that are excreted predominantly in unchanged form by the renal route (e.g. aminoglycosides, lithium, digoxin, H_2-receptor antagonists) should be reduced in the elderly according to the expected decrease in CL, as during multiple dosing, the mean steady-state plasma concentration – $C_{ss} = F \times D/CL \times \tau$, where D is the dose – is inversely related to CL, or alternatively the dosing interval τ might be expanded [8].

A routinely applied way to estimate renal function, especially the glomerular filtration rate (GFR), is by the measurement of the endogenous creatinine clearance (CL_{cr}). More recent studies assessing the 'true' GFR have indicated that in healthy elderly subjects (up to the age of 75 years), the decrease in GFR is minor and that disease factors such as hypertension and congestive heart failure are primarily responsible for the modest decline in GFR from normally 120 ml/min to about 90 ml/min [9, 10].

Before final renal excretion, the vast majority of drugs have to be biotransformed to more polar (hydrophilic) metabolites by several cytochrome P450 (CYP)-dependent so-called phase I reactions and/or phase II pathways, such as glucuronidation, acetylation or sulfatation [3, 6]. This drug metabolism takes place mainly in the liver; however, recently the small bowel has received much attention as a site of drug metabolism and transport [11].

It is generally accepted that liver size (mass) and hepatic blood flow both decrease with age (table 1). Overall, any age-related microscopic changes are subtle and hepatic fine structure is markedly similar in both young and old subjects. Routine clinical tests of liver function do not change significantly with age [3, 12].

In the past, the model drug antipyrine (phenazone) has been extensively used in characterizing the hepatic metabolic capacity, and several CYP isoforms (e.g. CYP3A4, CYP1A2, CYP2C8/9) are involved in its metabolism. Similarly, the aminopyrine breath test has been widely applied as a kind of 'global' liver function test. With both tests, equivocal results (decrease, increase, no change in CL) have been observed in regard to differences between various age groups, suggesting that any age effects are at best minor [3].

Recently, the different CYP isoforms could be assigned to more specific metabolic pathways of certain probe drugs (table 2). Thereby, it was realized that CYP3A4 and the polymorphically expressed CYP2D6 represent the most important isoforms, as at least 50 and about 25%, respectively, of all drugs are metabolized by these two enzymes [3, 4, 13, 14]. The various pharmacokinetic results are somewhat contradictory, indicating sometimes a minor decrease in the hepatic elimination. However, in general, no clinically relevant changes have been observed.

Following oral administration, systemic drug exposure depends on drug absorption and presystemic metabolism. The multidrug efflux pump, P-glycoprotein, which limits oral bioavailability, is present at the site of absorption (villi of enterocytes) [11]. It was postulated that expression and function of P-glycoprotein is increased in lymphocytes of aging humans [17]. Whether these in vitro effects observed with subpopulations of lymphocytes have any clinical relevance remains to be investigated. As P-glycoprotein is also present in renal and liver-biliary systems as well as representing a major constituent of the blood-brain barrier, any age-dependent changes in this drug transporter (and other systems) could affect drug distribution and elimination [18].

Drugs Used in Upper Gastrointestinal Tract Disorders

Peptic ulcer and gastroesophageal reflux disease are quite common in the elderly, and complications are more often seen in this population at risk. Clinical efficacy and tolerability of the most frequently used antisecretory drugs [e.g. H_2-receptor antagonists, proton pump inhibitors (PPIs)], prokinetic agents and cytoprotective compounds are similar in the elderly to those observed in younger patients. Whereas age-related changes in drug disposition might contribute to the interindividual variability in drug action, poor compliance and consumption of antiinflammatory drugs are thought to cause more therapeutic problems in the elderly [19–21].

Sucralfate is a 'nonabsorbable', topically acting aluminium (Al) salt of sucrose octasulfate containing approximately 21% Al by weight. A daily dose of 4 g of sucralfate represents an Al intake of 800 mg, and small amounts are absorbed, resulting in Al blood levels ranging from 8 to 49 µg/l in subjects with normal kidney function. As Al is eliminated by the renal route, progressive loss

Table 2. Important CYP isoforms involved in human drug metabolism and their typical substrates whose pharmacokinetics (elimination) has been studied also in the elderly [3, 4, 13, 14]

CYP isoform (% of all drugs metabolized)	Drugs (examples)	Pharmacokinetic effects seen in the elderly
CYP1A2 (11%)	caffeine	no changes
	theophylline	no significant changes if smoking habits are taken into account
CYP2C8/9 (15%)	diclofenac	no change
	ibuprofen	16% ↓ and 12% ↑ in CL
	celecoxib	no change
	phenytoin	6% ↓ and 62% ↑ in CL
	S-warfarin	25% ↓ and no change in CL
CYP2C19 (4%)	omeprazole ⎫	25% ↓ in oral CL
	lansoprazole ⎪	45% ↓ in oral CL
	pantoprazole ⎬ + (CYP3A4)	no change
	rabeprazole ⎪	50% ↓ in oral CL
	diazepam ⎭	$t_{1/2}$ ↑ 3-fold, V ↑, CL unchanged
CYP2D6 (25%)	sparteine	no change ⎫ in
	dextromethorphan	no change ⎬ metabolic
	amitriptyline	no change ⎭ ratio
	propafenone (+ CYP3A4, CYP1A2)	no changes
CYP2E1 (7.5%)	chlorzoxazone	no changes
	paracetamol (+ conjugation)	8–35% ↓ in oral CL
CYP3A4 (52%)	midazolam	no changes
	erythromycin	50% ↓ in oral CL
	lidocaine	35% ↓ in CL and no changes
	nifedipine	25% ↓ in CL
	verapamil (+ CYP1A2, CYP2C)	no changes
glucuronidation	paracetamol	no changes
	morphine	45% ↓ in V, 33 and 18% ↓ in CL
	oxazepam, lorazepam	no changes
	lormetazepam, temazepam	no changes
N-acetylation	sulfamethazine	no changes

↓ = Decrease; ↑ = increase.

of GFR will inevitably lead to accumulation of Al and possible CNS toxicity, which tends to occur in patients with Al serum levels greater than 100–200 µg/l [22]. Thus, any age-related decline in GFR has to be taken into account when dosing sucralfate.

Several formulations of bismuth salts (Bi) are used to treat peptic ulcer and for the eradication of *Helicobacter pylori*. Most commonly, tripotassium dicitrato bismuthate (colloidal bismuth subcitrate) is applied [23]. Small amounts of Bi (0.2–0.3% of dose) are rapidly absorbed with a large interindividual variability [24, 25]. Bi is slowly eliminated from the body by both the urinary and fecal routes with a terminal $t_{1/2}$ of about 3 weeks and a renal clearance of 22 ml/min. During multiple dosing, extensive accumulation of Bi will occur, especially in patients with impaired renal function [24, 25]. Thus, to avoid Bi-induced CNS toxicity, any age-related impairments in GFR must be counteracted by a reduction in the doses of the various Bi salts.

The synthetic prostaglandin E analogue misoprostol is primarily used for the prevention of nonsteroidal antiinflammatory drug-induced ulcerations [26]. Following oral administration, the cytoprotective agent is rapidly absorbed and metabolized ($t_{1/2}$ of about 1.5 h) to the active metabolite misoprostol acid, which subsequently is further biotransformed to a number of metabolites that are excreted in the urine. Pharmacokinetic properties would suggest that the age of the patient has no major impact on the disposition of misoprostol [27].

The effect of metoclopramide in gastroesophageal reflux disease is thought to be partly due to an increase in the rate of gastric emptying and an increase in lower esophageal sphincter tone. Despite complete absorption, oral bioavailability is only about 75% because of hepatic first-pass elimination. Most of the dose is metabolized by conjugation, while 30% is excreted unchanged. In patients with renal failure, CL is reduced by about 70% [20]. This would suggest that any major decrease in GFR should be accompanied by a corresponding decrease in dosage. In the fit elderly, bioavailability, plasma levels and clearance of metoclopramide were similar to those in young controls. However, in the frail elderly, a significant decline in CL was observed [28].

The prokinetic drug domperidone has a low bioavailability of around 15% because of an extensive presystemic elimination. Metabolism includes hydroxylation and N-dealkylation [29]. It might be anticipated that oral bioavailability could be increased in the elderly.

H_2-receptor antagonists have been widely studied in different populations, including the elderly. The various compounds (cimetidine, ranitidine, famotidine, nizatidine, roxatidine) are excreted mainly ($\leq$70% of ingested drug) in an unchanged form in the urine. Thus, renal function (GFR) determines the elimination rate and drug accumulation during multiple dosing. Depending on the severity of renal impairment, total or renal CL of H_2-receptor antagonists are

Table 3. Pharmacokinetic parameters (mean values) of H_2-receptor antagonists in the elderly

Drug	$t_{1/2}$, h		AUC, mg/l · h		Reference
	young	elderly	young	elderly	
Cimetidine	1.9	–	7.5	11.7	30
Ranitidine	2.4	3.2	1.9	2.8	31
Famotidine	2.9	4.1	6.6 ml/min/kg (CL)	3.2 ml/min/kg (CL)	32
Nizatidine	1.6	1.9	3.0	3.3	33
Roxatidine	6.0	–	250 ml/min (CL_R)	100 ml/min (CL_R)	34

AUC = Area under the curve; CL_R = renal CL.

reduced and dosage should be adjusted according to CL_{cr} [20]. In the elderly (table 3), a minor prolongation of $t_{1/2}$ and a decrease in renal CL resulting in a slight increase in plasma levels (area under the curve) have been observed with all H_2-receptor antagonists, which indicates that no dosage reductions are necessary as long as CL_{cr} is above 75 ml/min [35].

Today, PPIs represent the drugs of first choice for the treatment of gastroesophageal reflux disease and peptic ulcer. All marketed PPIs (omeprazole or its S-enantiomer, lansoprazole, pantoprazole, rabeprazole) are metabolized in the liver by CYP2C19 and CYP3A4 [36, 37]. The published pharmacokinetic data in the elderly are summarized in table 4. While omeprazole [37, 38] and lansoprazole [37, 39] exhibit a slower elimination in the elderly which causes an increased bioavailability of omeprazole, the disposition of pantoprazole seems to be independent of the age of the patient [37, 40]. With the new agent rabeprazole, a slightly longer $t_{1/2}$ and almost 2-fold higher values for the area under the curve have been observed in healthy elderly individuals [37, 41]. As all PPIs have a relatively wide margin of safety, no dosage adjustments seem to be necessary in the elderly as long as hepatic function is not severely impaired such as in cirrhotic patients [37].

Most *H. pylori* eradication schemes include, in addition to an acid inhibitory agent (PPI or ranitidine), two different antibacterials, primarily amoxicillin, clarithromycin or metronidazole. The effect of age on the disposition of these antimicrobial agents has been investigated in clinical and pharmacokinetic studies. Age per se seems to have a minor impact, but renal function is a more important factor to be considered for any dosage adjustments [42].

Table 4. Pharmacokinetic parameters (mean values) of PPIs in the elderly

PPI	$t_{1/2}$, h		CL, ml/min		F, %		Reference
	young	elderly	young	elderly	young	elderly	
Omeprazole	0.5	0.8	620	230	46	79	37, 38
Lansoprazole	1.4	2.9	187[1]	96[1]	85		37, 39
Pantoprazole	1.4	1.5	107	95	80	95	37, 40
Rabeprazole	0.9	1.2	517[1]	275[1]	52		37, 41

F = Oral bioavailability, [1]Oral clearance.

The pharmacokinetic parameters of the renally eliminated amoxicillin in the elderly (CL 191 ml/min, renal CL 154 ml/min, $t_{1/2}$ 2.1 h) were similar to those in younger healthy controls [43]. Elimination of clarithromycin (partly renally, partly metabolized by CYP3A4) is slower in the elderly (oral CL 300 ml/min, renal CL 84 ml/min, $t_{1/2}$ 7.7 h) than in young controls (oral CL 476 ml/min, renal CL 168 ml/min, $t_{1/2}$ 4.9 h), which was primarily caused by a decrease in CL_{cr} (67 vs. 116 ml/min) [44]. Metronidazole is oxidatively metabolized with subsequent conjugation, and no age-related differences in its pharmacokinetics have been observed [45].

Drugs Used in the Treatment of Inflammatory Bowel Disease

Corticosteroids still form a mainstay of short-term treatment in patients with active inflammatory bowel disease, and prednisone/prednisolone are standard substances in use [46]. Both are metabolically interconvertible, and prednisolone represents the pharmacologically active species. In a very informative review, the nonlinear (dose-dependent) pharmacokinetic properties of prednisolone have been comprehensively summarized [47]. In elderly individuals, a decrease (37%) in the CL of unbound drug was observed, which was attributable to decreased renal and nonrenal CL of prednisolone [47]. In contrast to prednisone/prednisolone, methylprednisolone exhibits linear (dose-independent) plasma protein binding and elimination characteristics. In elderly adults, CL (4 ml/min/kg) was somewhat lower than in young adults (6 ml/min/kg) [48]. With budesonide, there is extensive presystemic elimination by CYP3A4-mediated metabolism in the intestinal wall and liver. Consequently, oral bioavailability is only approximately 10–15% [49]. It is not known whether $t_{1/2}$ (2.8 h) and CL (1,395 ml/min) will be altered in elderly subjects [50]. Because budesonide represents a typical high clearance drug (CL dependent on hepatic blood flow), it could be anticipated that in older patients, a higher bioavailability might be present [51].

Aminosalicylates, either in the form of the 'prodrug' sulfasalazine or as the active (in inflammatory bowel disease) metabolite 5-aminosalicylate (5-AS), are widely used in inflammatory bowel disease, especially ulcerative colitis. 5-AS is rapidly eliminated ($t_{1/2}$ 0.5–2 h, CL varies dose dependently from 300 to 610 ml/min) by intestinal and hepatic acetylation. The disposition of the topically acting 5-AS has been studied in many different patient populations, however, apparently without emphasis on aging [51]. Sulfasalazine is effective in rheumatoid arthritis, and multiple doses of sulfasalazine are eliminated more slowly in the elderly ($t_{1/2}$ 13.7 h) than in young subjects ($t_{1/2}$ 6.5 h) of fast acetylator phenotype. There was no effect of age on any sulfapyridine disposition parameters, and only the steady-state plasma levels of the acetylated, inactive metabolite of 5-AS were about 50% higher in the elderly because of a decrease in GFR and renal CL of acetylated 5-AS [52].

The immunomodulators 6-mercaptopurine and azathioprine are increasingly applied. Both are actually inactive and must be converted in vivo to active compounds (6-thioguanine nucleotides). Again, several populations have been pharmacokinetically investigated, but apparently putative age effects have been neglected [51]. Likewise, no special pharmacokinetic data in the elderly are available for the renally eliminated methotrexate [51]; its dosage should be guided according to the actually estimated GFR. The influence of age on the pharmacokinetics of cyclosporine, which is metabolized by CYP3A4, has been studied in healthy elderly individuals, elderly patients with rheumatoid arthritis and young adults. Neither peak plasma concentrations (1–1.1 µg/ml), oral CL (16.6 ml/min) or $t_{1/2}$ (10.7–12.7 h) differed significantly [53]. These data indicate that an age-adjusted regimen of cyclosporine is not necessary for the elderly.

Pharmacokinetic data on the specific TNF-α antibody infliximab are limited. The new compound is predominantly distributed to the vascular compartment (V 3–4 liters), and elimination is very slow ($t_{1/2}$ 9–14 days, CL 0.17 ml/min). As no accumulation of infliximab was observed when the agent was administered at intervals of 4 or 8 weeks [51, 54], the age of the patient is probably of minor importance.

Conclusions

The elderly often suffer from multiple chronic illnesses and consequently they require treatment with a variety of drugs, including such that act on the gastrointestinal tract. Age-related changes in physiology and drug disposition might complicate the clinical problem. When prescribing drugs, basic principles of pharmacokinetics (e.g. type and characteristics of elimination, enzymes involved in drug metabolism, actual GFR) should be known and applied. Most drugs have to be metabolized before final excretion and this hepatic elimination seems to be quite normal in advanced age, at least in the fit elderly. Likewise, the age-dependent decline in kidney function (GFR) is less marked and well preserved in the healthy elderly. Apparently, frailty (e.g. impaired liver and/or kidney function) contributes more than age per se to impairments in drug elimination [55]. In addition, more systematic clinical studies addressing both the pharmacokinetics and pharmacodynamics at the same time are needed to differentiate the reasons for any putative age-dependent drug action.

In conclusion, because of the complexity of aging and concomitant diseases and because of some inconsistencies, no definite predictions regarding whether or not the disposition of a particular drug will be affected by aging can be provided. However, in general, any influence of advanced age on pharmacokinetics is minor or at best modest. Nevertheless, the 'old' clinical principle 'start low, go slow' should still be applied when initiating drug therapy in populations with special risks.

Acknowledgements

This work was supported by the Robert Bosch Foundation, Stuttgart, Germany. The secretarial assistance of Mrs. Bonilla Torres is highly appreciated.

References

1   Winkler MA: Aging: A global issue. JAMA 1997;278:1377.
2   Crome P, Flanagan RJ: Pharmacokinetic studies in elderly people – are they necessary? Clin Pharmacokinet 1994;26:243–247.
3   Herrlinger C, Klotz U: Drug metabolism and drug interactions in the elderly. Best Pract Res Clin Gastroenterol 2001;15:897–918.
4   Turnheim K: Drug dosage in the elderly. Is it rational? Drugs Aging 1998;13:357–379.
5   Wilkinson GR: The effects of diet, aging and disease-states on presystemic elimination and oral drug bioavailability in humans. Adv Drug Deliv Rev 1997;27:129–159.
6   Hämmerlein A, Derendorf H, Lowenthal DT: Pharmacokinetics and pharmacodynamic changes in the elderly. Clinical implications. Clin Pharmacokinet 1998;35:49–64.
7   Klotz U, Avant GR, Hoyumpa A, Schenker S, Wilkinson GR: The effect of age and liver disease on the disposition and elimination of diazepam in adult man. J Clin Invest 1975;55:347–359.
8   Mörike K, Schwab M, Klotz U: Use of aminoglycosides in elderly patients. Pharmacokinetic and clinical considerations. Drugs Aging 1997;10:259–277.
9   Fliser D, Franek E, Joest M, Block S, Mutschler E, Ritz E: Renal function in the elderly: Impact of hypertension and cardiac function. Kidney Int 1997;51:1196–1204.
10 Fliser D, Bischoff I, Hanses A, Block S, Joest M, Ritz E, Mutschler E: Renal handling of drugs in the healthy elderly. Creatinine clearance underestimates renal function and pharmacokinetics remain virtually unchanged. Eur J Clin Pharmacol 1999;55:205–211.

11   Zhang Y, Benet LZ: The gut as a barrier to drug absorption. Combined role of cytochrome P450 3A and P-glycoprotein. Clin Pharmacokinet 2001;40:159–168.

12   Schmucker DL: Aging and the liver: An update. J Gerontol A Biol Sci Med Sci 1998;53: B315–B320.

13   Kinirons MT, Crome P: Clinical pharmacokinetic considerations in the elderly. An update. Clin Pharmacokinet 1997;33:302–312.

14   Le Couteur DG, McLean AJ: The aging liver. Drug clearance and an oxygen diffusion barrier hypothesis. Clin Pharmacokinet 1998;34:359–373.

15   Brenner S, Herrlinger C, Dilger K, Mürdter TE, Hofmann U, Marx C, Klotz U: Influence of age and cytochrome P4502C9 genotype on the steady-state disposition of diclofenac and celecoxib. Clin Pharmacokinet 2003;42:283–292.

16   Kim RB, O'Shea D, Wilkinson GR: Interindividual variability of chlorzoxazone 6-hydroxylation in men and women and its relationship to CYP2E1 genetic polymorphisms. Clin Pharmacol Ther 1995;57:645–655.

17   Gupta S: P-glycoprotein expression and regulation. Age-related changes and potential effects on drug therapy. Drugs Aging 1995;7:19–29.

18   Tanigawara Y: Role of P-glycoprotein in drug disposition. Ther Drug Monit 2000;22:137–140.

19   Porro GB, Lazzaroni M: Prescribing policy for antiulcer treatment in the elderly. Drugs Aging 1993;3:308–319.

20   Hatlebakk JG, Berstad A: Pharmacokinetic optimisation in the treatment of gastro-oesophageal reflux disease. Clin Pharmacokinet 1996;31:386–406.

21   Lazzaroni M, Porro GB: Treatment of peptic ulcer in the elderly. Proton pump inhibitors and histamine H_2 receptor antagonists. Drugs Aging 1996;9:251–261.

22   Marks IN: Sucralfate – safety and side effects. Scand J Gastroenterol Suppl 1991;185:36–42.

23   Wagstaff AJ, Benfield P, Monk JP: Colloidal bismuth subcitrate – a review of its pharmacodynamic and pharmacokinetic properties, and its therapeutic use in peptic ulcer disease. Drugs 1988;36:132–157.

24   Slikkerveer A, de Wolff FA: Pharmacokinetics and toxicity of bismuth compounds. Med Toxicol Adverse Drug Exp 1989;4:303–323.

25   Treiber G, Gladziwa U, Ittel TH, Walker S, Schweinsberg F, Klotz U: Tripotassium dicitrato bismuthate: Absorption and urinary excretion of bismuth in patients with normal and impaired renal function. Aliment Pharmacol Ther 1991;5:491–502.

26   Agrawal NM, Roth S, Graham DY, White RH, Germain B, Brown JA, Stromatt SC: Misoprostol compared with sucralfate in the prevention of nonsteroidal anti-inflammatory drug-induced gastric ulcer. A randomized, controlled trial. Ann Intern Med 1991;115:195–200.

27   Nicholson PA, Karim A, Smith M: Pharmacokinetics of misoprostol in the elderly, in patients with renal failure and when coadministered with NSAID or antipyrine, propranolol or diazepam. J Rheumatol Suppl 1990;20:33–37.

28   Wynne HA, Yelland C, Cope LH, Boddy A, Woodhouse KW, Bateman DN: The association of age and frailty with the pharmacokinetics and pharmacodynamics of metoclopramide. Age Ageing 1993;22:354–359.

29   Brogden RN, Carmine AA, Heel RC, Speight TM, Avery GS: Domperidone. A review of its pharmacological activity, pharmacokinetics and therapeutic efficacy in the symptomatic treatment of chronic dyspepsia and as an antiemetic. Drugs 1982;24:360–400.

30   Vestal RE, Cusack BJ, Mercer GD, Dawson GW, Park BK: Aging and drug interactions. I. Effect of cimetidine and smoking on the oxidation of theophylline and cortisol in healthy men. J Pharmacol Exp Ther 1987;241:488–500.

31   Green DS, Szego PI, Anslow JA, Hooper AW: The effect of age on ranitidine pharmacokinetics. Clin Pharmacol Ther 1986;39:300–305.

32   Lin JH, Chremos AN, Yeh KC, Antonello J, Hessy GA II: Effects of age and chronic renal failure on the urinary excretion kinetics of famotidine in man. Eur J Clin Pharmacol 1988;34:41–46.

33   Callaghan JT, Rubin A, Knadler MP, Bergstrom RF: Nizatidine, an H_2-receptor antagonist: Disposition and safety in the elderly. J Clin Pharmacol 1987;27:618–624.

34   Lameire N, Rosenkranz B, Brockmeier D: Pharmacokinetics of histamine (H_2)-receptor antagonists, including roxatidine, in chronic renal failure. Scand J Gastroenterol Suppl 1988;146: 100–110.

35   Gladziwa U, Klotz U: Pharmacokinetic optimisation of the treatment of peptic ulcer in patients with renal failure. Clin Pharmacokinet 1994;27:393–408.

36   Ishizaki T, Horai Y: Cytochrome P450 and the metabolism of proton pump inhibitors – emphasis on rabeprazole. Aliment Pharmacol Ther 1999;13(suppl 3):27–36.

37   Klotz U: Pharmacokinetic considerations in the eradication of *Helicobacter pylori.* Clin Pharmacokinet 2000;38:243–270.

38   Cederberg C, Andersson T, Skånberg I: Omeprazole: Pharmacokinetics and metabolism in man. Scand J Gastroenterol Suppl 1989;166:33–40.

39   Flouvat B, Delhotal-Landes B, Cournot A, Dellatolas F: Single and multiple dose pharmacokinetics of lansoprazole in elderly subjects. Br J Clin Pharmacol 1993;36:467–469.

40   Breuel HP, Hartmann M, Bondy S, et al: Pantoprazole in the elderly: No dose-adjustment. Gut 1994;35(suppl 4):177.

41   Swan SK, Hoyumpa AM, Merritt GJ: The pharmacokinetics of rabeprazole in health and disease. Aliment Pharmacol Ther 1999;13(suppl 3):11–17.

42   Ammon S, Treiber G, Kees F, Klotz U: Influence of age on the steady state disposition of drugs commonly used for the eradication of *Helicobacter pylori*. Aliment Pharmacol Ther 2000;14: 759–766.

43   Sjövall J, Alván G, Huitfeldt B: Intra- and inter-individual variation in pharmacokinetics of intravenously infused amoxycillin and ampicillin to elderly volunteers. Br J Clin Pharmacol 1986;21:171–181.

44   Chu SY, Wilson DS, Guay DR, Craft C: Clarithromycin pharmacokinetics in healthy young and elderly volunteers. J Clin Pharmacol 1992;32:1045–1049.

45   Lau AH, Lam NP, Piscitelli SC, Wilkes L, Danziger LH: Clinical pharmacokinetics of metronidazole and other nitroimidazole anti-infectives. Clin Pharmacokinet 1992;23:328–364.

46   Sands BE: Therapy of inflammatory bowel disease. Gastroenterology 2000;118:S68–S82.

47   Frey BM, Frey FJ: Clinical pharmacokinetics of prednisone and prednisolone. Clin Pharmacokinet 1990;19:126–146.

48   Tornatore KM, Logue G, Venuto RC, Davis PJ: Pharmacokinetics of methylprednisolone in elderly and young healthy males. J Am Geriatr Soc 1994;42:1118–1122.

49   Hamedani R, Feldman RD, Feagan BG: Drug development in inflammatory bowel disease: Budesonide – a model of targeted therapy. Aliment Pharmacol Ther 1997;11(suppl 3):98–108.

50   Spencer CM, McTavish D: Budesonide. A review of its pharmacological properties and therapeutic efficacy in inflammatory bowel disease. Drugs 1995;50:854–872.

51   Schwab M, Klotz U: Pharmacokinetic considerations in the treatment of inflammatory bowel disease. Clin Pharmacokinet 2001;40:723–751.

52   Taggart AJ, McDermott BJ, Roberts SD: The effect of age and acetylator phenotype on the pharmacokinetics of sulfasalazine in patients with rheumatoid arthritis. Clin Pharmacokinet 1992;23:311–320.

53   Kovarik JM, Koelle EU: Cyclosporin pharmacokinetics in the elderly. Drugs Aging 1999;15: 197–205.

54   Sandborn WJ, Hanauer SB: Antitumor necrosis factor therapy for inflammatory bowel disease: A review of agents, pharmacology, clinical results, and safety. Inflamm Bowel Dis 1999;5: 119–133.

55   Holt PR: Gastrointestinal drugs in the elderly. Am J Gastroenterol 1986;81:403–411.

Prof. Dr. Ulrich Klotz
Dr. Margarete Fischer-Bosch-Institut für Klinische Pharmakologie,
Auerbachstrasse 112, D–70376 Stuttgart (Germany)
Tel. +49 711 8101 3702, Fax +49 711 859295, E-Mail ulrich.klotz@ikp-stuttgart.de

Pilotto A, Malfertheiner P, Holt PR (eds): Aging and the Gastrointestinal Tract.
Interdiscipl Top Gerontol. Basel, Karger, 2003, vol 32, pp 40–56

....

Aging of the Esophagus and Stomach

Adhip P.N. Majumdar[a-d], *Richard Jaszewski*[a,b]

[a]Veterans Affairs Medical Center and [b]Department of Internal
Medicine and [c]Department of Biochemistry and Molecular Biology and
[d]Karmanos Cancer Institute, Wayne State University School of Medicine,
Detroit, Mich., USA

Esophagus: Disorders of Swallowing

Oropharyngeal

The normal swallowing mechanism is a complex coordinated interaction of neurologic, muscular and visceral components resulting in an orderly progression of a solid or liquid bolus from the mouth to the stomach. Initially, following mastication, the tongue exerts pressure on the hard and soft palates to propel the bolus from the oral cavity to the pharynx. Normally, the pharyngeal pressure consists primarily of a propagated contraction through the oropharynx and hypopharynx to facilitate clearance of the pharynx and to minimize residue in the valleculae and pyriform sinuses [1, 2]. The pharyngeal contraction ultimately delivers the bolus to the upper esophageal sphincter (UES). The resting pressure should rapidly decrease at the UES immediately prior to arrival of the bolus at the level of the pyriform sinus [3, 4]. Adjacent structures such as the larynx, as reflected by movements of the hyoid bone, can contribute to physiologic relaxation of the UES [5]. Opening and relaxation of the UES during swallowing is further influenced by the relaxation of the cricopharyngeus muscle as well as the traction forces imparted upon this muscle by contraction of the suprahyoid and thyrohyoid muscles [6]. These muscles also contribute to closure of the airway with reflexive inhibition of respiration, which is critical in the prevention of aspiration as the bolus proceeds to the UES.

Aging has been associated with a diversity of alterations in the oropharyngeal components of swallowing. In general, oropharyngeal segmental transit times [5, 6] as well as pharyngeal peristaltic pressure wave activity and amplitude [7, 8] have been found to be significantly increased in elderly patients [5, 6]. Peak pharyngeal pressures are higher in elderly patients [9] and the anteroposterior diameter of the UES as well as the anterior hyoid bone and laryngeal excursion was found to be significantly less in elderly individuals compared to their younger counterparts [6]. Although the mean UES resting pressure tends to decrease with aging [9], possibly as the result of striated muscle degeneration, the UES residual pressure following deglutition is increased [10]. Rapid anterior movements of the hyoid normally observed in younger patients were delayed in elderly patients as was the subsequent anticipated relaxation of the UES. Consequently, smooth passage of the bolus from the oropharynx to the esophagus would be compromised, rendering inefficient the mechanisms which normally preclude aspiration.

Esophageal Body

During the esophageal phase of swallowing, the ingested bolus is propelled through the esophagus by primary peristaltic waves and, subsequently, with a coordinated relaxation of the lower esophageal sphincter (LES), is delivered into the stomach. There have been numerous studies examining the effects of aging on esophageal motility in patients with dysphagia as well as healthy asymptomatic controls. A variety of abnormalities have been described in both subgroups; however, the consistency of these aberrant findings has been the subject of debate. For example, Grande et al. [11] studied 79 healthy subjects and noted an inverse correlation of age with LES pressure as well as peristaltic wave amplitude and velocity. Alternatively, Richter et al. [12] did not detect any differences in LES pressure between young and elderly subjects using either the rapid or stationary pull-through methods. This finding has been confirmed by others [13], who further noted that the total length of the LES high-pressure zone was similar between young and elderly subjects. Several investigators have found an age-related decrease in the amplitude of peristaltic wave pressure [11, 14]. These studies also noted a decrease in peristaltic velocity and an increase in wave duration, while Hollis and Castell [15] found no age-related differences in these parameters. Secondary peristalsis, which is essentially a peristaltic wave which is not induced by a swallow, occurs less frequently in elderly subjects and may contribute to reduced clearance of residual as well as refluxed esophageal contents [14]. Finally, several investigators have shown an increased frequency of tertiary or spontaneous nonperistaltic contractions in elderly subjects [10, 11, 16].

Gastroesophageal Reflux Disease

The antireflux barrier at the gastroesophageal junction is generally believed to be attributable to the intrinsic LES tone and the crural diaphragm which exerts extrinsic pressure on the LES, as well as the length and thoracic-abdominal distribution of the LES [17, 18]. Xie et al. [19] found that elderly subjects had increased gastroesophageal reflux events after pharyngeal water swallows significantly more often than their younger counterparts. This increase in reflux events was further associated with a decreased intra-abdominal segment of the LES in the elderly. Other investigators [20–22] have noted an increased duration of reflux episodes in elderly patients. Interestingly, however, elderly patients seem to perceive reflux episodes less frequently than younger patients [15, 22, 23].

Barrett's Esophagus

Barrett's esophagus, a premalignant lesion, involves the replacement of normal stratified squamous epithelium with intestinal metaplastic epithelium at the distal esophagus [24]. The prevalence of Barrett's esophagus increases with age and plateaus in the seventh decade [25]. Although this increasing prevalence with aging certainly reflects the cumulative effect of protracted esophageal exposure to acid, aging may independently contribute to the evolution and progression of Barrett's epithelium through age-related reduction in perception of acid reflux [22, 23, 26]. Similarly, elderly patients would also be more likely to require certain medications which potentially diminish LES pressure, such as calcium channel blockers, β-adrenergic agonists and nitrates, thereby increasing the likelihood of acid reflux disease [27].

It is well recognized that Barrett's esophagus is a premalignant lesion with the potential to transform into adenocarcinoma of the esophagus. The presence of Barrett's esophagus is associated with a 30- to 40-fold increased risk of esophageal adenocarcinoma [28]. The development of adenocarcinoma in Barrett's esophagus is a multistep process during which the metaplastic epithelium ultimately transforms into low-grade and subsequently high-grade dysplasia. There is evidence that continuous acid exposure can induce differentiation and reduced proliferation, whereas short bursts of acid exposure increase proliferation [29]. More importantly, normalization of intraesophageal pH can reduce esophageal mucosal cell proliferation. Interestingly, complete eradication of symptoms does not guarantee normalization of intraesophageal pH [30]. Therefore, it is certainly conceivable that elderly individuals with intrinsically enhanced reflux but compromised sensitivity to reflux would be particularly susceptible to induction of mucosal cell proliferation.

Cyclooxygenase-2 (COX-2), a membrane-bound protein involved in the generation of prostaglandins from arachidonic acid, mediates prostanoid release involved in inflammatory as well as tumorigenic responses [31]. Recent evidence suggests that COX-2 protein expression is significantly higher in Barrett's metaplastic and dysplastic epithelium as well as adenocarcinoma and is correlated with progressive morphologic changes [32]. Certainly, nonselective COX inhibitors (nonsteroidal antiinflammatory agents) as well as newer selective COX-2 inhibitors may have a role in cancer chemoprevention for patients with Barrett's esophagus.

Finally, mutations in the tumor suppressor gene p53, one of the most common genetic alterations in human cancer, have been described in the majority of cases of Barrett's esophagus with high-grade dysplasia or adenocarcinoma [33]. Similarly, immunohistochemical staining of p53 has been demonstrated in low-grade dysplasia associated with Barrett's esophagus and may be predictive of future evolution to high-grade dysplasia. Elderly patients with comorbid conditions precluding definitive surgical intervention for Barrett's dysplasia are often considered for a variety of endoscopic ablative techniques. Despite the effectiveness of many of these techniques to destroy Barrett's mucosa, there is still evidence that the genetic aberrations associated with Barrett's esophagus may persist [34].

Stomach

Since most of the information pertaining to the age-related changes in the structure and function of the stomach is restricted to the mucosa, we will briefly review the structural and functional changes in the gastric mucosa during aging.

Structural Changes

Like other parts of the gastrointestinal tract, the gastric mucosa is composed of numerous exocrine and endocrine cells [35] which renew at different rates. In the oxyntic gland area of the stomach, most of the newly produced cells migrate rapidly to the surface while differentiating into mucus cells. The migration time, which represents the time for replacement of the total cell population above the dividing zone, is about 3 days in adult rats [36] and 4–6 days in the adult dog and human [37]. Most studies have indicated that parietal cells are unable to divide, and some newly formed cells slowly migrate down the gland to differentiate into acid-producing cells [37]. In the adult mouse, zymogen (chief) cells are replaced by mitosis [38], but after injury, they have been found to originate from undifferentiated cells.

Aging is associated with marked changes in the structural and functional properties of the gastric mucosa. In rats, aging is found to be associated with gastric atrophy, as evidenced by a significant reduction in mucosal glandular height, gland density (number of glands per cm^2) and total mucosal DNA content [39, 40], and may lead to a reduction in the number of glandular epithelial cells of all types. In aged rats, gastric epithelial cells also show evidence of decreased secretory activity, with a decreased number of intracytoplasmic secretory granules and decreased cell size [39]. In contrast, the connective tissues of the lamina propria of aged rats, especially between the glands and the muscularis, are found to be thickened due to massive collagen deposition [39]. Electron microscopy studies in rats have further demonstrated ultrastructural degenerative changes in both parietal and chief cells [39, 41].

Although earlier studies have suggested that the gastric mucosa remains normal in older human subjects, several reports have documented a marked rise in the incidence of atrophic gastritis among the elderly [42, 43]. Earlier studies by Andrews et al. [42] demonstrated some degree of chronic atrophic gastritis in 23 of 24 subjects over 60 years of age. Bird et al. [43], who analyzed 201 gastric biopsy specimens from individuals aged between 65 and 90 years, observed signs of atrophy in most of the specimens. Hradsky et al. [44] also found an increased incidence of gastritis with aging by comparing the results of gastric biopsy examinations in groups of patients under 44 years of age, between 45 and 59 years and between 60 and 84 years of age. Although the regulatory mechanism(s) underlying the development of gastric atrophy is unknown, one plausible explanation could be that with aging, the ability of the gastric mucosa to replenish the lost surface cells decreases. Indeed, we have observed that in aged rats, reepithelialization of the gastric mucosa following hypertonic saline-induced mucosal erosion is markedly delayed compared to young animals [45].

Aging is also associated with increased susceptibility of the gastric mucosa to damaging agents [46]. This, together with impediments to the repair process, may contribute to the increased incidence of gastric and duodenal ulcers observed among the elderly. Since the intake of aspirin and other nonsteroidal antiinflammatory drugs (NSAIDs) is generally higher among the elderly, studies have been performed to determine the frequency of NSAID-induced injury in elderly subjects. Epidemiological data suggest that aging is associated with increased NSAID-induced gastric mucosal injury [47]. Our investigation with hypertonic saline, which virtually eliminates the surface epithelium, revealed a 67% higher lesion index (percent damaged area) in the gastric mucosa of 24-month-old Fischer-344 rats compared to their 4-month-old counterparts [48]. Microscopic examination also revealed that although administration of hypertonic saline virtually eliminated the surface epithelium in both young and aged rats, the injury in older animals extended beyond the surface epithelium [45]. In aged rats, epithelial cells in deeper parts of the gastric glands demonstrated severe swelling with vacuolization and disintegration of the cell organelles and dying and dead cells [45]. Aspirin and ethanol have also been shown to produce a greater number of lesions in the gastric mucosa of aged rats than in young rats [49]. Taken together, these observations suggest that aging is associated with a reduction in mucosal protective mechanisms that may predispose aged animals to mucosal injury. Although the underlying biochemical mechanisms for this increased susceptibility are poorly understood, several investigators have demonstrated that gastric mucosal prostaglandin content, which provides cytoprotection to the surface epithelium, decreases with aging in humans [50]. Gronbech and Lacy [51] have suggested that impaired mucosal defense and reduced restitution in aged rats is partly due to decreased density of calcitonin gene-related peptide in nerve fibers and the prostaglandin biosynthetic capacity of the mucosa. A decline in mucosal blood flow in aged rats has also been suggested as another causative factor for the age-related decline of mucosal repair [52]. In addition, *Helicobactor pylori* infection, which is increased among diabetics and the elderly, is thought to be an important causative factor for duodenal and gastric ulcers [53]. Clearly, further studies are needed to evaluate the roles of various endogenous and exogenous factors in the age-related rise in the frequency of gastric mucosal injury.

Functional Changes

Although the major constituents of the gastric juice are hydrogen ion, pepsin, mucus and intrinsic factor, the only indispensable ingredient is intrinsic factor, which is required for absorption of vitamin B_{12} by the ileal mucosa. Pernicious anemia resulting from vitamin B_{12} deficiency has been observed in the aging population [54]. A decreased mucosal cell mass and, in turn, a diminished production of intrinsic factor by the parietal cells could, in part, be responsible for the development of pernicious anemia observed in the aging population. However, an association of atrophic gastritis with pernicious anemia has been disputed. Considering that a severe reduction in intrinsic factor is required before vitamin B_{12} absorption by the ileal mucosa is impaired, evidence has been presented to show that in atrophic gastritis, appreciable quantities of intrinsic factor may still be produced when acid production is greatly diminished [54].

At times, atrophic gastritis is also associated with intestinal metaplasia, and both conditions are age related and considered to be precancerous lesions [55]. Thus, aged individuals with gastritis are statistically at risk of developing gastric cancer, but precise measurement of this risk has not been carried out. Furthermore, endoscopic examination in asymptomatic individuals who had undergone partial gastrectomy for duodenal ulcer 15 years previously or earlier revealed unsuspected mucosal abnormalities, including atrophic gastritis, intestinal metaplasia or carcinoma of the gastric stump [56]. We analyzed time-dependent changes in ornithine decarboxylase (ODC) activity, an indicator of the proliferative process, in the gastric mucosa of subjects who underwent Billroth I or II gastrectomy [57]. We reported that ODC was significantly higher in Billroth II patients in whom gastrectomy had been performed >15 years earlier compared with those in whom it had been performed <15 years earlier or normal controls [57]. We suggested that patients who underwent gastrectomy >15 years earlier may be at risk of developing cancer [57].

In view of the fact that one of the main functions of the stomach is to secrete acid, considerable work has been done to examine the age-related changes in acid output by the gastric mucosa. Earlier studies demonstrated a decline in both basal and histamine-stimulated acid output in aging humans [58], which was related to the degree of gastric mucosal atrophy and the parietal cell number. In Fischer-344 rats, we also observed an age-related decline in basal and gastrin-induced acid secretion [40], which could partly be due to a reduced number of acid secretory cells [39, 41]. In contrast, recent studies on healthy humans revealed no significant change in either basal or stimulated gastric acid output with aging [59, 60]. Similarly, the pentagastrin-induced stimulation of acid output was found to be only slightly decreased among the elderly [61]. Thus, the findings of earlier studies, which reported a decline in both basal and maximal gastric acid output in aging human populations, could be the result of inclusion of subjects with atrophic gastritis, a condition which is recognized to be common among the elderly, affecting 25% of those over 60 years of age [43, 61, 62]. Another factor that may affect gastric acid secretion in humans is *H. pylori* infection [59, 63], the incidence of which is also increased with aging [53, 64]. *H. pylori* has been recognized as a causative factor in the development of chronic antral gastritis [65] and may be associated with the development of gastric carcinoma [66, 67]. Whether aging alone results in gastric mucosal atrophy or whether chronic antral gastritis associated with *H. pylori* evolves over time into chronic atrophic gastritis is the subject of continuing debate. However, the prevalence of gastric and duodenal ulcers is high in patients with *H. pylori* infection, suggesting an involvement of the bacterium in peptic ulcer formation [68–70]. Persistent *H. pylori* infection also delays ulcer healing [69]. Although the precise mechanism(s) is not fully understood, the cytotoxin Vac A produced by this bacterium may inhibit proliferation and migration of epithelial cells [71, 72], processes that are essential for mucosal healing. Moreover, Vac A interferes with the binding of epidermal growth factor (EGF) to its receptor, thereby inhibiting EGF- or transforming growth factor (TGF)-α-induced proliferation and migration of epithelial cells during ulcer healing [72, 73]. Delay in ulcer healing in *H. pylori*-infected patients is likely to expose the damaged mucosa to further cellular injury and DNA damage and thus may induce the processes of carcinogenesis, the incidence of which increases with aging.

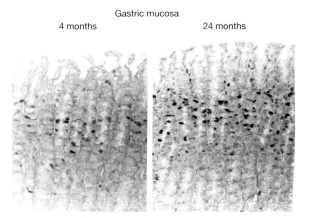

Gastric mucosa

4 months   24 months

Fig. 1. Photomicrograph showing changes in gastric mucosal proliferative activity, as assessed by bromodeoxyuridine immunoreactivity, in 4- and 24-month-old rats.

Basal pepsin secretion as well as the mucosal pepsinogen concentration have also been found to be lower in aged than in young rats [40]. The regulatory mechanism(s) for the age-related decline in mucosal pepsinogen content in rats is not known. We reported a decline in steady-state mRNA levels of several gastric proteases including pepsinogen C with aging [74]. Whether this could result in decreased synthesis of the enzyme remains to be determined. In humans, aging has also been shown to decrease both basal and stimulated gastric pepsin output, and was found to be independent of atrophic gastritis, *H. pylori* infection or smoking [60]. On the other hand, serum pepsinogen I levels in normal females, but not in males, were shown to increase with age [75]. A similar observation was also made in duodenal ulcer patients aged 50 or over [76].

Maintenance of Structural and Functional Integrity

Since the structural and, in turn, the functional integrity of the mucosa of various parts of the gastrointestinal tract, including that of the stomach, are maintained by constant renewal of cells, a number of laboratories, including our own, have studied the age-related changes in gastrointestinal mucosal cell proliferation and the regulation of this process at different stages of life. Earlier, we reported that gastric mucosal proliferative activity in rats, as assessed by DNA synthesis and thymidine kinase activity, remained elevated during the first 2 weeks of postnatal life then decreased over the next 2–3 weeks [77]. Conversely, morphological as well as biochemical studies from this laboratory indicate that in the Fischer-344 rat model, aging is associated with increased gastric mucosal proliferative activity (fig. 1), as evidenced by increased mitotic

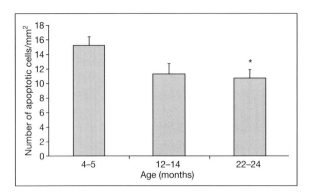

Fig. 2. Changes in the number of apoptotic cells, as assessed by TUNEL assay, in the gastric mucosa of overnight-fasted 4- to 5-, 12- to 14- and 22- to 24-month-old Fischer-344 rats.

labeling of the rate of DNA synthesis, thymidine kinase activity and ODC [78]. Others have also reported a similar phenomenon in both the small and large intestine [79], where these investigators found a greater level of crypt cell production relative to villus cell populations [79]. However, this was not accompanied by increased growth of the organs. Therefore, the reported increased production of crypt cells could not be explained by formation of more crypts, which suggests that in the small and large intestine of aged rats, DNA replication occurred without cytokinesis. A similar explanation could also be offered for our observation in the gastric mucosa in which increased mucosal proliferative activity was not accompanied by a concomitant rise in mucosal growth, but rather aging resulted in atrophy of the tissue, as evidenced by the decreased mucosal height as well as DNA and RNA content in 24-month-old Fischer-344 rats compared with their 4-month-old counterparts [40, 41]. Whether this is the result of increased cell loss or a block in mitotic or other cell cycle regulatory events remains to be determined. However, recent data from our laboratory have demonstrated that the age-related rise in gastric mucosal proliferative activity is associated with increased expression and activity of cyclin-dependent kinase 2, accompanied by an increase in cyclin E but not D1 levels and inhibition of p21$^{Waf1/Cip1}$ [80]. These and other relevant observations have led us to suggest that aging enhances the transition from G1 to S phase as well as progression through the S phase in the gastric mucosa [80]. Interestingly, the age-related rise in gastric mucosal proliferative activity in Fischer-344 rats was not accompanied by an increase in apoptosis. In fact, the number of gastric mucosal cells in Fischer-344 rats undergoing apoptosis was found to be lower in older animals (fig. 2).

Over the past three decades, numerous reports have appeared which indicate that several gastrointestinal hormones/growth factors, including gastrin, bombesin, EGF and TGF-α, stimulate gastrointestinal mucosal cell proliferation in young adult animals [81, 82]. However, at least in the gastric mucosa, the age-related rise in mucosal proliferative activity cannot be attributed to either gastrin or bombesin [83, 84]. Although the underlying mechanisms for the age-related loss of the growth-stimulatory effect of either gastrin or bombesin remain to be fully elucidated, at least for gastrin, this could in part be attributed to the loss of functional receptors [85]. In contrast to what has been observed for gastrin and bombesin, pharmacological doses of EGF and its structural and functional analogue TGF-α have been shown to inhibit gastric mucosal proliferative activity in aged rats [86, 87]. Our data suggest that this inhibition could in part be due to increased sensitivity of aged gastric mucosa to these peptides such that low doses of these peptides are stimulatory, whereas high doses inhibit proliferative processes [87]. In support of this postulation, we have observed that the concentration of TGF-α needed to induce maximal stimulation of EGF receptor (EGF-R) tyrosine kinase activity in gastric mucosal membrane preparations from aged rats is considerably lower than that required for the same level of induction in young rats [87].

In addition to hormones, nutritional factors are also known to regulate gastrointestinal mucosal cell proliferation. In the stomach, food deprivation decreases mucosal cell proliferation and refeeding reverses the situation [88]. A similar phenomenon has also been observed in the small and large intestine [89, 90]. However, the food-induced stimulation of proliferative activity in the small intestine in aged but not in young rats has been shown to be associated with broadening of the proliferative zone [89, 90]. In fasted aged rats, proliferative responsiveness of the large intestine to food was found to be blunted [90]. Although these observations indicate that nutritional regulation of mucosal cell proliferation is affected by aging, little information is available about the role of different nutrients in gastrointestinal mucosal cell proliferation during advancing age. However, calorie restriction has been shown to prevent the age-related rise in intestinal crypt hyperplasia in rats [91].

In evaluating the intracellular events regulating the age-related rise in gastric mucosal cell proliferation, we have assessed the role of tyrosine kinases, which are known to play a critical role in cell proliferation and differentiation [92]. Tyrosine kinases are associated with the products of many protooncogenes as well as with receptors of several growth factors, including EGF-R, the common receptor for EGF and TGF-α [92], which is a 170-kD transmembrane glycoprotein that spans the plasma membrane. High-affinity binding sites for the EGF family of peptides, specifically EGF and TGF-α, have been detected in much of the gastrointestinal tract, with highest concentrations in the esophagus, stomach and colon [93, 94]. Moreover, mRNAs for TGF-α as well as its receptor have also been detected in gastric and colonic mucosal cells [95, 96].

Overexpression of EGF-R with increased tyrosine kinase activity has been associated with many human malignancies, including gastric cancer [97]. We have reported that the age-related rise in gastric mucosal proliferative activity is associated with increased expression and activation of EGF-R [98, 99]. Additionally, we have observed that increased gastric mucosal proliferation after injury is accompanied by a concomitant rise in EGF-R tyrosine kinase activity and that these increases can be greatly attenuated by prior administration of tyrphostin, an inhibitor of EGF-R tyrosine kinase [100]. These and other relevant observations suggest a role for EGF-R tyrosine kinase in gastric mucosal cell proliferation. Further support for this postulation comes from the observation that the age-related rise in EGF-R activation in the gastric mucosa results in stimulation of the EGF-R signaling pathways as evidenced by induction of extracellular signal-regulated kinases and c-Jun NH_2-terminal/stress-activated kinases as well as the transcriptional activity of activator protein-1 and nuclear factor-κB [101].

Ligand binding is one of the primary causes for activation of the intrinsic tyrosine kinase activity of EGF-R, triggering a complex array of enzymatic and biological events leading to stimulation of cell proliferation. There is considerable evidence to show that TGF-α, which is synthesized in the mucosa of much of the gastrointestinal tract including the stomach, may play a key role in regulating EGF-R tyrosine kinase activity in different pathophysiological conditions [102]. However, results from cell surface and biochemical studies have demonstrated that the presence of the transmembrane TGF-α is a normal consequence of TGF-α synthesis, and in most cases, the peptide is present on the cell surface in its precursor form, which can also activate EGF-R [103, 104]. We have observed that the age-related rise in EGF-R tyrosine kinase in the gastric mucosa is accompanied by a marked rise in 16- to 20-kD precursor forms of TGF-α in the mucosal membrane fraction, but not in the cytosol [98, 99]. In addition, our recent in vitro studies showed that the membrane-bound precursor form(s) of TGF-α from the gastric and colonic mucosa of aged rats induces greater stimulation of EGF-R tyrosine kinase activity than that from young rats [99], which could partly be attributed to a greater amount of TGF-α bound to EGF-R [99]. Since TGF-α, but not EGF, is synthesized in much of the gastrointestinal mucosa of normal adult rats [105, 106], we postulate that TGF-α plays a key role in regulating gastric mucosal proliferation during aging, probably through an autocrine/juxtacrine mechanism.

Carcinogenesis

One of the most consistent pathological observations in senescent animals is an increased incidence of many types of malignancies, including gastric and colorectal cancers. Gastric cancer rarely occurs before the age of 40 years, but its incidence increases subsequently, with peak incidence occurring in the seventh decade. Many probable explanations, including altered carcinogen metabolism and long-term exposure to cancer-causing agents, have been offered for the age-dependent rise in malignancies [107].

Carcinogenesis, which is a multistep process, results from the accumulation of mutations during progression from normal epithelium to carcinoma [108]. Genetic changes that occur at different stages of epithelial cell carcinoma have been extensively studied by Fearon and Vogelstein [108] in human colon cancer. At least for colon cancer, it has been suggested that the loss or inactivation of the tumor suppressor gene adenomatous polyposis coli (APC) initiates genomic instability that may produce the phenotypic appearance of an adenoma. Advanced tumors, however, possess mutations and/or deletion of a number of oncogenes and tumor suppressor genes not seen in early adenoma [108]. Although such detailed analysis of genetic alterations has not been performed for gastric cancer, inactivation of several tumor suppressor genes, including APC, p53 and deleted in colorectal cancer (DCC), has been observed in gastric cancer [109]. However, little information is available as to whether aging, which is thought to predispose the gastrointestinal tract to carcinogenesis, is associated with increased inactivation of tumor suppressor genes. We have recently demonstrated that in humans, the incidence of mutations of several tumor suppressor genes, specifically APC, DCC and p53, in the gastric mucosa is higher in older subjects [110].

Hyperproliferation is considered central to the initiation of carcinogenesis in the gastrointestinal tract [111]. Activation of certain growth factor receptor signal transduction pathways, including that of the EGF-R, is also evident in both pre-neoplastic and neoplastic lesions [109]. In the gastrointestinal tract, a positive relationship between the hyperproliferative state and increased tyrosine kinase activity has been demonstrated in various premalignant and malignant lesions [112–114]. We have observed that aging is not only associated with increased tyrosine kinase activity of EGF-R but also pp60^{c-src} in the gastric mucosa of Fischer-344 rats [115]. This, together with the observation of increased incidence of inactivation of a number of tumor suppressor genes and increased mucosal proliferative activity of the stomach in the aged suggests that aging may predispose the stomach to carcinogenesis. Moreover, the fact that aging is associated with a modest decrease in the number of apoptotic cells in the gastric mucosa raises the possibility that aberrant survival of a small group of cells or a single cell could increase the susceptibility of the tissue to certain carcinogen(s) or tumor promoter(s) that may initiate the process of carcinogenesis in the stomach.

Acknowledgments

The work described in this communication was supported by the National Institutes of Health/National Institute on Aging (AG 14343) and the Department of Veterans Affairs.

References

1 Kahrilas PJ, Logemann JA, Lin S, Ergun GA: Pharyngeal clearance during swallowing: A combined manometric and videofluorographic study. Gastroenterology 1992;103:128–136.
2 Cerenko D, McConnel FMS, Jackson RT: Quantitative assessment of pharyngeal bolus driving forces. Otolaryngol Head Neck Surg 1989;100:57–63.
3 McConnel FMS: Analysis of pressure generation and bolus transit during pharyngeal swallowing. Laryngoscope 1988;98:71–78.
4 Sokol EM, Heitmann P, Wolf BS, Cohen BR: Simultaneous cineradiographic and manometric study of the pharynx, hypopharynx and cervical esophagus. Gastroenterology 1966;51: 960–974.
5 Yokoyama M, Mitomi N, Tetsuka K, Tayama N, Niimi S: Role of laryngeal movement and effect of aging on swallowing pressure in the pharynx and upper esophageal sphincter. Laryngoscope 2000;110:434–439.
6 Kern M, Bardan E, Arndorfer R, Hofmann C, Ren J, Shaker R: Comparison of upper esophageal sphincter opening in healthy asymptomatic young and elderly volunteers. Ann Otol Rhinol Laryngol 1999;108:982–989.
7 Sears VW, Castell JA, Castell DO: Radial and longitudinal asymmetry of human pharyngeal pressures during swallowing. Gastroenterology 1991;101:1559–1563.
8 Shaker R, Ren J, Podvrsan B, Dodds WJ, Hogan WJ, Kern M, Hoffmann R, Hintz J: Effect of aging and bolus variables on pharyngeal and upper esophageal sphincter motor function. Am J Physiol 1993;264:G427–G432.
9 Meier-Ewert HK, van Herwaarden MA, Gideon RM, Castell JA, Achem S, Castell DO: Effect of age on differences in upper esophageal sphincter and pharynx pressures between patients with dysphagia and control subjects. Am J Gastroenterol 2001;96:35–40.
10 Ribeiro AC, Klingler PJ, Hinder RA, DeVault K: Esophageal manometry: A comparison of findings in younger and older patients. Am J Gastroenterol 1998;93:706–710.
11 Grande L, Lacima G, Ros E, Pera M, Ascaso C, Visa J, Perra C: Deterioration of esophageal motility with age: A manometric study of 79 healthy subjects. Am J Gastroenterol 1999;94: 1795–1801.
12 Richter JE, Wu WC, Johns DN, Blackwell JN, Nelson JL 3rd, Castell JA, Castell DO: Esophageal manometry in 95 healthy adult volunteers. Dig Dis Sci 1987;32:583–592.
13 Bardan E, Xie P, Brasseur J, Dua K, Ulualp SO, Kern M, Shaker R: Effect of aging on the upper and lower esophageal sphincters. Eur J Gastroenterol Hepatol 2000;12:1221–1225.
14 Ren J, Shaker R, Kusano M, Podvrsan B, Metwally N, Dua KS, Sui Z: Effect of aging on the secondary esophageal peristalsis: Presbyesophagus revisited. Am J Physiol 1995;268: G772–G779.
15 Hollis JB, Castell DO: Esophageal function in elderly men: A new look at 'presbyesophagus'. Ann Intern Med 1974;80:371–374.
16 Grishaw EK, Ott DJ, Frederick MG, Gelfand DW, Chen MYM: Functional abnormalities of the esophagus: A prospective analysis of radiographic findings relative to age and symptoms. AJR Am J Roentgenol 1996;167:719–723.
17 Dent J, Dodds WJ, Friedman RH, Sekguchi T, Hogan WJ, Arndorfer RC, Petrie DJ: Mechanism of gastroesophageal reflux in recumbent asymptomatic human subjects. J Clin Invest 1980;65: 256–267.
18 Mittal RK, Rochester DF, McCallum RW: Effect of the diaphragmatic contraction on lower oesophageal sphincter pressure in man. Gut 1987;18:1564–1568.
19 Xie P, Ren J, Bardan E, Mittal RK, Sui Z, Shaker R: Frequency of gastroesophageal reflux events induced by pharyngeal water stimulation in young and elderly subjects. Am J Physiol 1997; 272:G233–G237.
20 Ter RB, Johnston BT, Castell DO: Influence of age and gender on gastroesophageal reflux in symptomatic patients. Dis Esophagus 1998;11:106–108.
21 Ferriolli E, Oliveira RB, Matsuda NM, Braga JFHN, Dantas RO: Aging, esophageal motility, and gastroesophageal reflux. J Am Geriatr Soc 1998;46:1534–1537.

---

22 Fass R, Pulliam G, Johnson C, Garewal HS, Sampliner RE: Symptom severity and oesophageal chemosensitivity to acid in older and young patients with gastro-oesophageal reflux. Age Ageing 2000;29:125–130.

23 Lasch H, Castell DO, Castell JA: Evidence for diminished visceral pain with aging: Studies using graded intraesophageal balloon distention. Am J Physiol 1997;272:G1–G3.

24 Spechler SJ, Goyal RK: Barrett's esophagus. N Engl J Med 1986;315:362–371.

25 Benipal P, Garewas HS, Sampliner RE, Martinez P, Hayden CW, Fass R: Short segment Barrett's esophagus: Relationship of age with extent of intestinal metaplasia. Am J Gastroenterol 2001; 96:3084–3088.

26 Grade A, Pulliam G, Johnson C, Garewal H, Sampliner RE, Fass R: Reduced chemoreceptor sensitivity in patients with Barrett's esophagus may be related to age and not to the presence of Barrett's epithelium. Am J Gastroenterol 1997;92:2040–2043.

27 Lagergren J, Bergstrom R, Adami H, Nyren O: Association between medications that relax the lower esophageal sphincter and risk for esophageal adenocarcinoma. Ann Intern Med 2000; 133:165–175.

28 Pera M, Cameron AJ, Trastek VF, Carpenter HA, Zinsmeister AR: Increasing incidence of adeno-carcinoma of the esophagus and esophagogastric junction. Gastroenterology 1993;104:510–513.

29 Ouatu-Lascar R, Fitzgerald RC, Triadafilopoulos G: Differentiation and proliferation in Barrett's esophagus and the effects of acid suppression. Gastroenterology 1999;117:327–335.

30 Ouatu-Lascar R, Triadafilopoulos G: Complete elimination of reflux symptoms does not guaran-tee normalization of intraesophageal acid reflux in patients with Barrett's esophagus. Am J Gastroenterol 1998;93:711–716.

31 Crofford LJ: COX-1 and COX-2 tissue expression: Implications and predictions. J Rheumatol 1997;24(suppl 49):15–19.

32 Shirvani VN, Ouatu-Lascar R, Kaur BS, Omary MB, Triadafilopoulos G: Cyclooxygenase 2 expression in Barrett's esophagus and adenocarcinoma: Ex vivo induction by bile salts and acid exposure. Gastroenterology 2000;118:487–496.

33 Neshat K, Sanchez CA, Galipeau PC, Blount PL, Levine DS, Joslyn G, Reid BJ: P53 mutations in Barrett's adenocarcinoma and high-grade dysplasia. Gastroenterology 1994;106:1589–1595.

34 Krishnadath KK, Wang KK, Taniguchi K, Sebo TJ, Buttar NS, Anderson MA, Lutzke LS, Liu W: Persistent genetic abnormalities in Barrett's esophagus after photodynamic therapy. Gastroenterology 2000;119:624–630.

35 Lipkin M: Proliferation and differentiation of normal and diseased gastrointestinal cells; in Johnson LR (ed): Physiology of the Gastrointestinal Tract. New York, Raven, 1987, pp 255–284.

36 Creamer E, Shorter EG, Bamforth J: The turnover and shedding of epithelial cells. I. The turnover in the gastrointestinal tract. Gut 1961;2:110–118.

37 Willems G, Vansteenkiste Y, Lambosch JM, Verbeustel S: Autoradiographic study of cell renewal in fundic mucosa of fasting dogs. Acta Anat (Basel) 1971;80:23–32.

38 Lawson HH: The origin of chief and parietal cells in regenerating gastric mucosa. Br J Surg 1970;57:139–141.

39 Majumdar APN, Jasti S, Hatfield JS, Tureaud J, Fligiel SEG: Morphological and biochemical changes in gastric mucosa of aging rats. Dig Dis Sci 1990;35:1364–1370.

40 Maitra RS, Edgerton EA, Majumdar APN: Gastric secretion during aging in pyloric-ligated rats and effects of pentagastrin. Exp Gerontol 1988;23:463–472.

41 Hollander D, Tarnawski A, Stachura J, Gregely H: Morphologic changes in gastric mucosa of aging rats. Dig Dis Sci 1989;34:1692–1700.

42 Andrews GR, Haneman B, Arnold BJ, Booth JC, Taylor K: Atrophic gastritis in the aged. Australas Ann Med 1967;16:230–235.

43 Bird T, Hall MRP, Schade ROK: Gastric histology and its relation to anemia in the elderly. Gerontology 1977;23:309–321.

44 Hradsky M, Groh J, Langr F, Herout V: Chronische Gastritis bei jungen und alten Personen: Histologische und histochemische Untersuchung. Gerontol Clin (Basel) 1966;8:164–171.

45 Fligiel SEG, Relan NK, Dutta S, Tureaud J, Hatfield J, Majumdar APN: Aging diminishes gastric mucosal regeneration: Relationship to tyrosine kinases. Lab Invest 1994;70:764–774.

46 Majumdar APN, Fligiel SEG, Jaszewski R: Gastric mucosal injury and repair: Effect of aging. Histol Histopathol 1997;12:492–501.

47 Fries JF, Miller SR, Spitz PW, Williams CA, Hubert HB, Bloch DA: Toward an epidemiology of gastropathy associated with nonsteroidal anti-inflammatory drug use. Gastroenterology 1989;96: 647–655.

48 Majumdar APN, Moshier JA, Arlow FL, Luk GD: Biochemical changes in the gastric mucosa after injury in young and aged rats. Biochim Biophys Acta 1989;992:35–40.

49 Gronbech JE, Lacy ER: Impaired gastric defense mechanisms in aged rats. Role of sensory neurons, blood flow, restitution and prostaglandins. Gastroenterology 1994;106:A84.

50 Lee M, Feldman M: Age-related reductions in gastric mucosal prostaglandin levels increase susceptibility to aspirin-induced injury in rats. Gastroenterology 1994;107:1746–1750.

51 Gronbech JE, Lacy E: Role of gastric blood flow in impaired defense and repair of aged rat stomachs. Am J Physiol 1995;269:G737–G744.

52 Lee M: Age-related changes in gastric blood flow in rats. Gerontology 1996;42:289–293.

53 Oldenburg B, Diepersloot RJA, Hoekstra JBL: High seroprevalence of *Helicobactor pylori* in diabetes mellitus patients. Dig Dis Sci 1966;41:458–461.

54 Geokas MC, Conteas CN, Majumdar APN: The aging gastrointestinal tract, liver, and pancreas. Clin Geriatr Med 1985;1:177–205.

55 Morson BC, Sobin LH, Grundman E, Johansen A, Nagayo T, Serck-Hanssen A: Precancerous conditions and epithelial dysplasia in the stomach. J Clin Pathol 1980;33:711–721.

56 Pickford IR, Craven JL, Hall R, Thomas G, Stone WD: Endoscopic examination of the gastric remnant 3–39 years after subtotal gastrectomy for peptic ulcer. Gut 1984;25:393–397.

57 Jaszewski R, Katta S, Zaki N, Majumdar APN: Changes in gastric mucosal ornithine decarboxylase and tyrosine phosphorylation of proteins in postgastrectomy patients. Scand J Gastroenterol 1993;28:609–612.

58 Baron JH: Studies of basal and peak acid output with an augmented histamine meal. Gut 1963;4: 136–144.

59 Goldschmiedt M, Barnett CC, Schwartz BE, Karnes WE, Redfern JS, Feldman M: Effect of age on gastric acid secretion and serum gastrin concentrations in healthy men and women. Gastroenterology 1991;101:977–990.

60 Feldman M, Cryer B, McArthur KE, Huet BA, Lee E: Effects of aging and gastritis on gastric acid and pepsin secretion in humans: A prospective study. Gastroenterology 1996;110:1043–1052.

61 Giacosa A, Cheli R: Corrélations anatomo-sécrétoires gastriques en fonction de l'âge chez des sujets ayant une muqueuse fundique normale. Gastroentérol Clin Biol 1979;3:647–650.

62 Cox AJ: Gastric mucosal changes in peptic ulcer. Gastroenterology 1963;45:558–561.

63 Katelaris PH, Seow F, Lin BPC, Ngu MC, Jones DB: Effect of age, *Helicobacter pylori* infection, and gastritis with atrophy on serum gastrin and gastric acid secretion in healthy men. Gut 1993;34:1032–1037.

64 Faisal MA, Russell RM, Samloff IM, Holt PR: *Helicobacter pylori* infection and atrophic gastritis in the elderly. Gastroenterology 1990;99:1543–1544.

65 Dixon MF: *Campylobacter pylori* and chronic gastritis; in Rathbone BJ, Heatley RV (eds): *Campylobacter pylori* and Gastrointestinal Disease. Oxford, Blackwell Scientific, 1989, pp 106–116.

66 Parsonnet GD, Friedman DP, Vandersteen Y, Chang JH, Vogelman N, Orentreich Y, Sibley RK: *Helicobacter pylori* infection and risk of gastric carcinoma. N Engl J Med 1991;325:1127–1131.

67 Forman A: An association between *Helicobacter pylori* and gastric cancer. Lancet 1993;341: 1359–1362.

68 Cover TL, Blaser MJ: *Helicobacter pylori* infection, a paradigm for chronic mucosal inflammation: Pathogenesis and implications for eradication and prevention. Adv Intern Med 1996;41: 85–117.

69 Marshall BJ, Warren JR: Unidentified curved bacilli in the stomach of patients with gastritis and peptic ulceration. Lancet 1984;i:1311–1315.

70 Graham DY, Go MF: *Helicobacter pylori:* Current status. Gastroenterology 1993;105:279–282.

71 Wyle F, Chang KJ, Stachura J, Tarnawski A: *Helicobacter pylori* cytotoxin and healing of experimental gastric ulcer. Eur J Gastroenterol 1993;12(suppl 1):S99–S103.

72 Fujiwara Y, Wyle F, Arakawa T, Domek MJ, Fukuda T, Kobsyashi K, Tarnawski A: *Helicobacter pylori* culture supernatant inhibits binding and proliferative response of human gastric cells to epidermal growth factor: Implications for *H. pylori* interference with ulcer healing? Digestion 1997;58:299–303.

73 Tarnawski A: Cellular mechanisms of gastric ulcer healing; in Domschke W, Konturek S (eds): The Stomach. Berlin, Springer, 1993, pp 177–192.

74 Moshier JA, Cornell T, Majumdar APN: Expression of protease genes in the gastric mucosa during aging. Exp Gerontol 1993;28:249–258.

75 Kekki M, Samloff IM, Sipponen P, Ihamaki T, Siurala M: Increase of serum pepsinogen I with age in females with normal gastric mucosa but not in males, possibly due to increase in acid-pepsin secreting area. Scand J Gastroenterol Suppl 1991;186:62–64.

76 Pilotto A, Vianello F, Di Mario F, Plebani M, Farinati F, Azzini CF: Effect of age on gastric acid, pepsin, pepsinogen group A and gastrin secretion in peptic ulcer patients. Gerontology 1994;40:253–259.

77 Majumdar APN, Johnson LR: Gastric mucosal cell proliferation during development in rats and effects of pentagastrin. Am J Physiol 1982;242:G135–G139.

78 Majumdar APN, Jaszewski R, Dubick MA: Effect of aging on the gastrointestinal tract and pancreas. Proc Soc Exp Biol Med 1997;215:134–144.

79 Attillasoy E, Holt PR: Gastrointestinal proliferation and aging. J Gerontol 1993;48:B43–B49.

80 Xiao Z-Q, Yu Y, Khan A, Jaszewski R, Ehrinpreis MN, Majumdar APN: Induction of G1 checkpoint in the gastric mucosa of aged rats. Am J Physiol 1999;277:G917–G921.

81 Johnson LR: Regulation of gastrointestinal growth; in Johnson LR (ed): Physiology of the Gastrointestinal Tract. New York, Raven, 1987, pp 301–333.

82 Majumdar APN: Growth and maturation of the gastric mucosa; in Solomon TE, Morisset J (eds): Growth of the Gastrointestinal Tract: Gastrointestinal Hormones and Growth Factors. Boca Raton, CRC, 1991, pp 119–130.

83 Majumdar APN, Edgerton EA, Dayal Y, Murthy SNS: Gastrin: Levels and trophic action during advancing age. Am J Physiol 1988;254:G538–G542.

84 Majumdar APN, Tureaud J: Role of tyrosine kinases in bombesin regulation of gastric mucosal proliferative activity in young and aged rats. Peptides 1992;13:795–800.

85 Singh P, Rae-Venter B, Townsend CM Jr, Khalil T, Thompson JC: Gastrin receptors in normal and malignant gastrointestinal mucosa: Age-associated changes. Am J Physiol 1985;249:G761–G769.

86 Majumdar APN, Arlow FL: Aging: Altered responsiveness of gastric mucosa to epidermal growth factor. Am J Physiol 1989;257:G554–G560.

87 Turner JD, Liu L, Fligiel SEG, Jaszewski R, Majumdar APN: Aging alters gastric mucosal responses to epidermal growth factor and transforming growth factor α. Am J Physiol Gastrointest Liver Physiol 2000;278:G805–G810.

88 Majumdar APN: Regulation of gastric mucosal DNA synthesis during fasting and refeeding in rats. Digestion 1983;27:36–43.

89 Holt PR, Yeh KY: Small intestinal crypt cell proliferation rates are increased in senescent rats. J Gerontol 1989;44:B9–B14.

90 Holt PR, Yeh KY: Colonic proliferation is increased in senescent rats. Gastroenterology 1988;95: 1556–1563.

91 Heller TD, Holt PR, Richardson A: Food restriction retards histological changes in rat small intestine. Gastroenterology 1990;98:387–391.

92 Yarden T, Ullrich A: Growth factor receptor tyrosine kinases. Annu Rev Biochem 1988;57: 443–487.

93 Gallo-Payet N, Hugon JS: Epidermal growth factor receptors in isolated adult mouse intestinal cells: Studies in vivo and organ culture. Endocrinology 1985;116:161–201.

94 Thompson JF: Specific receptors for epidermal growth factor in rat intestinal microvillous membranes. Am J Physiol 1988;254:G429–G435.

95 Bennett C, Paterson IM, Corbishiev CM, Lugamani YA: Expression of growth factor and epidermal growth factor receptor encoded transcripts in human gastric tissues. Cancer Res 1989; 49:2104–2111.

96 Malden LT, Novak U, Burgess AW: Expression of transforming growth factor alpha messenger RNA in the normal and neoplastic gastrointestinal tract. Int J Cancer 1989;43:380–384.

97 Khazaie K, Schirrmacher V, Lichtner RB: EGF receptor in neoplasia and metastasis. Cancer Metastasis Rev 1993;12:255–274.

98 Tureaud J, Sarkar FH, Fligiel SEG, Kulkarni S, Jaszewski R, Reddy K, Yu Y, Majumdar APN: Increased expression of EGFR in gastric mucosa of aged rats. Am J Physiol 1997;273: G389–G398.

99 Xiao Z-Q, Majumdar APN: Increased in vitro activation of EGFR by membrane-bound TGF-α from gastric and colonic mucosa of aged rats. Am J Physiol Gastrointest Liver Physiol 2001;281: G111–G116.

100 Majumdar APN, Fligiel SEG, Jaszewski R, Tureaud J, Chelledurai B: Inhibition of gastric mucosal regeneration by tyrphostin: Evaluation of the role of epidermal growth factor receptor tyrosine kinase. J Lab Clin Med 1996;128:173–178.

101 Xiao Z-Q, Majumdar APN: Induction of transcriptional activity of AP-1 and NF-κB in the gastric mucosa during aging. Am J Physiol Gastrointest Liver Physiol 2000;278:G855–G865.

102 Coffey R Jr, Shipley GD, Moses HL: Production of transforming growth factors by human colon cancer cell lines. Cancer Res 1986;46:1164–1169.

103 Brachmann R, Lindquist PB, Nagashima M, Kohr W, Lipari T, Napier M, Derynck R: Transmembrane TGF-α precursors activate EGF/TGF-α receptors. Cell 1989;56:691–700.

104 Massague J: Epidermal growth factor-like transforming growth factor. II. Interaction with epidermal growth factor receptors in human placenta membranes and A431 cells. J Biol Chem 1983; 258:13614–13620.

105 Cartlidge SA, Elder JB: Transforming growth factor alpha and epidermal growth factor levels in normal human gastrointestinal mucosa. Br J Cancer 1989;60:657–660.

106 Relan NK, Saeed A, Ponduri K, Fligiel SEG, Dutta S, Majumdar APN: Identification and evaluation of the role of endogenous tyrosine kinases in azoxymethane induction of proliferative processes in the colonic mucosa of rats. Biochim Biophys Acta 1995;1244:368–376.

107 De Jong T, Skinner SA, Malcontenti-Wilson C, Vogiagis D, Bailey M, Van Driel IR, O'Brian PE: Inhibition of rat colon tumors by sulindac and sulindac sulfone is independent of k-ras (codon 12) mutation. Am J Physiol Gastrointest Liver Physiol 2000;278:G266–G272.

108 Fearon ER, Vogelstein B: A genetic model for colorectal tumorigenesis. Cell 1990;61:759–767.

109 Yokozaki H, Yasui W, Tahara E: Genetic and epigenetic changes in stomach cancer. Int Rev Cytol 2001;204:49–95.

110 Moragoda L, Jaszewski R, Kukarni P, Majumdar APN: Age-associated loss of heterozygosity of tumor suppressor genes in the gastric mucosa of humans. Am J Physiol Gstrointest Liver Physiol 2002;282:G932–G936.

111 Lipkin M: Biomarkers of increased susceptibility to gastrointestinal cancer. Their development and application to studies of cancer prevention. Gastroenterology 1987;92:1083–1086.

112 Cartwright CA, Coad CA, Egbert BM: Elevated c-src tyrosine kinase activity in premalignant epithelia of ulcerative colitis. J Clin Invest 1994;93:509–515.

113 Colarian J, Arlow FL, Calzada R, Luk GD, Majumdar APN: Differential activation of ornithine decarboxylase and tyrosine kinase in the rectal mucosa of patients with hyperplastic and adenomatous polyps. Gastroenterology 1991;100:1528–1532.

114 Lans JI, Jaszewski R, Arlow FL, Luk GD, Majumdar APN: Supplemental calcium suppresses colonic mucosal ornithine decarboxylase activity in elderly patients with adenomatous polyps. Cancer Res 1991;51:3416–3419.

115 Majumdar APN, Tureaud J, Relan NK, Kessel A, Dutta S, Hatfield J, Fligiel SEG: Increased expression of pp60[c-src] in gastric mucosa of aged rats. J Gerontol 1994;49:B110–B116.

A.P.N. Majumdar, PhD, DSc
Research Service – 151, VA Medical Center,
4646 John R Street, Detroit, MI 48201 (USA)
Tel. +1 313 576 4460, Fax +1 313 576 1112, E-Mail a.majumdar@wayne.edu

Pilotto A, Malfertheiner P, Holt PR (eds): Aging and the Gastrointestinal Tract.
Interdiscipl Top Gerontol. Basel, Karger, 2003, vol 32, pp 57–64

······················

Effect of Aging upon the Small Intestine and Colon

Peter R. Holt

St. Luke's Hospital Center, and Institute for Cancer Prevention,
New York, N.Y., USA

In this chapter, the physiologic changes in the small and large intestine that can be ascribed to the aging process and not to diseases will be discussed. In contrast to the effect of aging upon many other organ systems, relatively few such changes have been clearly demonstrated in the gastrointestinal tract.

In which gastrointestinal tissues should we look for effects of advancing age? The small and large intestinal wall consists of the mucosa, principally epithelial cells, muscle, nerves, blood vessels and submucosal connective tissue. The functions of the bowel are also dependent upon afferent and efferent nerve impulses and bioactive peptides, such as neurotensin and glucagon-like peptides, as well as the lymphoid tissue of the bowel wall and surrounding lymph nodes (the gut-associated lymphoid tissue) that act as an immunologic barrier to extraneous ingested toxins. The overall physiology of the gut also requires coordinated control of motility and evacuation, absorption and secretion. These structures and functions are too extensive to be covered in a single chapter and many have not been investigated in detail in aging animals or in humans.

Early authors who evaluated the anatomy and physiology of the gastrointestinal tract during aging confirmed their expectations that major abnormalities must occur in all tissues with the aging process. Thus, they speculated that if there were fewer absorbing epithelial cells and less intestinal surface area then, surely, decrements in intestinal nutrient absorption were bound to follow. The aging bowel surely had to be defective.

From the early studies of Mathis published in 1928 to those of Baker and coworkers in 1963, progressive pathological changes were described in the anatomic appearance of the small intestine. In the 1970s, altered structure of the gastrointestinal tract was described as modest or absent. In the 1980s, an increase in jejunal crypt epithelial cells was noted. Data from biopsies obtained from the human intestine show no loss of villus epithelial cells with advancing age [1]. The pancreas does suffer from a loss of acinar cells, which causes a widening of the pancreatic duct system similar to changes seen in chronic pancreatitis, which presumably is due to a loss of the parenchymal supporting tissues [2]. Liver size also decreases, probably resulting from a reduced blood supply [3]. These changes are not clinically important if they do not result in significant changes in physiologic function and it is clear that many do not.

Carbohydrate Absorption

Many early studies demonstrated modest changes in carbohydrate absorption with advancing age [summarized in ref. 4]. In one study using breath hydrogen production as an indicator of impaired carbohydrate absorption, some decrement in overall transport was described in older individuals [5]. To this author's knowledge, more precise experiments have not been performed in elderly persons. The important studies of Ferraris et al. [6] demonstrated that glucose transporter density per epithelial cell was reduced in older rats but epithelial cell hyperplasia appeared to compensate for this reduction.

Where shall we look for more data in the future? The precise functions of most of the GLUT transporter proteins in the intestine and other tissues have been defined. Furthermore, the control of these transporters is under active study. However, to date, few investigators have defined possible changes in these transporters and, more importantly, their modulation in older animals or humans [7]. For example, it is known that Na^+/glucose transporter 1 expression is increased in the intestine of obese animals; on the other hand, cholecystokinin reduces the abundance of SGLT protein and may impair the absorption of a glucose analog (3 methyl D glucose) [8]. Since blood levels of cholecystokinin are known to be elevated during aging, would this alter glucose absorption?

There is little evidence for a reduction in brush border intestinal disaccharidase enzymes with aging. Of course, the exception is lactase (lactase-phloridzin hydrolase), the activity of which falls dramatically in the majority of the world's population with age. The genetic difference responsible for a polymorphism which determines high or low lactase-phloridzin hydrolase mRNA expression is cis acting to the lactase gene. The genetic downregulation of the lactase gene may be found as a early as the second year of life but the phenotype may not be expressed until much later. What determines the switching off of this system late in life is still unclear.

Fat Absorption

Studies of intestinal fat absorption during aging have been reviewed previously [9] and little new information has been published since. Although orlistat has been developed as an inhibitor of pancreatic and other lipases for the treatment of obesity, no specific studies in older individuals have been described. Novel data have recently been obtained defining several putative proteins involved in ileal bile acid transport. These transport proteins may be modulated by experimental manipulation of the lumenal concentrations of bile acids. There is evidence that idiopathic bile acid malabsorption may accompany unexplained chronic diarrhea, which is commonly associated with alterations in bile acid transporter proteins [10]. However, to this author's knowledge, there have been no studies of these transporter proteins as a function of age, nor is it known whether idiopathic diarrhea due to bile acid absorption occurs more commonly in the elderly.

Recent work has also focussed upon the biology of fatty acid binding proteins in the gut and the liver and the possible importance of these proteins in altering intramucosal pathways of triglyceride synthesis and causing changes in plasma lipoprotein responses to the feeding of different diets [11]. Again, no data on the effect of age upon this process have been described. Furthermore, the assembly of intestinal chylomicrons and the incorporation of individual apoproteins into these lipid molecules is better understood than previously. Whether aging per se alters the distribution of intestinal apoproteins or lipoproteins is unknown.

Minerals and Vitamins

Modern cloning techniques have defined a range of putative metal iron transporters in the intestine. Many of these transporters have broad ranges of substrates, explaining how the presence of one metal may impair the intestinal absorption of another. There is little evidence for changes in metal absorption as a function of age but the concentration and distribution of intestinal transport proteins have not been examined.

It is well known that calcium absorption falls with advancing age, which may contribute to age-associated osteopenia. The current hypothesis for this effect suggests that reduced calcium absorption results from alterations of vitamin D metabolites or their effects at the intestinal levels. Many data have shown that plasma 1,25 dihydroxy vitamin D [1,25(OH)2 D] levels are lower in elderly subjects than in the young, and the unique studies of Ireland and Fordtran [12] showed that calcium absorption failed to respond appropriately to changes in calcium intake. Some studies have demonstrated that the mucosal vitamin D-dependent calbindin concentration may be lower, but stimulation of mRNA for this calcium binding protein by 1,25(OH)2 D is unaltered, suggesting a translational defect. Some studies have shown a change in intestinal 1,25(OH)2 D receptor sites in the intestine and bone. There is also evidence for reduced capacity of the human skin to produce vitamin D from sunlight in advanced age [13], although more recent data raise new questions that deserve further study. Classical teaching stated that the active metabolite of vitamin D, 1,25 dihydroxy vitamin D (calcitriol), is formed in the kidney and that circulating levels of calcitriol determine the action of this hormone through interaction with vitamin D receptors in peripheral tissues. However, recently, increasing evidence points to the presence of a 1-α hydroxylase enzyme in many peripheral tissues including the gastrointestinal tract, bone and prostate [14]. Thus, it becomes likely that autocrine or paracrine formation of the active metabolite of vitamin D, calcitriol, at the organ level determines its ultimate tissue concentration. The intestine also contains a vitamin D 24,25 hydroxylase enzyme that can break down calcitriol [15]. In the future, it will be important to study the levels of these enzymes as well as their receptors in the small and large intestine of aging animals and humans in order to expand our knowledge of mechanisms of bone loss in the elderly.

In addition to vitamin D, changes in vitamin B_{12} (cobalamin) are increasingly recognized as important during the aging process. Vitamin B_{12} depletion is quite common in the elderly. Previously, it was believed that pernicious anemia was the commonest cause of cobalamin deficiency. However, now it is recognized that malabsorption of cobalamin from food is much more common [16]. Hypochlorhydria secondary to chronic atrophic gastritis interferes with vitamin B_{12} by impairing the release of free cobalamin from food protein complexes. Such impairment may also occur in individuals who are taking proton pump inhibitors for extended periods of time. Under these circumstances, not only might food-bound cobalamin not be released, but, in addition, bacterial overgrowth in the upper small intestine might contribute to the depletion of vitamin B_{12}. It is pertinent to point out that since the intestinal absorption of free cobalamin is not impaired in the elderly, vitamin B_{12} depletion or deficiency can be prevented not only by systemic but also by oral administration of large amounts of this vitamin. Oral therapy has been used successfully for many years, and may be more acceptable to the elderly than monthly injections [17].

Drugs

Drug transport from the intestinal lumen into the circulation occurs through or between enterocytes. Changes in drug absorption as a function of age have been reviewed previously [18]. However, there appear to be few studies of several important systems that may alter drug transport. The multidrug resistant

P-glycoprotein and other multidrug resistance proteins are expressed in the gastrointestinal tract as well as in many other tissues. P-glycoprotein is an ATP-dependent reflux pump that increases the outward transport of some drugs from the blood into the intestinal lumen [19]. Thus, P-glycoprotein may limit oral drug absorption. Classically, this protein causes resistance to cancer chemotherapeutic drugs by pumping these agents out of target cells. However, the protein is also a substrate for other agents that require absorption, such as beta-blockers. The author is unaware of studies of these proteins in subjects of advanced age.

Several intestinal cytochrome P450s are involved in the biotransformation of absorbed toxins and xenobiotics. Again, little is known about the effect of age on these systems, which may either limit or induce the transport of toxic agents into the body. Furthermore, first-pass metabolism may be greatly altered at the level of the small and large intestine. Many of the enzymes that determine the metabolism of drugs in the liver are also present in the intestine [20]. A good example involves changes in circulating levels of 5-fluorouracil because of variation in first-pass metabolism. Little work has been directed at the effects of age upon these processes.

Proliferation

Data obtained in the last two decades clearly indicate that proliferation in the gastrointestinal tract in aging animals [21] and at least in the colon in humans [22] is increased when compared to younger individuals. The precise reason for this has not been established but data point to increases in tyrosine kinase phosphorylation as one mechanism [23]. Much of the interest in increased proliferation relates to the possibility that this may enhance the susceptibility of gastrointestinal tissues to carcinogenesis.

A further defect which could account for an age-related change in intestinal proliferation would be alterations in cell death. One study of apoptosis in the small intestine in young and aging animals fed ad libitum and calorie-restricted diets detected that food restriction was accompanied by a significantly higher intestinal apoptotic rate [24]. This study suggests that enhanced apoptosis with caloric restriction might protect the gastrointestinal tract from the accumulation of DNA-altered cells during the aging process.

Motor Function and Motility

It is important to recognize that older healthy active subjects do not have any differences in their rate of intestinal transit from mouth to anus compared to that measured in the young. Furthermore, overall, small intestinal motor patterns appear to be maintained in the elderly. Some reduction in the frequency and strength of contractions in the small bowel was described in early studies in humans and in animals and some preliminary studies found changes in interdigestive motility patterns, but the significance of this is still unclear.

Responses to Stress

A general physiologic phenomenon which occurs during the aging process is that responses to stress, i.e. adaptation to a new stimulus, are generally altered. This contrasts with the observation that basal organ functions may often be maintained in the elderly as well as in the young. Small intestinal responses to stress are classically evaluated by determining the effect of intestinal resection or the responses to changes in food intake in rodents. Such responses have been found to be decreased in elderly animals [25].

One of the major controls of the adaptive response involves responses by circulating hormones. The small and large intestine produce a wide variety of peptides which might be responsible for such impaired responses to stress. Circadian rhythms of peptide activity may be altered. The responses of the pancreas to several hormonal stimuli are known to be impaired or delayed.

An intriguing and as yet not well explained observation is that fasting and postprandial concentrations of serum pancreatic polypeptide are dramatically higher in the elderly and that circulating motilin and neurotensin concentrations also may be elevated in the elderly [26]. Both hyperglucagonemia and increased concentrations of cholecystokinin have also been noted. The precise reason for these elevated serum levels of peptides in the elderly is unknown.

Nitric oxide has been recognized as a crucial molecule altering many small intestinal functions, including stimulation of ion channels and activation of protein kinase C as well as activation of soluble guanyl cyclase in myenteric neurons. This leads to inhibition of the release of the excitatory transmitter substance P. Nitric oxide is present in myenteric plexuses independent of vagal nerves and appears to be negatively regulated by the splanchnic nerves in the small intestine [27]. No studies have been performed on the effect of aging upon endogenous nitric oxide formation or distribution.

Colon

Much less research has been directed to evaluating age-related changes in the structure and function of the colon as compared to studies in the small intestine.

Anatomic changes that occur with aging include increased internal anal thickness associated with increased echogenicity as studied by ultrasonography, due in part to increased fibrosis. Internal anal sphincter elasticity is reduced; in contrast, external anal thickness is usually found to be decreased. These anatomic changes are accompanied by a decrease in anal canal resting and squeeze pressure and a reduction in rectal reservoir function [28]. Neurologic changes that have been described include a decrease in mucosal electrosensitivity and sensation to rectal distension and an increase in nerve motor latency and single-fiber electromyography of the sphincter fibers [29].

There is no evidence that colonic transit changes with age unless intractable constipation develops. Anatomic studies do show a reduction in the number of neurons from the myenteric plexus with some replacement by fibrosis but it seems likely that these changes are not accompanied by significant functional effects [30]. Whether some of these changes cause decreased colonic circular muscle inhibitory junction potentials is unknown. Neither colonic mucosal absorptive function, nor the metabolic activity of the colonic flora, have been evaluated in humans.

The commonest anatomic abnormality found in the elderly colon is colonic diverticulosis. Diverticula typically occur in groups, commonly in gaps in the muscle layers of the colon between the longitudinal fibers of the taenia coli or between rings of circular smooth muscle fibers. They occur particularly at entry points of the vasa recti where the bowel wall is weakest. Diverticula consist of only mucosa and submucosa and are usually located between the mesentery and antimesenteric taenia where the submucosal vessels penetrate.

References

1   Corazza GR, Frazzoni M, Gatto MRA, Gasbarrini G: Ageing and small-bowel mucosa: A morphometric study. Gerontology 1986;32:60–65.
2   Aoyama S, Kawamura S, Nishio K, Harima K, Aibe T, Takemoto T: Histopathological study on aging of the pancreas from 423 autopsy cases (in Japanese). Nippon Ronen Igakkai Zasshi 1979; 16:574–579.
3   Zoli M, Magalottti D, Bianchi G, Gueli C, Orlandini C, Grimaldi M, Marchesini G: Total and functional hepatic blood flow decrease in parallel with ageing. Age Ageing 1999;28:29–33.
4   Holt PR: The gastrointestinal tract; in Masoro EJ (ed): Handbook of Physiology. Section 11: Aging. New York, Oxford University Press, 1995, pp 505–554.
5   Feibusch JM, Holt PR: Impaired absorptive capacity for carbohydrate in the aging human. Dig Dis Sci 1982;27:1095–1100.
6   Ferraris RP, Hsiao J, Hernandez R, Hirayama B: Site density of mouse intestinal glucose transporters declines with age. Am J Physiol 1993;264:G285–G293.
7   Thomson ABR, Keelan M, Thiesen A, Clandinin MT, Ropeleski M, Wild GE: Small bowel review: Normal physiology part 1. Dig Dis Sci 2001;46:2567–2587.
8   Hirsh AJ, Cheeseman CI: Cholecystokinin decreases intestinal hexose absorption by a parallel reduction in SGLT1 abundance in the brush-border membrane. J Biol Chem 1998;273:14545–14549.
9   Holt PR, Balint J: The effects of aging upon intestinal lipid absorption. Am J Physiol 1993;264: G1–G6.

10 Montagnani M, Aldini R, Roda A, Roda E: New insights in the physiology and molecular basis of the intestinal bile acid absorption. Ital J Gastroenterol Hepatol 1998;30:435–440.

11 Niot I, Poirier H, Besnard P: Regulation of gene expression by fatty acids: Special reference to fatty acid-binding protein (FABP). Biochimie 1997;79:129–133.

12 Ireland P, Fordtran JS: Effect of dietary calcium and age on jejunal calcium absorption in humans studied by intestinal perfusion. J Clin Invest 1973;52:2673–2681.

13 MacLaughlin J, Holick MF: Aging decreases the capacity of human skin to produce vitamin D3. J Clin Invest 1985;76:1536–1538.

14 Tangpricha V, Flanagan JN, Whitlatch LW, Tseng CC, Chen TC, Holt PR, Lipkin MS, Holick MF: 25-Hydroxyvitamin D-1α-hydroxylase in normal and malignant colon tissue. Lancet 2001;357: 1673–1674.

15 Cross HS, Bareis P, Hofer H, Bischof MG, Bajna E, Kriwanek S, Bonner E, Peterlik M: 25-Hydroxyvitamin D3-1α-hydroxylase and vitamin D receptor gene expression in human colonic mucosa is elevated during early cancerogenesis. Steroids 2001;66:287–292.

16 Bareis P, Bises G, Bischof MG, Cross HS, Peterlik M: 25-Hydroxyvitamin D metabolism in human colon cancer cells during tumor progression. Biochem Biophys Res Commun 2001;285:1012–1017.

17 Van Asselt DZB, de Grott LCPGM, van Staveren WA, Blom HJ, Wevers RA, Biemond I, Hoefnagels WHL: Role of cobalamin intake and atrophic gastritis in mild cobalamin deficiency in older Dutch subjects. Am J Clin Nutr 1998;68:328–334.

18 Emi Y, Tsunashima D, Ogawara K-I, Higaki K, Kimura T: Role of P-glycoprotein as a secretory mechanism in quinidine absorption from rat small intestine. J Pharm Sci 1998;87:295–299.

19 Suzuki H, Sugiyama Y: Role of metabolic enzymes and efflux transporters in the absorption of drugs from the small intestine. Eur J Pharm Sci 2000;12:3–12.

20 Attilasoy E, Holt PR: Gastrointestinal proliferation and aging. J Gerontol 1993;48:B43–B49.

21 Roncucci L, Ponz De Leon M, Scalmati A, Malagoli G, Pratissoli S, Perini M, Chahin NJ: The influence of age on colonic epithelial cell proliferation. Cancer 1988;62:2373–2377.

22 Xiao Z-Q, Majumdar APN: Increased in vitro activation of EGFR by membrane-bound TGF-alpha from gastric and colonic mucosa of aged rats. Am J Physiol Gastrointest Liver Physiol 2001;281:G111–G116.

23 Holt PR, Moss SF, Heydari AR, Richardson A: Diet restriction increases apoptosis in the gut of aging rats. J Gerontol A Biol Sci Med Sci 1998;53:B168–B172.

24 Poston GJ, Saydjari R, Lawrence J, Alexander RW, Townsend CM Jr, Thompson JC: The effect of age on small bowel adaptation and growth after proximal enterectomy. J Gerontol 1990;45:B220–B225.

25 Khalil T, Walker JP, Wiener I, Fagan CJ, Townsend CM Jr, Greeley GH Jr, Thompson JC: Effect of aging on gallbladder contraction and release of cholecystokinin-33 in humans. Surgery 1985;98:423–429.

26 Khalil T, Thompson JC: Aging and gut peptides; in Thompson JC, Greeley CH, Rayford PL, Townsend CM (eds): Gastrointestinal Endocrinology. New York, McGraw-Hill, 1987, pp 147–157.

27 Hebeiss K, Kilbinger H: Nitric oxide-sensitive guanylyl cyclase inhibits acetylcholine release and excitatory motor transmission in the guinea-pig ileum. Neuroscience 1998;82:623–629.

28 Papachrysostomou M, Pye SD, Wild SR, Smith AN: Anal endosonography in asymptomatic subjects. Scand J Gastroenterol 1993;28:551–556.

29 Roig JV, Villoslada C, Lledo S, Solana A, Buch E, Alos R, Hinojosa J: Prevalence of pudendal neuropathy in fecal incontinence: Results of a prospective study. Dis Colon Rectum 1995;38: 952–958.

30 Klosterhalfen B, Offner F, Topf N, Vogel P, Mittermayer C: Sclerosis of the internal anal sphincter – a process of aging. Dis Colon Rectum 1990;33:606–609.

Peter R. Holt, MD, St. Luke's Hospital Center,
1111 Amsterdam Avenue, New York, NY 10025 (USA)
Tel. +1 212 523 3679, Fax +1 212 523 3683, E-Mail pholt@chpnet.org

Pilotto A, Malfertheiner P, Holt PR (eds): Aging and the Gastrointestinal Tract.
Interdiscipl Top Gerontol. Basel, Karger, 2003, vol 32, pp 65–73

....

Effect of Aging on the Liver and Pancreas

Giorgio Annoni[a], *Nicoletta Gagliano*[b]

[a] Internal Medicine and Gerontology, DIMEP, University of Milan-Bicocca and
[b] Department of Human Anatomy, University of Milan, Milan, Italy

Liver

Aging affects various organs, tissues and cell types of the same organism in different ways, resulting in different rates of decline in their function. The aging of the mammalian liver has not been fully defined, but morphofunctional studies suggest that, compared with other organs, it seems to age fairly well. Age-related changes in hepatic morphology and functions have been described, but these observations are often conflicting [1], probably because of major species, strain and sex differences in the liver's response to aging.

Here, we summarize the main knowledge about the morphology, function, regeneration and drug metabolism of the liver as it ages.

Morphology

Liver morphology has been studied mostly in rodents, and the few studies in humans suffer from some limitations regarding the experimental conditions, including the difficulty of distinguishing changes that are clearly a consequence of senescence from those caused by maturation.

In human liver, the most frequent change is a reduction in size [2]. Some authors report that its mass decreases by up to 40% only during the first two or three decades of life, whereas others found a similar reduction but only during maturation and senescence [3]. In elderly people, the hepatocytes are fewer and larger, also with larger nuclei, and often display polyploidy [4].

These data have not been completely confirmed in animal models. In inbred Fisher 344 rats, there was no clear demonstration of a correlation between aging and the increased number of binuclear hepatocytes [5]. In general, studies in rodents have provided no evidence of marked age-related alterations in hepatocytes. At the ultrastructural level, during aging, both rodent and human hepatocytes have mitochondria that are larger, but the total number is smaller [6]. The consequences of these ultrastructural modifications have not been fully elucidated, but they are believed to cause respiratory rate deficits [7].

In 1997, Sakai et al. [8] assessed liver longevity in a rat transplant model. Livers from young donors (5 months old) were transplanted into two groups of syngeneic recipients, one aged 5 and the other 28 months. Recipient survival after transplantation was similar, independently of age. Late deaths (more than 1 year) after surgery were mainly caused by heart failure or tumors and none of the animals died of liver failure. At autopsy, the main morphological changes were in the heart and kidney, which became fibrotic, while in the liver the main histological features were hepatocyte degeneration, bile duct proliferation, pigment deposition and a mild to moderate fibrosis.

From a morphological point of view, fibrosis is, without any doubt, a hallmark of aging of various organs, including the heart and kidney [9, 10], and reflects increased deposition of the physiological components of the extracellular matrix (ECM). The liver ECM is not merely a passive structural support, since it provides a structural framework and is important for maintaining the differentiated phenotype and normal function of hepatocytes, sinusoidal, endothelial and stellate cells [11]. ECM turnover is vital in the tissue remodeling that accompanies physiological and pathological processes, so any quantitative changes can result in deranged hepatic function. Although liver fibrosis has been extensively studied in normal and pathological livers and in several experimental models, data about age-associated liver fibrosis is still scant and incomplete since mainly biochemical aspects have been investigated, including the increased content of cross-linked proteins.

A recent study [12] in young, adult and senescent Sprague-Dawley rats provides a comprehensive description of this aspect using different approaches. Since interstitial collagens are the major components of liver ECM, constituting about 80% of the total [13], and since collagen content is governed by the balance between its synthesis and degradation, we focussed particularly on collagen metabolism. The results confirm that aging is associated with moderate hepatic sclerosis, mainly involving the portal tracts (fig. 1). Interestingly, fibrosis is due to accumulation of interstitial collagen type III, type I remaining almost unchanged. This occurs without a predominant role of any one of the mechanisms that control ECM turnover, and appears to be the consequence of a dissociation between collagen type I and III gene regulation and decreased collagenolytic activity, enhanced by inhibition of tissue inhibitor of metalloproteinases-1. The gene expression of the pluripotent transforming growth factor

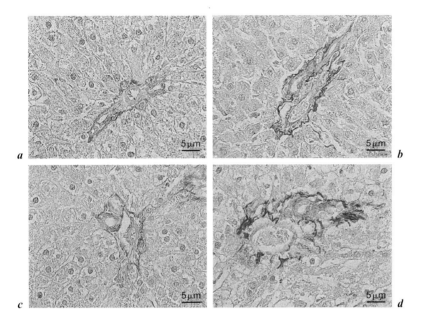

Fig. 1. Microphotographs showing Sirius red staining of portal areas in liver sections of rats aged 2 (*a*), 6 (*b*), 12 (*c*) and 19 (*d*) months. Scale bars show the magnification.

(TGF)-β1, whose upregulation in active fibroplasia is well established, does not change during liver aging, suggesting that this factor does not play a major role in the development of age-related liver fibrosis, as previously evidenced in the heart and kidney [9, 10].

Hepatic Function

Aging affects some hepatic functions, but here too the picture is uncertain. No significant changes in conventional liver function tests have been identified, excluding the wider interindividual variability in many parameters usual in elderly people. This was clearly shown by Tietz et al. [14], who evaluated 15,000 laboratory variables in more than 200 subjects and concluded that many hepatic functions are well preserved in the elderly, although with wide variability among subjects. Only biliary function seems to be influenced, with deficits in bile flow and bile acid secretion. Collectively, these findings probably account for the higher frequency of gallstones in elderly people.

Liver Regeneration

Although the aged liver shows no major morphological changes and functional tests remain almost unchanged [14, 15], the regenerative potential appears to decline with age [16]. This statement is based on the observation that partially resected livers in old animals take longer to return to their original size than in young animals. From a clinical point of view, this is a vital factor in deciding whether to perform liver resection in elderly patients and in relation to donor age in liver transplantation. However, how the mechanisms that control liver regeneration are affected by aging has still not been completely described [16, 17].

The complex machinery that controls hepatocyte proliferation has been investigated in the senescent phenotype, with analysis of some aspects of the triggering mechanisms involved in the early phase of this process by histological, biochemical and molecular techniques.

Liver regeneration can be elicited experimentally by surgical removal of a large proportion of the parenchyma or by acute chemical treatment such as with CCl_4 [18, 19]. In young and adult rodents, reduction of the liver mass induces cell proliferation. During this process, hepatocytes pass through two phases: a 'priming' phase that gives them replicative competence and a 'progression' phase in which primed cells undergo DNA replication [18, 20]. This transition requires the expression of some genes whose products regulate key events during the G0 and G1 phases, many of which have been identified as proto-oncogenes, including c-fos and c-myc [18, 21]. These early genes act as transcription factors, encoding nuclear phosphoproteins believed to function as regulators of cell proliferation.

The process of regeneration is regulated by growth factors and cytokines, which control the transition from the normal quiescent state of adult hepatocytes to the proliferative condition of regenerating cells. Hepatocyte growth factor and TGF-α exert a positive control on this process [19, 20], acting, respectively, in an autocrine and paracrine fashion. They promote hepatocyte proliferation [18, 21] and their mRNA is upregulated in replicating hepatocytes both in vitro and in vivo [22].

Regeneration ends when the liver mass has been restored, so important negative regulatory influences are needed; a stop signal is encoded by the TGF-β1 gene.

In the study mentioned above [22], liver regeneration was induced in young (2 months), adult (6 and 12 months) and aged rats (19 months) by a single intraperitoneal injection of CCl_4, and the response was analyzed in livers obtained 2 and 24 h after intoxication, compared to age-matched untreated rats. Albumin, c-fos, c-myc, hepatocyte growth factor, TGF-α and TGF-β1 gene expression were analyzed, together with transaminases and histological patterns (fig. 2). During aging, the liver regenerative machinery was preserved but its activation was reduced and delayed.

In the same study, besides the regenerative response, heat shock protein (HSP)70 gene expression was also investigated in order to assess the aged

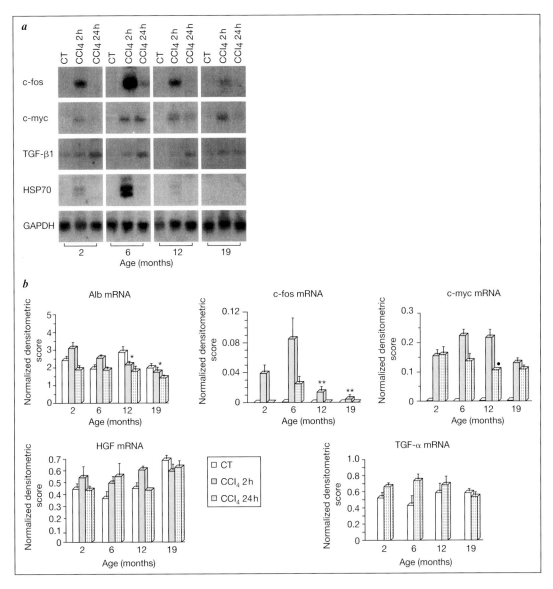

Fig. 2. *a* Northern blot hybridizations of total RNA from controls (CT) or rats killed 2 and 24 h after CCl_4 treatment. RNA was hybridized with the ^{32}P-labeled probes indicated. Glyceraldehyde 3-phosphate dehydrogenase (GAPDH) expression served as internal control. *b* Bar graphs illustrating the mRNA steady-state levels (means ± SEM) in liver homogenates from control (CT) and CCl_4-treated rats aged 2, 6, 12 and 19 months. Changes are seen in mRNA signals of albumin (Alb), c-fos, c-myc, hepatocyte growth factor (HGF) and TGF-α. *p < 0.05 versus 2-month-old rats, CCl_4 2 h; **p < 0.05 versus 6-month-old rats, CCl_4 2 h; •p < 0.05 versus 12-month-old rats, CCl_4 2 h.

Effect of Aging on the Liver and Pancreas

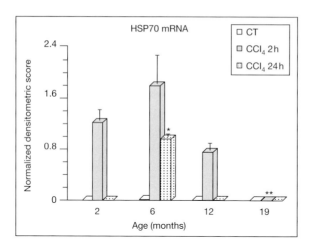

Fig. 3. HSP70 mRNA steady-state levels (means ± SEM) in liver homogenates from controls (CT) and CCl$_4$-treated rats aged 2, 6, 12 and 19 months. *p $<$ 0.05 versus 6-month-old rats, CCl$_4$ 2 h; **p $<$ 0.05 versus 2-, 6- and 12-month-old rats, CCl$_4$ 2 h.

liver's defenses against a noxious stimulus. CCl$_4$, as expected, increased HSP70 mRNA levels, most markedly in 2- and 6-month-old rats, while aged animals had less prompt defense responses and were not able to maintain the stress response for a long time (24 h; fig. 3).

The heat shock response is a universal phenomenon observed in a variety of cell types [23]. All organisms synthetize a group of HSPs in response to certain stress factors such as hyperthermia and xenobiotics.

The HSPs, particularly HSP70, play a role in protecting cells against the adverse effects of stress; changes in their expression could be important in aged organisms, since senescence is characterized physiologically by a decrease in the ability to respond to environmental stress. A decline in the induction of HSP70 by hyperthermia is observed in senescent isolated fibroblasts and hepatocytes [24].

Drug Metabolism

With age, hepatic mass and blood flow both decrease, as demonstrated by ultrasound and Doppler examination. The decrease in hepatic blood flow affects the elimination of drugs in rare situations, for instance when lidocaine, a drug with high clearance, is given intravenously.

Although the expression of drug-metabolizing enzymes in the cytochrome P450 system does not appear to decrease with age, overall hepatic metabolism of many drugs by these enzymes typically drops by 30–40%. However, the rate of hepatic metabolism of drugs can vary greatly from person to person, and careful individual titration is required. The clearance of drugs that undergo phase I hepatic metabolism by the cytochrome P450 system (diazepam, amitriptyline, chlordiazepoxide) is often reduced in the elderly. By contrast, age less often affects the clearance of drugs that are metabolized by glucuronate or sulfate conjugation (phase II reaction), such as lorazepam, desipramine and oxazepam.

Reduced drug clearance predisposes older subjects to a higher rate of adverse drug reactions, especially because many such patients require multiple drugs.

Clinical Considerations

Recent information from basic research clearly suggests that the liver ages fairly well compared with other organs. This is of special interest in relation to liver transplantation. The donor's age is one of the criteria used for the selection of liver grafts, and an upper limit of 50 years has been arbitrarily set for donation [25]. However, the limited supply of grafts has led to the use of older donors (up to 65 years) for liver transplantation [25], and old donors have become an important source of organs, accounting for 17% of the total liver transplantations in the United States. Livers from donors older than 50 years can be transplanted with the same success rate as those from younger donors. Nevertheless, the age of potential recipients has both clinical and ethical implications including tolerance of the surgical stress associated with liver transplantation.

Finally, recent findings on the reduced defense mechanisms and delayed regenerative response of the aged liver offer new insights to explain the well-known fact that hepatitis C causes much worse liver disease in people as they get older.

Pancreas

There is still some uncertainty about the effects of age on pancreatic secretion. The literature is limited and the few studies there are give the impression that aging per se does not affect exocrine function.

However, several morphological changes occur with aging; the findings mostly come from autopsies. The main changes include a decrease in the weight and size of the organ, adipose tissue invasion and atherosclerosis of the pancreatic vasculature [26]. Periductular, intralobular and perilobular fibrosis is also reported [27]. Pancreatic atrophy may be severe and can cause pancreatic insufficiency. Calcified stones are present in the majority of these patients, who, at autopsy, have a high incidence of pancreatic lithiasis [28]. A theory about the formation of pancreatic stones in old people holds that a major factor is the defective production of a stabilizing protein, lithostatin, in pancreatic fluid [29].

Ultrasound techniques show an increase in the echogenicity of the pancreas starting in the fourth decade of life; anatomical findings such as fibrosis and fatty infiltration could contribute to this pattern. Ultrasound scan can also reveal dilatation of the pancreatic duct as a common feature of the aging pancreas. Since both the increased echogenicity and ductal dilatation are hallmarks of both chronic pancreatitis and normal aging, sometimes it is difficult to distinguish these two conditions.

Uncertainty also remains about the effect of age on pancreatic secretion. Serum levels of the major enzymes, such as amylase, remain constant, whereas others (lipase, trypsin) decrease [30]. The reasons for this functional decline are not clear, but vascular sclerosis and organ fibrosis may be involved.

In general, these age-related changes do not seriously affect pancreatic function, but depending on their severity they may increase the incidence of some pancreatic diseases including acute and chronic pancreatitis and also cancer.

References

1 Schmucker DL: Do hepatocytes age? Exp Gerontol 1990;25:403–412.
2 Munro HN, Young VR: Protein metabolism in the elderly: Observations relating to dietary needs. Postgrad Med 1978;63:143–148.
3 Wynne HA, Cope LH, Mutch E, Rawlins MD, Woodhouse KW, James OFW: The effect of age upon liver volume and apparent liver blood flow in healthy man. Hepatology 1989;9:297–301.
4 Watanabe T, Tanaka Y: Age-related alterations in the size of human hepatocytes. A study of mononuclear and binucleate cells. Virchows Arch B Cell Pathol Incl Mol Pathol 1982;39:9–20.
5 Schmucker DL, Mooney J, Jones AL: Stereological analysis of hepatic fine structure in the Fisher 344 rat. Influence of sublobular location and animal age. J Cell Biol 1978;78:319–337.
6 Sastre J, Pallardo FV, Pla R, Pellin A, Juan G, O'Connor JE, Estrema JM, Miquel J, Vina J: Aging of the liver: Age associated mitochondrial damage in intact hepatocytes. Hepatology 1996;24: 1199–1205.
7 Yen TC, Chen YS, King KL, Yeh SH, Wei YH: Liver mitochondrial respiratory functions decline with age. Biochem Biophys Res Commun 1989;165:994–1003.
8 Sakai Y, Zhong R, Garcia B, Zhu L, Wall WJ: Assessment of the longevity of the liver using a rat transplant model. Hepatology 1997;25:421–425.
9 Annoni G, Luvarà G, Arosio B, Gagliano N, Fiordaliso F, Santambrogio D, Jeremic G, Mircoli L, Latini R, Vergani C, Masson S: Age-dependent expression of fibrosis-related genes and collagen deposition in the rat myocardium. Mech Ageing Dev 1998;101:57–72.
10 Gagliano N, Arosio B, Santambrogio D, Balestrieri MR, Padoani G, Tagliabue J, Masson S, Vergani C, Annoni G: Age-dependent expression of fibrosis-related genes and collagen deposition in rat kidney cortex. J Gerontol 2000;55:B365–B372.
11 Martinez-Hernandez A: The hepatic extracellular matrix. I. Electron immunohistochemical studies in normal rat liver. Lab Invest 1984;51:57–74.
12 Gagliano N, Arosio B, Grizzi F, Masson S, Tagliabue J, Dioguardi N, Vergani C, Annoni G: Reduced collagenolytic activity of metalloproteinases and development of liver fibrosis in the aging rat. Mech Ageing Dev 2002;123:413–425.

13   Biagini G, Ballardini G: Liver fibrosis and extracellular matrix. J Hepatol 1989;8:115–124.

14   Tietz NW, Shuey DF, Wekstein DR: Laboratory values in fit aging individuals – sexagenarians through centenarians. Clin Chem 1992;38:1167–1185.

15   Schmucker DL: Aging and the liver: An update. J Gerontol 1998;53:B315–B320.

16   Beyer HS, Sherman R, Zieve L: Aging is associated with reduced liver regeneration and diminished thymidine kinase mRNA content and enzyme activity in the rat. J Lab Clin Med 1991;118:101–108.

17   Bucher NLR, Swaffeld N, Di Troia JF: The influence of age upon the incorporation of thymidine-2-14C into DNA of regenerating rat liver. Cancer Res 1964;24:509–512.

18   Fausto N, Mead JE: Biology of disease. Regulation of liver growth: Protooncogenes and transforming growth factors. Lab Invest 1989;60:4–13.

19   Michalopulos GK: Liver regeneration: Molecular mechanisms of growth control. FASEB J 1990;4:176–187.

20   Fausto N: Liver regeneration. J Hepatol 2000;32:19–31.

21   Thompson NL, Mead JE, Braun L, Goyette M, Shank PR, Fausto N: Sequential protooncogene expression during rat liver regeneration. Cancer Res 1986;46:3111–3117.

22   Webber EM, Fitzgerald MJ, Brown PI, Bartlett MH, Fausto N: Transforming growth factor-α expression during liver regeneration after partial hepatectomy and toxic injury, and potential interactions between transforming growth factor-α and hepatocyte growth factor. Hepatology 1993;18:1422–1431.

23   Lindquist S: The heat-shock response. Annu Rev Biochem 1986;55:1151–1191.

24   Heydari AR, Wu B, Takahashi R, Strong R, Richardson A: Expression of heat shock protein 70 is altered by age and diet at the level of transcription. Mol Cell Biol 1993;13:2909–2918.

25   Adam R, Astarcioglu I, Azoulay D, Morino M, Bao YM, Castaing D, Bismuth H: Age greater than 50 years is not a contraindication for liver donation. Transplant Proc 1991;23:2602–2603.

26   Gullo L, Ventrucci M, Naldoni P, Pezzilli R: Aging and the exocrine pancreatic function. J Am Geriatr Soc 1986;34:790–792.

27   Schmitz-Moormann P, Himmelmann GW, Brandes JW, Folsch UR, Lorenz-Meyer H, Malchow H, Soehendra LN, Wienbeck M: Comparative radiological and morphological study of human pancreas. Pancreatitis-like changes in post-mortem ductograms and their morphological pattern. Possible implication for ERCP. Gut 1985;26:406–414.

28   Nagai H, Ohtsubo K: Pancreatic lithiasis in the aged. Its clinicopathology and pathogenesis. Gastroenterology 1984;86:331–338.

29   Multigner L, Sarles H, Lombardo D, De Carlo A: Pancreatic stone protein. II. Implication in stone formation during the course of chronic calcifying pancreatitis. Gastroenterology 1985;89:387–391.

30   Meyer J, Necheles H: Studies in old age. IV. The clinical significance of salivary, gastric, and pancreatic secretion in the aged. JAMA 1940;115:2050–2055.

Prof. Giorgio Annoni
Department of Clinical Medicine, Prevention and Biotechnology
University of Milano-Bicoccia
Via Cadore 48, I–20052 Monza, Milan (Italy)
Tel. +39 335 804 92 90, E-Mail giorgio.annoni@unimib.it

Pilotto A, Malfertheiner P, Holt PR (eds): Aging and the Gastrointestinal Tract.
Interdiscipl Top Gerontol. Basel, Karger, 2003, vol 32, pp 74–99

....

Dysphagia in the Elderly

Prashanthi N. Thota, Joel E. Richter

Department of Gastroenterology and Hepatology,
Center for Swallowing and Esophageal Disorders, The Cleveland
Clinic Foundation, Cleveland, Ohio, USA

With advances in medical care, life expectancy has improved steadily so that the aging population has a major impact on the health care system. Digestive diseases are a common cause of morbidity and mortality in the elderly. Symptoms related to esophageal dysfunction are particularly common. When evaluating an elderly patient for esophageal diseases, the following principles should be considered:

(1) Elderly patients are more susceptible to complications. For example, erosive esophagitis, peptic stricture and Barrett's esophagus are more common in elderly patients with gastroesophageal reflux disease (GERD).

(2) Diseases may present with atypical symptoms or the symptoms may be attributed to other coexisting disorders. For example, chest pain due to GERD can be confused with angina with coronary artery disease. In addition, few elderly patients seek medical care as they tolerate symptoms better. All these factors lead to delay in diagnosis.

(3) Some diseases such as Zenker's diverticulum, cervical osteophytes and dysphagia aortica may occur exclusively in the elderly.

(4) Elderly patients may be more prone to side effects from medications such as metoclopramide or H_2-receptor blockers.

(5) The frequency of diseases change as one ages. For example, when an elderly patient presents with features suggestive of achalasia, one has to be more suspicious about pseudoachalasia associated with malignancy.

In this chapter, we will discuss the physiological changes observed with aging, followed by the clinical presentation, diagnostic approach and management of common swallowing disorders in the elderly.

Physiological Changes with Aging

In 1964, Zboralske et al. [1] used the term 'presbyesophagus' to describe the degenerative changes in the aging esophagus characterized by diminished amplitude of peristaltic contractions, frequent tertiary waves, incomplete lower esophageal sphincter (LES) relaxation and esophageal dilatation. In later years, these changes were found to be secondary to common coexisting illnesses in elderly patients, such as diabetic neuropathies or other neurological disorders and medications, but not due to aging per se. However, minor changes in esophageal function and structure are relatively common as we age, especially into the eighties and nineties, but rarely lead to clinically significant esophageal dysfunction and symptoms. Familiarity with these changes is important for accurate interpretation of manometric data and to prevent the overdiagnosis of disease states.

Changes in the Pharynx and Upper Esophageal Sphincter
Most studies examining subjects in their eighties and nineties show a decrease in the resting pressure of the upper esophageal sphincter (UES) with age but a normal UES response to distension [2]. However, there is reduced opening of the UES and a delay in UES relaxation after deglutition as one ages due to a decrease in the compliance of the sphincter [2]. Compared to younger subjects, the amplitude and duration of the pharyngeal contractions are increased in healthy elderly persons [2]. These changes increase the propulsive force of the pharyngeal pump and reflect an adaptive response to increased resistance across the UES. These physiological changes with aging contribute to the development of cricopharyngeal bars and Zenker's diverticulum.

Esophageal Body
Hollis and Castell [3] reported a decrease in the amplitude of peristaltic waves in elderly patients over 80 years of age. In a study by Richter et al. [4], the amplitude of the distal esophageal peristaltic waves increased with each decade and peaked in the fifties, with a subsequent decline afterwards. However, the amplitude of the proximal esophageal peristaltic waves did not vary with age [4].

Lower Esophageal Sphincter
The mean length and the resting pressure of the LES are preserved as we age. However, abnormalities in LES relaxation, such as failure to contract after initial relaxation or complete absence of relaxation, are 4–6 times more frequent in the elderly when compared to younger subjects [5].
Morphological changes in the pharynx and esophagus contribute to these age-related changes in esophageal physiology. The morphological changes reported include a decrease in the density and number of striated muscle fibers in the

pharynx, cricopharyngeus and upper esophagus [6], a reduction in the number of myenteric plexus cells [7] and weakness of the smooth muscle of the esophagus [7].

Dysphagia in the Elderly

Dysphagia is a sensation of impaired passage of food from the esophagus to the stomach. It is a common complaint in the elderly. The prevalence of dysphagia has been reported to be around 12–13% in short-term care hospitals [8] and as high as 60% in nursing home residents [9]. Dysphagia can result from various defects affecting the oral, pharyngeal or esophageal phases of deglutition. For clinical purposes, dysphagia can be classified into two distinct categories: oropharyngeal dysphagia and esophageal dysphagia. Oropharyngeal dysphagia is the inability to initiate the act of swallowing. It is a 'transfer problem' due to impaired ability to transfer food from the mouth to the upper esophagus. On the other hand, esophageal dysphagia is a 'transport problem' and is defined as the sensation of difficult passage of solids or liquids from the mouth to the stomach. Both are involuntary processes.

A careful history and physical examination can provide clues to the diagnosis of dysphagia in over 80% of cases. Patients with oropharyngeal dysphagia present with complaints such as trouble initiating a swallow, nasal regurgitation, choking, dysarthria, coughing, nasal speech and aspiration. In patients with esophageal dysphagia, the crucial points are (1) if the dysphagia is with solids, liquids or both, (2) if the symptoms are intermittent or progressive, and (3) if there is any associated heartburn or weight loss. Motility disorders usually present with dysphagia with both solids and liquids from the onset, whereas obstructing anatomic lesions cause dysphagia with solids initially which may progress over time to dysphagia with liquids.

Physical examination may reveal findings such as neurological deficits in patients with oropharyngeal dysphagia, ptosis in myasthenia gravis, cachexia in advanced malignancies and signs of calcinosis, Raynaud's phenomenon, esophageal dysmotility, sclerodactyly and telangectasia (CREST) syndrome in scleroderma. An algorithm for the diagnostic approach to a patient with dysphagia [10] is summarized in figure 1.

Oropharyngeal Dysphagia

Oropharyngeal dysphagia is very common in the elderly, with neuromuscular disorders accounting for nearly 80% of the cases. The major causes of oropharyngeal dysphagia are listed in table 1 [10].

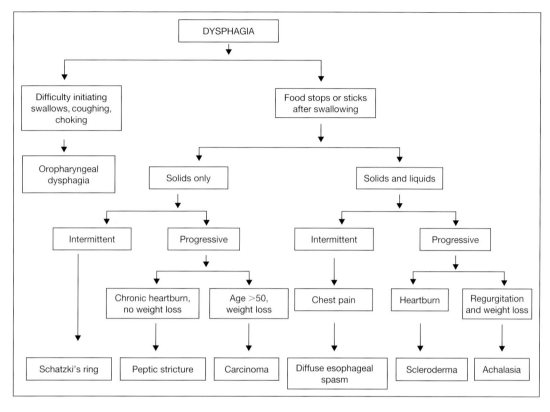

Fig. 1. Diagnostic approach to a patient with dysphagia [10].

Cerebrovascular Accidents

Oropharyngeal dysphagia is one of the common neurological manifestations associated with cerebrovascular accidents. It can be caused by anything affecting the swallowing center in the brain stem or the nerves regulating the swallowing process, i.e. cranial nerves 5, 7, 9, 10 and 12. In addition, hemispheric strokes can lead to dysphagia due to brain stem distortion from concomitant cerebral edema. Symptoms are typically abrupt in onset and associated with other neurological deficits. However, patients with deep lacunar infarcts may present with dysphagia as the sole manifestation of a stroke. A modified barium swallow may show inability to initiate a swallow, generalized motor incoordination, reduced pharyngeal peristalsis and aspiration of barium. A CT scan or MRI of the brain can help localize the infarcts, although the latter test is more sensitive for the evaluation of acute, small or posterior fossa infarcts. The majority of patients showing recovery do so within 2 weeks, but

Table 1. Causes of oropharyngeal dysphagia [10]

(1) Neurological disorders
    Cerebrovascular accidents
    Parkinson's disease
    Brain stem tumors
    Multiple sclerosis
    Amyotrophic lateral sclerosis
    Peripheral neuropathy
(2) Skeletal muscle disorders
    Inflammatory myopathies
      Polymyositis/dermatomyositis
      Inclusion body myositis
    Muscular dystrophies
      Myotonic dystrophy
      Oculopharyngeal dystrophy
    Myasthenia gravis
    Metabolic myopathies
      Hyperthyroidism
      Hypothyroidism
      Steroid myopathy
(3) Mechanical obstruction
    Inflammatory states
    Extrinsic compression (thyromegaly, cervical
      osteophytes, lymphadenopathy)
    Postsurgical change
(4) Motility disorders
    Zenker's diverticulum
    Cricopharyngeal bar
(5) Sialoporia
    Medications
    Sjögren's syndrome
    Secondary to radiation
(6) Cognitive dysfunction
    Alzheimer's disease
    Depression

some patients may take up to 6 months to regain normal swallowing. Aspiration pneumonias are particularly common (20–50%) in stroke patients with oropharyngeal dysphagia [11]. Brain stem strokes, especially those with bilateral involvement, portend a poor prognosis.

Parkinson's Disease

Patients affected with Parkinson's disease may present with tremor of the tongue, trouble initiating a swallow or pooling of saliva in the mouth. Nearly half the patients with Parkinson's disease have dysphagia to some degree [12], and 95% of these individuals have impairment in the oral and pharyngeal phases on videofluorography [13]. Common abnormalities are abnormal tongue control, piecemeal deglutition, a delayed swallowing reflex, bolus pooling in the vallecular space and pyriform fossa and aspiration [14]. On esophageal manometry, incomplete relaxation of the UES is frequently observed. Other changes such as simultaneous or increased-amplitude contractions in the esophageal body and low LES pressure have been reported. Treatment with antiparkinsonian drugs alone leads to inconsistent results. A combination of swallowing therapy and drug therapy has been shown to be effective [15].

Polymyositis and Dermatomyositis

Polymyositis is a diffuse inflammatory disease of the striated muscle which involves the pharynx and the upper one third of the esophagus. About 30–60% of patients present with oropharyngeal dysphagia, nasopharyngeal regurgitation or aspiration [16]. Modified barium swallow shows poor contraction of the pharyngeal constrictors, pooling, retention of barium in the vallecular, nasal regurgitation and disordered pharyngeal emptying [17]. Manometric abnormalities reported include a low UES pressure and decreased amplitude of pharyngeal and proximal esophageal contractions [17]. Decreased frequency and amplitude of peristaltic waves of the distal esophagus have also been described. Treatment with immunosuppressive agents, such as steroids, azathioprine or methotrexate, is effective in relieving symptoms in a significant number of patients [16].

Myotonic Dystrophy and Oculopharyngeal Dystrophy

Myotonic dystrophy is a familial disease characterized by progressive muscle weakness, myotonia, cataracts, hypersomnia, cardiac dysrhythmias, frontal baldness, testicular atrophy and other endocrine abnormalities. Oculopharyngeal dystrophy is an autosomal dominant disease presenting after the age of 60 in patients with French-Canadian ancestry. These disorders involve the striated muscles of the pharynx and esophagus, manifesting with decreased resting and contraction pressures of the UES and upper esophagus as well as incomplete UES relaxation (cricopharyngeal achalasia) [18]. The response to cricopharyngeal myotomy is consistently favorable in these disorders [19].

Myasthenia Gravis

This disorder is characterized by weakness on repetitive contractions and typically presents with dysphagia, ptosis and diplopia. Myasthenia can occur at any age, with the peak incidence in men occurring during the seventh decade and in women during the third decade of life. Diagnosis is made by the characteristic clinical history, presence of antiacetylcholine receptor antibodies, decremental response to repetitive nerve stimulation on electromyography and an improvement in muscle strength with administration of edrophonium, an anti-choline esterase drug (Tensilon test). The response of dysphagia to drug therapy is highly variable [16].

Drugs can cause oropharyngeal dysphagia by acting on various sites along the transmission of the impulses from the brain to the muscle groups, such as at the central level (phenothiazines, metoclopramide), at the neuromuscular junction (procainamide, aminoglycosides) and at the muscle (HMG-coA reductase inhibitors). Treatment involves withdrawal of the offending drug. Endocrine disorders such as hypothyroidism and hyperthyroidism may present with dysphagia as the sole initial manifestation of the disease. Dysphagia due to these disorders responds well to specific drug therapy.

Local Obstructive Lesions

Oropharyngeal tumors, infections such as retropharyngeal abscess or extrinsic compression from cervical osteophytes, thyromegaly or lymphadenopathy may present with dysphagia. Although cervical osteophytes are relatively common, compression causing dysphagia is distinctly unusual. Cervical osteophytes can occur alone or as part of diffuse idiopathic skeletal hyperostosis. The most common complaint is solid food dysphagia, but patients may also complain of odynophagia, foreign body sensation, cough, hoarseness and frequent throat clearing. The diagnosis is made by lateral views on a barium swallow showing delayed transport of tablets or a marshmallow by the osteophytes, reproducing the patient's symptoms. Endoscopy should be performed to rule out intraluminal pathology.

Zenker's Diverticulum

Zenker's diverticulum is formed by the protrusion of hypopharyngeal mucosa posteriorly at the intersection of the transverse fibers of the cricopharyngeus muscle and the obliquely oriented fibers of the inferior pharyngeal constrictor (Killian's triangle). It is thought to be secondary to myositis and fibrosis of the cricopharyngeus muscle, resulting in reduced compliance of the UES. This leads to increased pressures being generated in the hypopharynx to push the bolus through the rigid UES, leading to dysphagia and formation of a diverticulum. The typical patient is an elderly woman with regurgitation of previously eaten foods, halitosis, solid and liquid dysphagia, fullness and gurgling in the neck and cough. Some Zenker's diverticula may become large enough to form a visible lump, usually in the left side of the neck, or compress the esophagus. The diagnosis is made by a barium swallow (fig. 2). Treatment consists of cricopharyngeal myotomy with or without diverticulectomy.

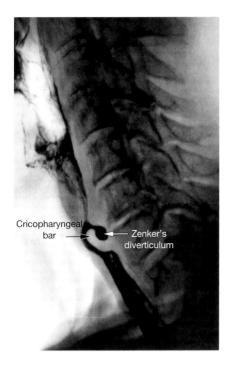

Fig. 2. Cricopharyngeal bar and Zenker's diverticulum.

Cricopharyngeal Dysfunction

Abnormalities of UES function include hypertensive UES, hypotensive UES, incomplete sphincter relaxation (cricopharyngeal achalasia), premature closure and delayed relaxation of the UES (familial dysautonomia).

Cricopharyngeal bar is a common radiological finding reported in 5–19% of patients undergoing pharyngeal evaluation [20]. Whether it is a cause of dysphagia is controversial. Lateral views on barium swallow show a prominent bar at the level of the cervical vertebrae C6 and C7 (fig. 2). Manometric studies show restricted sphincter opening and increased resistance to bolus transfer similar to those changes found in Zenker's diverticulum. In the absence of alternative esophageal or pharyngeal abnormalities accounting for symptoms, some patients with dysphagia and cricopharyngeal bar may be helped by cricopharyngeal myotomy. Alternatively, bougienage with large dilators provides temporary relief in some patients probably by stretching and possibly tearing the stiff sphincter.

Sialoporia

Lack of saliva (also known as xerostomia) can lead to poor lubrication of food with resulting impaired sensation and poor nutrition. It is most common secondary to drugs such as antihistamines, tricyclic antidepressants, phenothiazines, anticholinergics and antiparkinsonian drugs, or can be due to Sjögren's syndrome or secondary to radiation of the head and neck. Complications include dental caries and oral candidiasis. Mild to moderate symptoms can be managed by chewing sialogogues such as sugarless hard candy or chewing gum, frequent sips of water and use of saliva substitutes in the night. Severe symptoms require oral pilocarpine.

Treatment of Oropharyngeal Dysphagia

Management of oropharyngeal dysphagia depends on the underlying disorder. Unfortunately, many of the underlying conditions are not treatable and progressively deteriorate over time. However, most patients with cerebrovascular accidents improve with time. In those with residual deficits and other neuromuscular diseases, swallowing rehabilitation by a speech pathologist should be considered. Using a modified barium swallow to assess the patient's ability to safely swallow thin and thick liquids, pureed foods and solids, the speech pathologist can define relevant mechanisms of dysfunction and examine short-term effects of therapeutic strategies aimed at these dysfunctions [20]. The broad categories of oropharyngeal swallowing dysfunction are (1) an inability or excessive delay in the initiation of swallow, (2) aspiration of ingested foods, (3) nasopharyngeal regurgitation, and (4) food residue within the pharyngeal cavity after swallowing [20]. Swallowing therapies are intended to strengthen the weak oropharyngeal muscles and modify the swallowing mechanics to facilitate bolus transfer and prevent aspiration. These therapies include modification of diet, swallowing posture or swallowing technique. Changes in diet include the use of thin liquids when there is increased resistance to pharyngeal outflow and the use of thick liquids to decrease the risk of aspiration. Postural adjustments such as head tilt, chin tuck or head rotation can be tried in patients with unilateral pharyngeal weakness, which help in redirecting the bolus away from the weak side [20]. Various maneuvers can decrease the risk of aspiration by closing the vocal cords before and during the swallow (supraglottic swallow and supersupraglottic swallow), by increasing the posterior motion of the tongue base (effortful swallow) or by prolonging UES opening and clearing the pharynx (Mendelsohn's maneuver) [20]. If nutrition cannot be maintained orally without significant risk of aspiration, enteral feedings using a thin nasogastric tube, such as a Corpack or Dobhoff device, or eventually percutaneous endoscopic gastrostomy may be necessary. In some instances, surgical procedures aimed at minimizing aspiration such as epiglottoplasty, partial or total cricoid excision, laryngeal suspension or glottic closure may be needed.

Recently, botulinum toxin injections into the cricopharyngeus muscle have been reported to relieve symptoms of cricopharyngeal dysphagia. Botulinum A toxin (10–50 units) is injected into the UES under direct visualization with endoscopy or laryngoscopy or using electromyography for precise localization

Mechanical obstruction
  Intrinsic to the esophagus
    Complications of GERD
      Dysmotility
      Esophagitis
      Peptic stricture
    Lower esophageal ring
    Esophageal web
    Carcinoma
    Medication-induced injury
  Extrinsic to the esophagus
    Neoplasms
    Dysphagia aortica
    Mediastinal adenopathy
    Postsurgical changes
Motility disorders
  Achalasia
  Spastic disorders of the esophagus
Scleroderma

Table 2. Causes of esophageal dysphagia in the elderly [10]

of the UES. In various case series, improvement of dysphagia varied between 71 and 100%, with the duration of the response lasting from 4 to 7 months [21]. Patients with isolated cricopharyngeus dysfunction usually respond better than those with generalized neuromuscular diseases. In postlaryngectomized patients, improvement in voice quality may also be noted.

Cricopharyngeal myotomy is the most common surgical treatment for oropharyngeal dysphagia. It is most useful in patients with structural disorders that limit the opening of the cricopharyngeus in association with preserved pharyngeal muscle activity such as postcricoid stenosis, webs and Zenker's diverticulum. The efficacy of myotomy in patients with neurogenic dysphagia is highly variable, with an overall response rate of only 60% [20].

Esophageal Dysphagia

Esophageal dysphagia is caused by a variety of mechanical or motility disorders that inhibit the passage of food down the esophagus. The disorders capable of causing esophageal dysphagia are listed in table 2 [10].

Mechanical Obstruction

Mechanical obstruction can occur from disorders intrinsic to the esophagus or due to extrinsic compression from neoplasms, lymphadenopathy or an

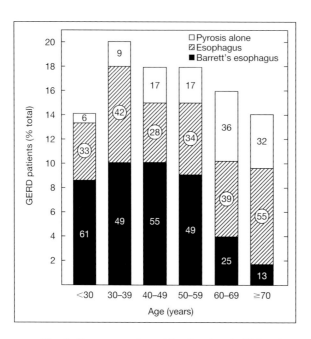

Fig. 3. Percentage of specific disorders in 228 patients with GERD according to age in decades [with permission from ref. 23].

atherosclerotic aorta. Intrinsic disorders causing esophageal dysphagia are severe or complicated GERD, rings or webs, malignancy and medication-induced injury.

Gastroesophageal Reflux Disease

GERD is a common disease in the elderly with an estimated prevalence of around 20% [22]. The incidence of GERD symptoms does not increase with age, but because of the cumulative acid injury to the esophagus over many years, the frequency of GERD complications, such as stricture and Barrett's esophagus, is significantly higher in older people (fig. 3) [23]. Although esophageal function is well preserved with aging, there are several minor factors predisposing to GERD in the elderly, including a decrease in the amplitude of peristaltic waves which may result in decreased clearance of refluxate, decreased salivary bicarbonate production in response to esophageal acid perfusion, increasing frequency of sliding hiatal hernia with age and the use of medications which lower LES pressure, such as anticholinergics, calcium channel blockers, theophylline and estrogens [24].

Heartburn is the classic symptom of GERD. In spite of the increased prevalence of GERD, the elderly complain of heartburn less because of an age-related decline in esophageal pain perception [25] and acid production from atrophic gastritis. On the other hand, symptoms such as dysphagia, chest pain and gastrointestinal bleeding are more common in elderly GERD patients when compared to younger subjects [26]. It may be particularly challenging for the clinician to differentiate chest pain of cardiac origin from that of esophageal origin. With severe esophagitis, patients may have esophageal dysmotility from hypotensive or simultaneous contractions, which further impair acid clearance and may cause dysphagia. In addition, dysphagia can be due to peptic strictures or a cancer in Barrett's esophagus. Extraesophageal symptoms, such as asthma, bronchitis, aspiration pneumonia, pulmonary fibrosis, hiccups and laryngitis, are also more common in elderly patients with GERD.

Because the severity of symptoms does not reliably predict the degree of esophagitis or the presence of complications, endoscopy should be the initial diagnostic test in all elderly patients regardless of the severity or duration of their symptoms. Esophageal manometry is reserved for locating the LES before 24-hour pH testing and for evaluating esophageal motility prior to antireflux surgery. Esophageal 24-hour pH testing is helpful before antireflux surgery and in patients not responding to medical therapy [24].

The elderly require an aggressive treatment approach for their reflux disease as they are more likely to have severe or complicated disease than younger patients. On the other hand, care must be taken when prescribing drugs as elder patients are more likely to have side effects and adverse drug interactions from concurrent use of various medications. Initial management involves avoidance of medications that decrease LES pressure and lifestyle modifications such as elevation of the head of the bed, avoiding refluxogenic foods (especially large, fatty meals), having meals at least 3–4 h before going to bed, smoking cessation and weight reduction. Intermittent use of antacids, alginic acid and over-the-counter H_2-receptor antagonists are useful for mild reflux disease. Antacids should be used cautiously in the elderly because of an increased risk of side effects from salt overload, constipation, diarrhea and interference with absorption of other drugs.

H_2 blockers are effective in treating nonerosive esophagitis. Side effects are rare but may include mental status changes in elderly patients with renal or hepatic dysfunction or interference with the metabolism of the drugs cleared by the hepatic cytochrome P450 system. Famotidine and nizatidine appear to be associated with the lowest rates of side effects in the elderly [27].

Prokinetic agents are effective in treating nonerosive esophagitis, especially in those patients with dyspeptic symptoms such as nausea, vomiting, epigastric pain and bloating. Metoclopramide must be used with caution in the elderly as side effects such as tremors, spasms, anxiety, insomnia, drowsiness or tardive dyskinesia can occur in up to one third of patients. If used, a low once-a-day dose may be preferable to minimize side effects. Cisapride and domperidone have no central side effects and may be preferred in the elderly. Cisapride has been withdrawn from the US markets and many others because it can cause serious cardiac arrhythmias such as torsade de pointes and ventricular fibrillation in people with cardiac or renal dysfunction or on drugs causing Q-T interval prolongation.

Proton pump inhibitors (PPIs) are especially useful in elderly patients for the treatment of erosive esophagitis or severe symptomatic reflux disease. A single daily dose will produce 67–95% symptom relief and esophagitis healing irrespective of the patient's age [28]. In elderly with swallowing difficulties, the capsules can be opened and taken with water, apple juice, applesauce or yogurt. PPIs are safe and well tolerated. Concerns have been raised about vitamin B_{12} malabsorption [29] and the development of carcinoid tumors with the long-term use of PPIs. So far, there are no reports of PPIs causing carcinoid or other gastric malignancies. In regards to vitamin B_{12} deficiency, vitamin B_{12} levels need to be monitored periodically in elderly patients on chronic PPI therapy.

Laparoscopic fundoplication is the surgical treatment of choice for GERD. Antireflux surgery should not be rejected solely on the basis of age because studies have shown no increase in the morbidity, mortality or length of hospital stay in elderly patients (over 65 years of age) compared to younger patients [30, 31]. A careful preoperative evaluation including endoscopy, esophageal manometry, 24-hour pH testing and, in selected cases, a gastric emptying study should be performed before referral for surgery.

Peptic Strictures

Peptic strictures are due to scarring from chronic acid-induced inflammation leading to narrowing of the esophagus [32]. They are seen with long-standing GERD and are typically smooth and less than 1 cm in length and occur most commonly in the distal esophagus, beginning at the squamocolumnar junction. Patients with peptic strictures are usually older than GERD patients without strictures. Patients present with progressive solid food dysphagia or sometimes with food impaction. As the stricture limits the amount of refluxate, heartburn may lessen in severity. Weight loss, if any, is minimal because of the preserved appetite. In patients with Barrett's esophagus, strictures can be seen in the mid-esophagus proximal to the Barrett's mucosa at the neo-squamocolumnar junction (fig. 4). Endoscopy should be performed to rule out Barrett's esophagus and malignancy and to assess the presence and severity of esophagitis. Treatment consists of excluding other aggravating factors such as pills, esophageal dilation with Maloney or Savary dilators and aggressive acid suppression, usually with PPIs. If strictures do not respond to conservative therapy, antireflux surgery may be necessary.

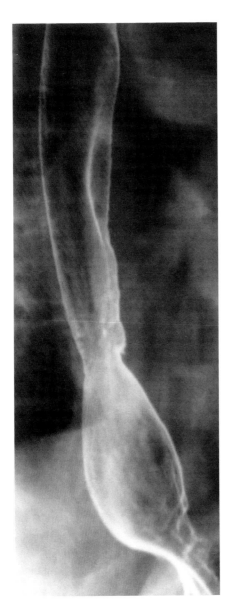

Fig. 4. A peptic stricture in the mid-esophagus associated with Barrett's esophagus.

Barrett's Esophagus

Barrett's esophagus is the most severe complication of GERD, wherein the squamous mucosa of the esophagus is replaced by specialized intestinal epithelium. The mean age of diagnosis is 60 years; most patients are white and male [24]. While most patients have long-standing reflux symptoms, 25% of the patients may be asymptomatic at the time of diagnosis. Elderly patients are typically less symptomatic than their younger counterparts [33]. The prevalence of Barrett's esophagus varies between 0.41 and 0.89% and increases with age until a plateau is reached by the seventh decade of life; however, the length of the Barrett's segment does not increase with age [34]. Barrett's esophagus and its associated dysplasia are the only recognized risk factors for esophageal adenocarcinoma. Patients with Barrett's esophagus are 30–125 times more likely to have adenocarcinoma of the esophagus than the general population. The estimated incidence of adenocarcinoma in patients with Barrett's esophagus is 0.2–2.1% per year [35].

We believe that all elderly patients, especially white men, should be screened for Barrett's esophagus, and if identified, patients should be placed in endoscopic surveillance programs and on aggressive antireflux therapy with PPIs. However, PPIs or, for that matter, antireflux surgery have not been shown to consistently cause regression of the Barrett's epithelium or prevention of esophageal cancer. Surveillance involves obtaining four-quadrant biopsies at 2-cm intervals in the Barrett's segment using a jumbo biopsy forceps as well as biopsies of any other mucosal abnormalities such as nodules or ulcers. If the biopsies are negative for dysplasia, endoscopy should be repeated within 1 year, followed by endoscopy every 2–3 years. If low-grade or indefinite dysplasia is identified, the surveillance interval is shortened to every 6 months for 1 year, followed by annual surveillance. If high-grade dysplasia is found, endoscopy is repeated at 1 month with four-quadrant biopsies at 1-cm intervals. If high-grade dysplasia is confirmed by two independent pathologists, options include esophagectomy or continued surveillance every 3 months [36]. Ablative therapies such as photodynamic therapy, laser, argon plasma coagulation and multipolar electrocoagulation appear to be very promising and merit consideration in patients who are poor surgical candidates.

Schatzki's Ring

This is a circumferential mucosal ring located at the gastroesophageal junction which is usually associated with a hiatal hernia [37]. It should not be confused with the muscular rings which occur more proximally in the esophagus and rarely cause dysphagia. Patients present with intermittent, nonprogressive dysphagia with solids. The first episode often occurs while the patient is eating a steak or bread hurriedly (steakhouse syndrome). Symptoms depend on the diameter of the ring. Patients rarely have symptoms when the ring is over 20 mm in diameter, but develop intermittent solid food dysphagia when the ring is 13 mm or less in diameter. The origin of Schatzki's ring is not known, but over half of the patients have evidence of GERD. Schatzki's ring is best demonstrated by a barium swallow, which shows a thin esophageal ring about 3–4 cm above the diaphragm. Treatment consists of a single session of dilation with a large bougie (52–60 Fr) followed by acid suppression therapy. Recurrence of the rings is unusual in the PPI era, but repeat dilation may be done if needed. Treatment options for refractory rings include endoscopic four-quadrant biopsy of the ring and electrosurgical incision of the ring using a papillotome. A concomitant motility disorder should be considered in cases of persistent symptoms.

Esophageal Webs

These are thin membranes of squamous epithelium that extend across the esophageal lumen. They most commonly occur in the anterior wall of the cervical esophagus. Cervical webs may be associated with iron deficiency anemia (Plummer-Vinson syndrome). Most patients are asymptomatic but may present with intermittent dysphagia. Symptomatic webs are treated with esophageal dilation.

Esophageal Cancer

Esophageal cancer is a common malignancy typically affecting elderly men, with either squamous cell carcinoma or adenocarcinoma accounting for more than 95% of the cases.

Squamous Cell Cancer

Esophageal squamous cell cancer accounts for 5–7% of all gastrointestinal malignancies. The annual incidence in the United States is 3–4 cases per 100,000 persons [38]. The incidence increases with age, being most common in men in their sixth and seventh decades of life. The incidence and mortality rates are much higher in elderly black men when compared to other groups. Risk factors for squamous cell cancer include alcohol and tobacco use, caustic esophageal injury, webs, chronic strictures, achalasia, squamous carcinoma of the nasopharynx, tylosis, partial gastrectomy and human papilloma virus [38].

Clinical features include dysphagia, initially with solids and later progressing to liquids, odynophagia and weight loss. Other manifestations include hoarseness, hemetemesis due to tumor invasion or aortoesophageal fistula. Endoscopy with biopsy and cytology is the best way to establish the diagnosis. The mid-esophagus is the most common site affected, followed by the distal esophagus. The majority of symptomatic lesions have ulcerated centers and heaped up margins and encroach on the lumen (fig. 5). However, early lesions may be subtle and almost normal in appearance. In vivo staining with Lugol's iodine or toluidine blue is helpful in delineating the abnormal mucosa. Barium esophagogram may show tumors but has low sensitivity in the detection of early tumors (fig. 6). Endosonography and CT scanning are useful for detection of local invasion and distant metastases, respectively.

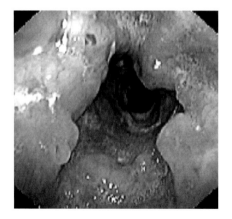

Fig. 5. Esophageal cancer: endoscopic appearance showing a narrowed and irregular esophageal lumen due to encroachment from the tumor.

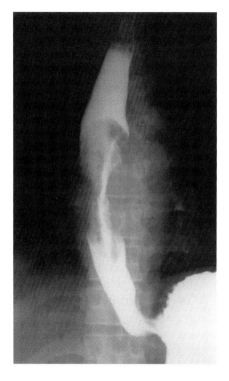

Fig. 6. Malignant stricture: barium esophagogram showing a long, narrow and irregular stricture in the mid-esophagus in a patient with squamous cell carcinoma of the esophagus.

Treatment and survival depends on the stage of the disease. Early cancers, such as those limited to the mucosa and the submucosa, can be cured by esophagectomy, but cure is not always possible due to presentation of cancers at a late stage. In patients with superficial cancers limited to the mucosa who are poor candidates for surgery, options include endoscopic mucosal resection or ablation with electrocautery, argon plasma coagulation, laser or photodynamic therapy. In locally advanced cancer, a multimodality approach involving surgery, radiation and chemotherapy provide the best chance for survival. Squamous cell cancer, unlike adenocarcinoma, is radiosensitive. A majority of patients have some response to radiation therapy but the response is brief, averaging about 3 months [39]. The most widely used combination for chemotherapy, cisplatin and 5-fluorouracil, has shown a response in 20–40% of cases, but has no impact on survival [40]. In patients with metastatic disease, treatment is mainly palliative. Palliative measures for dysphagia include esophageal dilation, stent placement or endoscopic tumor ablation. The 5-year survival rates for TNM stage I, II, III and IV cancers are 60.4, 31.3, 19.9 and 4.1%, respectively [38].

Adenocarcinoma

Adenocarcinoma of the esophagus has been increasing in frequency at an alarming rate over the past few decades, now accounting for more than 50% of the newly diagnosed esophageal cancers. The annual incidence of adenocarcinoma of the esophagus and gastric cardia is 5.1 cases per 100,000 persons [38]. Unlike squamous cell carcinoma, adenocarcinoma typically affects elderly white males. Barrett's esophagus secondary to long-standing reflux disease is the single most important risk factor for adenocarcinoma, but it is detectable in only 19–86% of the cases of adenocarcinoma [41, 42]. It is likely that all tumors arise from Barrett's mucosa but in some cases, the segment of specialized intestinal metaplasia is obscured due to tumor invasion or has regressed from acid suppressive therapy.

The clinical presentation is similar to that of squamous cell carcinoma, but malnutrition, fistulas and recurrent laryngeal nerve involvement are less common and extension into the stomach, diaphragm and the liver are more frequent. Over 80% of the tumors are in the distal esophagus. Most patients have a history of long-standing GERD.

The diagnostic evaluation, treatment modalities and prognosis are similar to those for squamous cell carcinoma. However, with increased use of endoscopic surveillance, cancers can be diagnosed at an early stage, offering the best chance of cure.

Medication-Induced Esophageal Injury

Elderly people take multiple medications for various ailments and hence are prone to drug-induced esophageal injury [43]. Common culprits are doxycycline, emepronium bromide, slow-release potassium chloride, quinidine, iron sulfate, bisphosphonates such as alendronate, aspirin and nonsteroidal antiinflammatory drugs. Although patients with structural abnormalities and motility disorders are more prone to develop medication-induced esophagitis, most patients have a normal esophagus. Predisposing factors are taking pills with only small amounts of liquids or just before bedtime. Patients present with acute onset of dysphagia, odynophagia and, rarely, heartburn. The commonest sites of drug-induced injury are at the mid-esophagus at the level of the aortic arch and just above the gastroesophageal junction. On endoscopy, discrete ulcers are seen ranging from pinpoint ulcers to circumferential lesions several centimeters long. These ulcers may be complicated by stricture formation or, rarely, perforation. Preventive strategies include taking medication only when sitting or standing, drinking an adequate amount of water, avoiding taking pills at bedtime and taking a liquid preparation if available. Treatment involves discontinuation of the offending medication or taking the drug in liquid or parenteral form, acid suppression and dilation in cases of strictures.

Dysphagia Aortica

Dysphagia aortica is a disorder of the elderly due to compression of the esophagus from a large thoracic aortic aneurysm or a rigid atherosclerotic aorta [44]. Patients have dysphagia with solids with a feeling of fullness in the chest and regurgitation. A barium swallow shows compression of the esophagus and delayed passage of the solid bolus. Esophageal manometry shows increased intraluminal pressures with superimposed cardiac pulsations. Management involves dietary modification and, in severe cases, surgical repair.

Motility Disorders

Based on the predominant manometric abnormality, the motility disorders of the esophagus are classified into aperistalsis (achalasia), uncoordinated motility (diffuse esophageal spasm), hypercontractility (nutcracker esophagus, hypertensive LES) and hypocontractility (ineffective esophageal motility, hypotensive LES). Except for achalasia, which is well characterized, the clinical significance of the other esophageal motility disorders is not known, as the manometric abnormalities do not necessarily correlate with the symptoms.

Achalasia

Achalasia is a primary esophageal motor disorder characterized by abnormal relaxation of the LES and esophageal aperistalsis. It is due to the loss of ganglion cells in the myenteric plexus (Auerbach's plexus), mainly the nitric oxide-containing inhibitory postganglionic neurons that mediate LES relaxation and the normal latency gradient along the esophageal body responsible for peristalsis. This leads to unopposed excitation of the smooth muscle by acetylcholine, causing incomplete relaxation of the LES and loss of peristalsis. The etiology of idiopathic achalasia is unknown; available data have suggested hereditary, autoimmune, infection-induced destruction or degeneration associated with neurological disorders [45].

The onset of symptoms in patients with achalasia is usually between the ages of 20 and 40, but a third of the cases present after 60 years of age [46]. Dysphagia with solids and liquids is the most common symptom, followed by regurgitation of bland material (undigested food and saliva), chest pain and weight loss. Fewer elderly patients complain of chest pain, which, when present, is usually mild [47]. Heartburn, if present, is due to fermentation of retained food and secretions in the dilated esophagus.

Esophageal motor abnormalities similar to achalasia are found in certain disorders such as Chagas' disease, adenocarcinoma of the gastroesophageal junction and, rarely, squamous cell carcinoma of the esophagus, lymphoma or cancer of the pancreas, lung or prostate. These latter malignant conditions are grouped under the term 'secondary achalasia' or 'pseudoachalasia'. This should be considered with older age at presentation, rapid progression of symptoms and profound weight loss [48]. A CT scan or endosonography are needed to rule out a neoplasm. A narrowed distal esophageal segment longer than 3.5 cm with little or no proximal dilatation of the esophagus on barium study is suggestive of pseudoachalasia [49].

The initial investigation in a patient with suspected achalasia should be a barium esophagogram, which will show lack of peristalsis and a dilated, sometimes tortuous esophagus with a smooth tapered narrowing at the gastroesophageal junction (bird beak appearance; fig. 7). A timed barium esophagogram (1-, 2- and 5-min barium X-rays after ingestion of 250 ml of barium) can be used to measure esophageal emptying before treatment and to assess objective improvement after therapy [50]. Esophageal manometry is used to confirm the diagnosis of achalasia. The manometric features include aperistalsis of the body, abnormal LES relaxation and high LES pressure. Most features are not affected by age except residual LES pressure, which is negatively correlated with age [47]. An upper endoscopy should be performed in all patients, especially the elderly, to rule out pseudoachalasia. On endoscopy, the body appears dilated, atonic and sometimes with food residue. The LES area is puckered and offers gentle resistance to the passage of the scope; if excessive pressure is required for the scope passage, pseudoachalasia should be suspected. Endoscopic ultrasound may be useful in patients with negative endoscopy and with a clinical suspicion of pseudoachalasia.

There is no treatment to reverse the motor abnormalities in achalasia. Current treatments are aimed at decreasing the resting LES pressure to relieve the obstruction from the poorly relaxing sphincter and improve esophageal emptying. Pneumatic dilation with large balloons is the most effective nonsurgical treatment for achalasia. Rigiflex balloons are most commonly used and are available

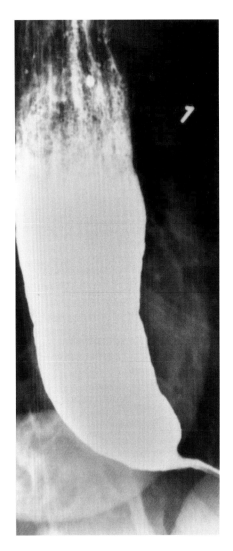

Fig. 7. Achalasia: barium esopha-gogram showing a dilated esophagus, retained secretions and smooth tapering at the gastroesophageal junction (bird beak appearance).

in 3-, 3.5- and 4-cm sizes. An alternative is the Witzel balloon dilator, which comes in a 4-cm size and is placed over the endoscope. Larger dilators are associated with a higher risk of perforation; hence, we recommend a graded approach in treating patients with the Rigiflex dilators, beginning with the smallest dilator and increasing the size as needed with subsequent dilations. Dilation with 3-, 3.5- and 4-cm balloon diameters results in good to excellent symptomatic relief in 74, 86 and 90% of the treated patients, respectively [51]. Patients over 40 years of age seem to have better long-term symptom relief than younger patients [52].

Symptomatic relief does not necessarily correlate with objective improvement. In one study, 31% of the patients with complete symptom resolution had a barium esophagogram showing less than 50% improvement in esophageal emptying [53]. The only predictor of this discordant response was older age. In such patients, dilation with a larger size balloon may be required to ensure long-term remission and prevent decompensation possibly requiring esophagectomy.

Surgical myotomy of the LES (modified Heller's approach) is another effective method for the treatment of achalasia. In the past, this was done by an open procedure through a thoracic or abdominal incision. With the advent of minimally invasive surgery, cardiomyotomy can be performed by a laparoscopic or, less commonly, thoracoscopic technique. Laparoscopic myotomy has a good to excellent clinical response rate of 83–100% [51]. GERD is reported in about 10% of these patients [51]. The choice of adding an antireflux procedure is controversial as it may decrease problems with secondary reflux disease but may also increase the incidence of postoperative dysphagia. Both pneumatic dilation and surgical myotomy are equally effective methods and hence the treatment chosen depends on the patient preference and the available skills.

In the elderly with other serious medical problems in whom pneumatic dilation and surgery are associated with a high risk, endoscopic injection of botulinum toxin into the LES is an attractive option. Botulinum toxin inhibits the calcium-dependant release of acetylcholine from the excitatory neurons that contribute to LES tone, thereby leading to a decrease in LES pressure. Botulinum toxin is injected endoscopically with a sclerotherapy needle into the LES region in each of the four quadrants to a total of 80–100 units. It leads to good short-term relief of symptoms and has a higher response rate in older patients (82% vs. 43% in patients less than 50 years of age) and in those with vigorous achalasia (100% vs. 52% in classic achalasia) [54].

Nitrates and calcium channel blockers are alternative therapies in older patients who are poor operative candidates. They are given in sublingual form immediately before meals and may produce side effects such as headaches, lightheadedness and pedal edema. In very rare patients in whom all therapies have failed, esophagectomy is the last resort.

Other Motility Disorders of the Esophagus

This group includes diffuse esophageal spasm, nutcracker esophagus, hypertensive LES, ineffective esophageal motility and hypotensive LES. Diffuse esophageal spasm is characterized by intermittent dysphagia with solids and liquids and chest pain. Symptoms may be brought on by ingesting cold or hot food or drinks and sometimes by stress. Esophageal manometry shows more than 10% simultaneous contractions mixed with normal peristalsis. Nutcracker esophagus is a manometric diagnosis characterized by increased peristaltic amplitude (>180 mm Hg) and prolonged duration (>6 s), usually associated with chest pain and sometimes with dysphagia. Ineffective esophageal motility is defined as a distal esophageal amplitude less than 30 mm Hg in at least 30% of the swallows and/or more than 30% nontransmitted peristalsis. It is seen commonly in GERD patients with respiratory symptoms. Treatment for all these disorders is unsatisfactory. Reassurance is important. Nitrates, calcium channel blockers and antidepressants can be tried. Esophageal dilation and myotomy may be required in severe, refractory cases.

Scleroderma

The esophagus is involved in 70–80% of patients with scleroderma or CREST syndrome [17]. There is muscular atrophy and fibrous replacement of the smooth muscle in the lower two thirds of the esophagus leading to impaired acid clearance, low LES pressure with poor motility and severe reflux esophagitis. The striated muscle in the UES and proximal esophagus is not affected. Patients present with severe heartburn, regurgitation and dysphagia. Mild dysphagia can be due to esophageal dysmotility but severe symptoms suggest severe esophagitis with a peptic stricture or a malignancy. 2–48% of patients with reflux due to scleroderma develop a peptic stricture [32]. The prevalence of Barrett's esophagus in scleroderma patients has varied between 16 and 37% in various case series [55, 56]. The barium esophagogram shows esophageal dilatation, aperistalsis of the distal esophagus and patulous LES with free reflux. Classic manometric features include low LES pressure and decreased or absent peristalsis in the lower two thirds of the esophagus. Treatment centers around aggressive treatment of the gastroesophageal reflux and its complications. Patients need lifelong treatment with PPIs and may require higher doses for adequate acid control. Strictures require esophageal dilation. Antireflux surgery may be warranted in severe cases.

Conclusion

Dysphagia in the elderly is due to a variety of diseases, some of which are unique to this group. Because of subtle and atypical presentation, coexistent illnesses and an interplay of various psychological factors in the elderly, esophageal diseases may pose a diagnostic challenge to the clinician. Management of esophageal diseases in the elderly is similar to that in the young; however, the clinician should be aware of the need for aggressive management, varying therapeutic response rates and a greater chance of drug interactions. Hence, as is true in all situations, treatment should be tailored to the individual needs of the patient.

References

1   Zboralske FF, Amberg JR, Soergel KH: Presbyesophagus: Cineradiographic manifestations. Radiology 1964;82:463–464.
2   Lock G: Physiology and pathology of the oesophagus in the elderly patient. Best Pract Res Clin Gastroenterol 2001;15:919–941.
3   Hollis JB, Castell DO: Esophageal function in elderly men: A new look at presbyesophagus. Ann Intern Med 1974;80:371–374.
4   Richter JE, Wu WC, John DN, Blackwell JN, Nelson JL III, Castell JA, Castell DO: Esophageal manometry in 95 healthy adult volunteers: Variability of pressures with age and frequency of 'abnormal' contractions. Dig Dis Sci 1987;32:583–592.
5   Khan TA, Shragge BW, Crsipin JS, Lind JF: Esophageal motility in the elderly. Am J Dig Dis 1977;22:1049–1054.
6   Leese G, Hopwood D: Muscle fibre typing in the human pharyngeal constrictors and oesophagus: The effect of ageing. Acta Anat (Basel) 1986;127:77–80.
7   Eckhardt VF, Le Compte PM: Esophageal ganglion and smooth muscle in the elderly. Am J Dig Dis 1978;23:443–448.
8   Groher ME, Bukatman R: The prevalence of swallowing disorders in two teaching hospitals. Dysphagia 1986;1:3–6.
9   Siebens H, Trupe E, Siebens A, Cook F, Anshen S, Hanauer R, Oster G: Correlates and consequences of eating dependency in the institutionalized elderly. J Am Geriatr Soc 1986;34:192–198.
10 Castell DO, Donner MW: Evaluation of dysphagia: A careful history is crucial. Dysphagia 1987;2:65–71.
11 Alberts JM, Horner J, Gray L, Brazer SR: Aspiration after stroke: Lesion analysis by brain MRI. Dysphagia 1992;7:170–173.
12 Leiberman AN, Horowitz L, Redmond P, Pachter L, Liberman I, Leibowitz M: Dysphagia in Parkinson's disease. Am J Gastroenterol 1980;74:157–160.
13 Ergun GA, Kahrilas PJ: Oropharyngeal dysphagia in the elderly. Pract Gastroenterol 1993;17:9–16.
14 Leopold NA, Kagel MC: Pharyngo-esophageal dysphagia in Parkinson's disease. Dysphagia 1997;12:11–20.
15 Bushmann M, Dobmeyer SM, Leeker L, Perlmutter JS: Swallowing abnormalities and their response to treatment in Parkinson's disease. Neurology 1989;39:1309–1314.
16 Cook IJ: Disorders causing oropharyngeal dysphagia; in Castell DO, Richter JE (eds): The Esophagus. Philadelphia, Lippincott Williams and Wilkins, 1999, pp 165–184.
17 Schroeder PL, Richter JE: Swallowing disorders in the elderly. Semin Gastrointest Dis 1994;5:154–165.
18 Novak TV, Ionasescu V, Anuras S: Gastrointestinal manifestations of the muscular dystrophies. Gastroenterology 1982;82:800–810.
19 Taillefer R, Duranceau AC: Manometric and radionuclide assessment of pharyngeal emptying before and after cricopharyngeal myotomy in patients with oculopharyngeal dystrophy. J Thorac Cardiovasc Surg 1988;95:868–875.
20 Cook IJ, Kahrilas PJ: AGA technical review on management of oropharyngeal dysphagia. Gastroenterology 1999;116:455–478.
21 Shaw GY, Searl JP: Botulinum toxin treatment for cricopharyngeal dysfunction. Dysphagia 2001;16:161–167.
22 Locke GR III, Talley NJ, Fett SL, Zinsmeister AR, Melton LJ III: Prevalence and spectrum of gastroesophageal reflux: A population-based study in Olmsted county, Minnesota. Gastroenterology 1997;112:1448–1456.
23 Collen MJ, Abdulian JD, Chen YK: Gastroesophageal reflux disease in the elderly: More severe disease that requires aggressive therapy. Am J Gastroenterol 1995;90:1053–1057.
24 Richter JE: Gastroesophageal reflux disease in the older patient: Presentation, treatment, and complications. Am J Gastroenterol 2000;95:368–373.
25 Lasch H, Castell DO, Castell JA: Evidence for diminished visceral pain with aging: Studies using graded intraesophageal balloon distension. Am J Physiol 1997;272:G1–G3.

26   Raiha IJ, Impivara O, Seppala M, Sourander LB: Prevalence and characteristics of symptomatic gastroesophageal reflux in the elderly. J Am Geriatr Soc 1992;40:1209–1211.
27   Lippy RJ, Fennerty B, Fagan TC: Clinical review of histamine-receptor antagonists. Arch Intern Med 1990;150:745–755.
28   Sontag S: The medical management of reflux esophagitis: Role of antacids and acid inhibition. Gastroenterol Clin North Am 1990;19:673–690.
29   Marcuard SP, Albernaz L, Khazamie PG: Omeprazole therapy causes malabsorption of cyanocobalamin (vitamin B_{12}). Ann Intern Med 1994;12:211–215.
30   Trus TL, Laycock WS, Wo JM, Waring JP, Branum GD, Mauren SJ, Katz EM, Hunter JG: Laparoscopic antireflux surgery in the elderly. Am J Gastroenterol 1998;93:351–353.
31   Allen R, Rappaport W, Hixson L, Sampliner R, Case T, Fennerty MB: Referral patterns and the results of antireflux operations in patients more than sixty years of age. Surg Gynecol Obstet 1991;173:359–362.
32   Richter JE: Peptic strictures of the esophagus. Gastroenterol Clin North Am 1999;28:875–890.
33   Johnson DA, Winters C, Spurling TJ, Chobanian SJ, Cattau EL Jr: Esophageal acid sensitivity in Barrett's esophagus. J Clin Gastroenterol 1987;9:23–27.
34   Cameron AJ, Lomboy CT: Barrett's esophagus: Age, prevalence, and extent of columnar epithelium. Gastroenterology 1992;103:1241–1245.
35   Falk GW: Barrett's esophagus. Gastrointest Endosc Clin N Am 1994;4:773–789.
36   Sampliner RE: Practice guidelines on the diagnosis, surveillance, and therapy of Barrett's esophagus. Am J Gastroenterol 1998;93:1028–1032.
37   Spechler SJ: AGA technical review on treatment of patients with dysphagia caused by benign disorders of the distal esophagus. Gastroenterology 1999;117:233–254.
38   Axelrad AM, Fleischer DE: Esophageal tumors; in Feldman M, Sleisenger MH, Scharschmidt BF (eds): Sleisenger & Fordtran's Gastrointestinal and Liver Disease, ed 6. Philadelphia, Saunders, 1998, pp 540–554.
39   Smalley SR, Gunderson LL, Reddy EK, Williamson S: Radiotherapy alone in esophageal carcinoma: Current management and future directions of adjuvant, curative and palliative approaches. Semin Oncol 1994;21:467–473.
40   Bhansali MS, Vaidya JS, Bhatt RG, Patil PK, Badwe RA, Desai PB: Chemotherapy for carcinoma of the esophagus: A comparison of evidence from meta-analyses of randomized trials and of historical control studies. Ann Oncol 1996;7:3555–3559.
41   Bytzer P, Christensen PB, Damkier P, Vinding K, Seersholm N: Adenocarcinoma of the esophagus and Barrett's esophagus: A population-based study. Am J Gastroenterol 1999;94:86–91.
42   Haggitt RC, Tryzelaar J, Ellis H, Colcher H: Adenocarcinoma complicating columnar epithelium-lined (Barrett's) esophagus. Am J Clin Pathol 1978;70:1–5.
43   Eng J, Sabanathan S: Drug-induced esophagitis. Am J Gastroenterol 1991;86:1127–1133.
44   Friedman LS, Castell DO: Esophageal diseases in the elderly; in Castell DO, Richter JE (eds): The Esophagus. Philadelphia, Lippincot Williams and Wilkins, 1999, pp 615–630.
45   Birgisson S, Richter JE: Achalasia: What's new in diagnosis and treatment? Dig Dis 1997; 15(suppl 1):1–27.
46   Mayberry JF, Atkinson M: Studies on the incidence and prevalence of achalasia in the Nottingham area. Q J Med 1985;56:451–456.
47   Clouse RE, Abramson BK, Todorczuk JR: Achalasia in the elderly. Effects of aging on clinical presentation and outcome. Dig Dis Sci 1991;36:225–228.
48   Tucker HJ, Snape WJ Jr, Cohen S: Achalasia secondary to carcinoma: Clinical and manometric features. Ann Intern Med 1978;89:315–318.
49   Woodfield CA, Levine MS, Rubesin SE, Langlotz CP, Laufer I: Diagnosis of primary versus secondary achalasia: Reassessment of clinical and radiographic criteria. AJR Am J Roentgenol 2000;175:727–731.
50   de Oliveira JM, Birgisson S, Doinoff C, Einstein D, Herts B, Davros W, Obuchowski N, Koehler RE, Richter JE: Timed barium swallow: A simple technique for evaluating esophageal emptying in patients with achalasia. AJR Am J Roentgenol 1997;169:473–479.
51   Vaezi MF, Richter JE: Current therapies for achalasia. Comparison and efficacy. J Clin Gastroenterol 1998;27:21–35.

52   Eckardt VF, Aignherr C, Bernhard G: Predictors of outcome in patients with achalasia treated by pneumatic dilation. Gastroenterology 1992;103:1732–1738.
53   Vaezi MF, Baker ME, Richter JE: Assessment of esophageal emptying post-pneumatic dilation: Use of the timed barium esophagogram. Am J Gastroenterol 1999;94:1802–1807.
54   Pasricha PJ, Rai R, Ravich WJ, Hendrix TR, Kalloo AN: Botulinum toxin for achalasia: Long-term outcome and predictors of response. Gastroenterology 1996;110:1410–1415.
55   Weston S, Thumshirn M, Wiste J, Camilleri M: Clinical and upper gastrointestinal motility features in systemic sclerosis and related disorders. Am J Gastroenterol 1998;93:1085–1089.
56   Recht MP, Levine MS, Katzka DA, Reynolds JC, Saul SH: Barrett's esophagus in scleroderma: Increased prevalence and radiographic findings. Gastrointest Radiol 1988;13:1–5.

Joel E. Richter, MD
Chairman, Center for Swallowing and Esophageal Disorders,
Department of Gastroenterology/A30, Cleveland Clinic Foundation,
9500 Euclid Avenue, Cleveland, OH 44195 (USA)
Tel. +1 216 445 9102, Fax +1 216 445 3889, E-Mail richtej@ccf.org

Pilotto A, Malfertheiner P, Holt PR (eds): Aging and the Gastrointestinal Tract.
Interdiscipl Top Gerontol. Basel, Karger, 2003, vol 32, pp 100–117

....

Gastroesophageal Reflux Disease in the Elderly

Alberto Pilotto, Marilisa Franceschi

Geriatric Unit, 'Casa Sollievo della Sofferenza' Hospital,
IRCCS, San Giovanni Rotondo, Italy

Gastroesophageal reflux disease (GERD) is defined by histopathological alterations and/or symptoms caused by the reflux of gastric contents into the esophagus. Manifestations of GERD range from mild episodes of heartburn and acid regurgitation, without esophagitis, to chronic mucosal inflammation and ulceration, accompanied in severe cases by stricture, bleeding and chronic anemia. Prolonged exposure of the esophageal mucosa to acid can also result in metaplasia and the development of columnar-lined mucosa in the lower esophagus (Barrett's esophagus), which is associated with a 20- to 40-fold increased risk of esophageal adenocarcinoma.

The prevalence of GERD increases with age; in older primary care outpatients, acid reflux may have an incidence as high as 20% [1]. A recent study from the United Kingdom reported an increase with age in the percentage of GERD patients who had consulted their general practitioner about their symptoms during the previous year [2]. Older age, male sex and white ethnicity were found to be the most important risk factors for the development of severe forms of GERD in a large epidemiological study involving 194,527 GERD patients followed from 1981 to 1994 in 172 hospitals of the Department of Veterans Affairs in the United States [3].

Pathophysiology

Pathophysiological changes in esophageal functions that occur with aging may, at least in part, be responsible for the high prevalence of GERD in old age. One study reported that a higher prevalence of gastroesophageal reflux events in the elderly was associated with a significantly shorter intra-abdominal segment of the lower esophageal sphincter (LES) [4]. Other changes that may be associated with GERD in the elderly are a reduction of secondary peristalsis [5], an increase in the prevalence of tertiary contractions [6] and a lower peristaltic contraction amplitude 5 and 10 cm above the LES [7]. A recent manometric study carried out in 79 healthy subjects reported that age correlated inversely with LES pressure and length, yet age correlated directly with the proportion of simultaneous contraction [8]. These data are in agreement with a previous finding of a marked failure of esophageal contraction after swallowing that resulted in incomplete esophageal emptying of both low- and high-viscosity liquids in elderly subjects [9]. Moreover, a manometric and scintigraphic study of healthy volunteers aged 20–80 years documented that older persons more frequently have abnormal peristalsis and a longer duration of gastroesophageal reflux episodes than young or middle-aged subjects [10]. The morphological origin of such functional alterations is not well established. It is known that even if the thickness of the human esophageal smooth muscle does not vary with aging [11], the number of myenteric neurons in the esophagus does decrease with age [12], especially in the superior third of the esophagus at the junction with the pharynx.

Other factors, often secondary to systemic diseases, may be involved in gastroesophageal reflux in the elderly, as well as alterations in salivary secretion or gastric emptying, decreased tissue resistance resulting from impaired epithelial cell regeneration or duodeno-gastroesophageal reflux of bile salts [13]. It is important to note that aging per se does not decrease gastric acid secretion in older subjects [14]. This pathophysiological feature is more likely related to a chronic *Helicobacter pylori* infection in which gastric mucosal atrophy has developed [15]. Currently, the significance of such pathophysiological changes in gastroesophageal function is not well defined, particularly in the elderly.

Undoubtedly, elderly subjects have a higher prevalence of risk factors that predispose the aging esophagus to lesions (table 1): (1) difficulty in maintaining an upright position after meals; (2) hiatus hernia associated with both repeat episodes of acid reflux and with more severe diseases [16] such as Barrett's esophagus [17]; (3) increased drug use, including drugs that may have a directly damaging effect on esophageal mucosa or an indirect effect on reducing LES pressure, and (4) delayed esophageal transit time of many drugs [18], creating a potentially dangerous situation in the presence of acid reflux, as recently reported for alendronate [19] and nonsteroidal antiinflammatory drugs (NSAIDs) [20].

Symptomatology

Particular attention has been given to the clinical presentation of GERD in the elderly since important differences between young and adult patients exist.

Table 1. Potential causes of GERD in the elderly

Functional causes
  Impaired motility of the esophagus
  Reduced LES pressure and length
  Normal gastric acid secretion
  Delayed gastric emptying transit time
  Reduced salivary secretion
  Decreased tissue resistance as a result of impaired
    epithelial cell regeneration
  Duodeno-gastroesophageal reflux of bile salts
Anatomical causes
  Hiatus hernia
  Difficulty in maintaining an upright position
Drug use
Direct effect on esophageal mucosa
  Aspirin
  NSAIDs
  Potassium salts
  Ferrous sulfate
  Corticosteroids
  Alendronate
Indirect effect of reducing LES pressure
  Theophylline
  Nitroderivates
  Calcium channel blockers
  Benzodiazepines
  Dopaminergics
  Tricyclic antidepressants
  Anticholinergics

In the elderly, heartburn is not frequent and acid regurgitation presents in less than 25% of patients [21]. In a study from North Europe, the primary symptoms in elderly patients with GERD were dysphagia, vomiting and respiratory difficulties, confirming the significant relationship of GERD with a restrictive ventilatory defect in the elderly [22]. This divergent symptomatology was also demonstrated by a recent large survey conducted on 775 patients with esophagitis divided into four groups according to age, i.e. young patients aged 16–49 years (mean age 36.5 years), adult patients aged 50–69 years (mean age 59.2 years), old patients aged 70–84 years (mean age 77.9 years) and very old patients over 85 years of age (mean age 88.2 years) [23]. Compared to young and adult subjects, elderly patients had a higher prevalence of severe esophagitis (3.1, 5.8, 13.3 and 23.4%, $p < 0.00001$) and hiatus hernia (44.8, 51, 51.9 and 62.1%, $p < 0.01$). Moreover, with advancing age, a significantly lower prevalence of

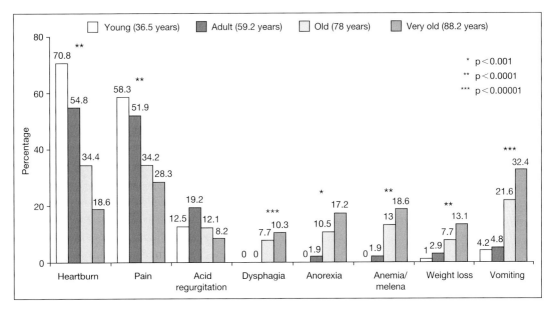

Fig. 1. Prevalence of symptoms in 775 subjects with esophagitis divided according to age (modified from Franceschi et al. [23]).

typical symptoms, i.e. heartburn (70.8, 54.8, 34.4 and 18.6%, $p < 0.0001$), acid regurgitation (12.5, 19.2, 12.1 and 8.2%, p = not significant) and pain (58.3, 51.9, 34.2 and 28.3%, $p < 0.0001$) was reported. In contrast, the prevalence of vomiting (4.2, 4.8, 21.6 and 32.4%, $p < 0.00001$), anorexia (0, 1.9, 10.5 and 17.2%, $p < 0.001$), weight loss (1, 2.9, 7.7 and 13.1%, $p < 0.0001$), dysphagia (0, 0, 7.7 and 10.3%, $p < 0.00001$) and anemia-melena (0, 1.9, 13 and 18.6%, $p < 0.0001$) increased significantly with age (fig. 1). The atypical nature of the symptomatology in elderly patients was confirmed by a previous study which reported esophagitis to be the cause of bleeding in 21% of patients over 80 years old [24]. The clinical consequence of the rarity of typical reflux symptoms in old age is that reflux esophagitis in the elderly may be missed, especially in the presence of a mild form of esophagitis, and that a substantial number of patients may suffer subclinical relapses of the disease [25].

The cause of such a different clinical expression of the disease in the elderly is not clear. A diminished sensitivity to visceral pain has been documented in the elderly by studies using esophageal balloon distension [26]. More recently, a study carried out using 24-hour esophageal pH monitoring and endoscopy documented an age-related reduction in acid chemosensitivity [27]. The same study confirmed that older patients with GERD had reduced symptom severity despite a tendency towards increased severity of esophageal mucosal injury and acid exposure.

Diagnosis

Endoscopy

In the younger patient, a clinical diagnosis of GERD can be made if typical symptoms are relieved with a therapeutic trial of antireflux therapy. Indeed, the current recommendations are to treat first and to reserve diagnostic testing, i.e. endoscopy, radiology and other functional tests, for those patients who have symptoms resistant to medical therapy, chronic relapsing or alarming symptoms (i.e. weight loss, anemia, dysphagia). Conversely, in the elderly, GERD very often presents with atypical and/or unspecific symptoms [24, 25] and usually is more severe despite milder symptoms [23, 28] because of the cumulative injury due to acid reflux over many years. For these reasons, endoscopy should be undertaken early as the initial diagnostic test in all elderly patients with typical symptoms (i.e. heartburn or acid regurgitation) regardless of the severity or duration of their complaints. Furthermore, elderly subjects without current typical symptoms but with a past history of reflux disease should be evaluated [29].

Early endoscopy is very useful in diagnosing the presence and severity of esophagitis and hiatus hernia. Indeed, the grade of severity of esophagitis and the presence of hiatus hernia are important prognostic factors to be considered in the long-term treatment of patients. Early endoscopy will also identify GERD complications, especially esophageal stricture and Barrett's esophagus, and concomitant gastroduodenal diseases, i.e. gastric or duodenal ulcers and/or *H. pylori* infection.

Barium Radiography, 24-Hour pH Testing and Manometry

Barium radiography of the esophagus is an excellent test to establish the presence of a hiatus hernia and is indicated as part of the evaluation of the patient with suspected motility abnormalities or peptic stricture. A barium study will identify rings and webs or other obstructive lesions. The barium swallow test is also a key test in identifying elderly patients with dysphagia, and it should be performed in conjunction with endoscopy in all elderly patients with this symptomatology. Barium studies are widely available and usually well tolerated by older people.

Esophageal 24-hour pH testing is helpful before antireflux surgery and in those patients not responsive to medical treatment. In the endoscopy-negative patient, an abnormal esophageal pH test may suggest the need for more aggressive drug therapy, whereas a normal test indicates the presence of a functional disorder. The elderly patient with persistent esophagitis warrants esophageal pH testing. A normal test could differentiate pathophysiological mechanisms, i.e. a drug-induced esophagitis from acid reflux disease.

Esophageal manometry is useful in identifying abnormalities of LES pressure or esophageal motility. In elderly patients, its major use is reserved for the localization of the LES before pH testing and for obtaining preoperative information on esophageal peristalsis.

The clinical significance of these functional findings may be at times not so evident in the elderly as in adult or young patients. 'Normal values' for currently used parameters of esophageal function may change with age, and thus, may not be directly comparable in young and old subjects. For example, a radiologic study performed in elderly, asymptomatic subjects found that only 16% had swallowing functions within the normal limits as defined in younger subjects [30]. A study of 24-hour esophageal pH monitoring demonstrated that 30% of asymptomatic elderly subjects were 'abnormal' when compared to conventional 24-hour pH-metric criteria [31]. More recently, identifying 'age-related normality limits' of esophageal pressures before establishing a manometric diagnosis in elderly patients has been suggested [8]. Our view of esophageal dysfunction derived from studies of younger populations may not always be applicable to the geriatric age group.

Therapeutic Trial with Proton Pump Inhibitors

A therapeutic trial with proton pump inhibitors (PPIs) has been recently suggested as a useful diagnostic test in patients with GERD. Treatment with omeprazole 40 mg daily for 14 days documented a 68% sensitivity and a 63% specificity for diagnosing GERD in patients with typical GERD symptoms [32]. High doses of omeprazole (40 mg in the morning plus 20 mg in the afternoon) for 7 days identified reflux disease in patients with noncardiac chest pain with a 78.3% sensitivity and 85.7% specificity, resulting in a 59% reduction in the number of diagnostic procedures [33]. Moreover, this PPI test proved to be as sensitive as ambulatory 24-hour esophageal pH monitoring in diagnosing GERD in patients with erosive esophagitis [32, 34]. However, none of these studies was performed in elderly subjects. Since typical (heartburn, acid regurgitation) and extraesophageal symptoms (asthma, chronic cough, noncardiac chest pain) of GERD are often absent in elderly patients, the patient's history is less reliable and a high prevalence of severe upper gastrointestinal diseases is very common despite mild symptomatology [35], a therapeutic trial with a PPI should be undertaken with great caution in older patients and possibly only after endoscopy as a first diagnostic test. This paradoxically more aggressive diagnostic approach in the elderly is recommended to avoid misleading and sometimes quite dangerous treatment approaches in this population.

Treatment

The main objectives of GERD treatment are: elimination of symptoms, healing of esophagitis, maintenance of remission of the disease and management of complications. To obtain these goals, the combined use of lifestyle modifications, medical therapy and surgery may be considered.

Lifestyle and Dietary Modifications
Studies with overnight pH monitoring have shown a significant decrease in total esophageal acid exposure after elevating the head of the bed 6 inches. A similar effect can be obtained by placing a foam rubber wedge (8–10 inches high) on top of the mattress under the patient's head [36]. Other potentially useful lifestyle modifications include weight loss, and avoiding tight-fitting garments, smoking and late meals before bedtime or recumbency early after eating. Recently, it was reported that chewing gum for 1 h after meals helps to reduce postprandial esophageal acid exposure, while the beneficial effect of walking for 1 h after meals was apparent only to a mild degree and only for a short duration [37]. Dietary modifications include eliminating or decreasing potential esophageal irritants, i.e. citrus juices, tomato products, coffee, alcohol, mint or chocolate, all of which may reduce LES pressure. Medications that decrease LES pressure and promote gastroesophageal reflux (theophylline, nitroderivates, calcium channel blockers, benzodiazepines, anticholinergics, tricyclic antidepressants) need to be avoided when possible. Other drugs may cause direct esophageal injury (potassium salts, iron sulfate, aspirin, NSAIDs and alendronate); these medications should be used with caution in older patients with GERD. In any case, these drugs must be taken while maintaining an upright position and with a full glass of water.

The importance of including these lifestyle modifications as part of a treatment program at a time when a highly successful antireflux therapy, such as PPIs, is available has been debated. Unfortunately, no studies have explored the role of such lifestyle and dietary modifications in GERD treatment in patients of different ages. However, from a clinical perspective, it is reasonable to suggest lifestyle and dietary modifications to patients with mild, infrequent symptoms who are motivated to follow these recommendations with a high grade of compliance. In patients with more severe disease, such lifestyle and dietary changes will have a lower impact on the outcome of the disease than medical treatment. In these cases, patients can decide for themselves, based on symptom control, how diligent they should be.

Short-Term Medical Treatment
Simple lifestyle modifications, antacids and alginic acid provide symptomatic relief in mild nonerosive esophagitis. Prokinetic drugs, either alone or in

combination with antisecretory drugs, are only moderately effective in GERD and require prolonged use before any benefit is seen. To date, no randomized and controlled clinical trials have evaluated the role of these drugs in the treatment of GERD in the elderly. Possible side effects of antacids include salt overload, constipation, hypercalcemia and interference with absorption of other drugs, particularly antibiotics such as tetracycline, azithromycin and quinolones. The prokinetic metoclopramide, a dopamine antagonist, may induce extrapyramidal effects, while cisapride has been retired from the market in the United States and Europe due to the appearance of ventricular arrhythmias, especially in patients who were taking cytochrome P4503A-metabolized drugs, such as ketoconazole or itraconazole and macrolides. In fact, these latter drugs may interfere with the metabolism of cisapride and may promote highly toxic blood levels [38]. For all these reasons, there are no evidence-based data to recommend the use of these drugs for the treatment of GERD in old age.

Antireflux therapy is focused largely on suppressing gastric acid secretion with H_2 blockers and PPIs. A retrospective analysis of two multicenter, randomized, double-blind clinical trials demonstrated no significant differences in healing rates of esophagitis between young and elderly patients. After 4 and 8 weeks of treatment, the PPI once daily, was more effective than the H_2 blockers twice daily [39]. These findings were confirmed in a meta-analysis of 43 articles including 7,635 patients aged 18–89 years (mean age 51 years) with grade 2–4 esophagitis treated for ≤ 12 weeks. The healing rate was found to be highest with PPIs ($83.6 \pm 11.4\%$) versus H_2 blockers ($51.9 \pm 17.1\%$), sucralfate ($39.2 \pm 22.4\%$) or placebo ($28.2 \pm 15.6\%$). Moreover, PPIs provided faster and more complete heartburn relief than H_2 blockers [40].

A study carried out in elderly patients with esophagitis confirmed that a 2-month therapy with omeprazole, lansoprazole or pantoprazole was highly effective in curing esophagitis and improving symptomatology in elderly patients without significant side effects and with excellent compliance [41]. More recently, a multicenter study reported excellent healing rates of esophagitis (94.5 and 82.5% by intention-to-treat and per protocol analyses, respectively) after a 2-month treatment with pantoprazole 40 mg daily in 167 elderly patients aged 65 years and over [42]. Healing rates were irrespective of the presence of concomitant diseases (76.2% of patients) or concomitant treatments (65.2% of patients). Moreover, out of the 22 patients who dropped out of the study, only 3 patients discontinued due to side effects (1 patient) or low compliance (2 patients).

These findings are in agreement with pharmacokinetic studies that reported pantoprazole to be associated with both a low percentage of drug interactions (table 2) and a minimal effect of age on its disposition [43]. In contrast, aging may influence oral bioavailability and renal clearance of omeprazole, and

Table 2. Drug interactions between PPIs and other drugs in humans (modified from Klotz [43])

Drug	Mechanism	Omeprazole	Lansoprazole	Pantoprazole	Rabeprazole
Digoxin	absorption	↑AUC	?	NO	↑AUC
Theophylline	CP4501A2	(↑CL)	(↑CL)	NO	NO
Warfarin®	CP4502C19	↓CL	NO	NO	NO
Nifedipine	CP4503A4	↓CL	?	NO	?
Carbamazepine	CP4503A4	↓CL	?	NO	?
Diazepam	CP4502C19	↓CL	NO	NO	NO
Phenytoin	CP4502C9	↓CL	NO	NO	NO
Ketoconazole	absorption	↓AUC	?	?	↓AUC
Metoprolol	CP4502D6	NO	?	NO	?
Alcohol	ADH + CP450	NO	?	NO	?
Oral contraceptives	CP4503A	?	NO	NO	?
Antipyrine	liver function	↓CL	(↑CL)	NO	?
Cyclosporin	CP4503A4	NO	?	NO	?

AUC = Area under the concentration-time curve; CP450 = cytochrome P450; CL = clearance; ADH = alcohol dehydrogenase; ↑ = increase; ↓ = decrease; NO = no significant interaction; ? = data not available; ( ) = data equivocal.

the elimination half-time and area under the concentration-time curve values for lansoprazole and rabeprazole [44]. Very recently, a pharmacokinetic study of esomeprazole, the newly developed S-isomer of omeprazole, carried out in 14 healthy elderly volunteers suggested that dosage adjustment should not be necessary in the elderly [45]. However, until now, no clinical experience has been reported with this PPI in elderly patients with GERD. Thus pantoprazole is the treatment of choice especially for elderly patients with comorbidities and comedications.

Long-Term Medical Treatment

GERD is a chronic relapsing condition and most patients require long-term management to control symptoms and maintain esophageal healing. The results of randomized clinical trials have documented that, after healing of esophagitis, 80–90% of patients treated with placebo or not treated at all may relapse during the following 6–12 months [46]. Furthermore, one long-term follow-up of GERD patients reported that 24–75% of patients were still under antisecretory treatment 3–10 years after diagnosis of esophagitis [47]. A recent study [48] reported that 68% of 138 acutely treated and healed patients with reflux esophagitis over 65 years of age were still in need of maintenance therapy after

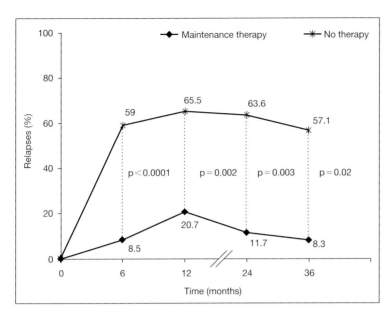

Fig. 2. Esophagitis relapse rates in elderly untreated patients compared to those in maintenance antisecretory therapy after 6 months to 3 years of follow-up (modified from Pilotto et al. [48]).

6 months, while 46% needed therapy after 3 years of follow-up. The same study reported that esophagitis relapse rates were significantly higher in untreated patients compared to those in maintenance antisecretory therapy after 6 months (59 vs. 8.5%, $p < 0.0001$), 1 year (65.5 vs. 20.7%, $p < 0.002$) and 3 years (57.1 vs. 8.3%, $p < 0.05$) (fig. 2). In this elderly population, the most effective measure for minimizing the occurrence of relapse was maintenance therapy with antisecretory drugs ($p < 0.00001$). Significant risk factors for relapse of esophagitis were the presence of typical symptoms ($p = 0.00001$), the presence of hiatus hernia ($p = 0.03$) and a high grade of severity of esophagitis at baseline ($p = 0.009$) [48]. These data were in agreement with the results of studies carried out in young or adult GERD patients [46, 47].

A great number of studies have shown higher efficacy of PPIs over H_2 blockers and prokinetics in maintaining healed esophagitis. Continuous therapy for 1 year with omeprazole at a dose of 20 mg daily was associated with an 80% healing rate [49]. Excellent healing rates were also observed after 1 year of treatment with rabeprazole 20 mg daily (86% healing rate) [50], lansoprazole 30 mg daily (80–90% healing rate) [51] and pantoprazole 20 mg daily (77–90% healing rate) [52].

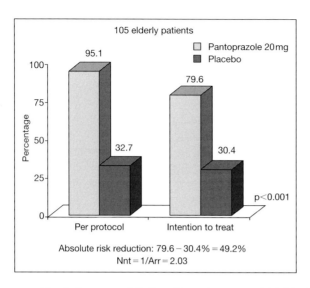

Fig. 3. Per protocol (left) and intention to treat (right) healing rates of esophagitis after 12 months of treatment with pantoprazole 20 mg daily or placebo in elderly subjects with esophagitis (modified from Pilotto et al. [56]). Nnt = Number needed to treat; Arr = absolute risk reduction.

In nonelderly populations, the use of low-dose PPIs is associated with a lower efficacy than standard-dose PPIs. A meta-analysis of five trials with omeprazole showed that omeprazole 20 mg daily maintained 82% of patients in remission over a 6-month period compared to 72% with omeprazole 10 mg daily and 43% with omeprazole 20 mg once daily for 3 days a week (on the weekend) [46]. A 6-month treatment with esomeprazole, the S-isomer of omeprazole, at the dosages of 40, 20 and 10 mg daily, maintained remission in 88, 79 and 54% of patients, respectively [53]. Treatment with pantoprazole 20 mg daily for 6 months maintained 84% of patients in remission compared to 93% with pantoprazole 40 mg daily [54], while after 1 year of treatment with lansoprazole, the healing rates were 72% with 15 mg daily versus 85% with 30 mg daily [55].

Unfortunately, long-term controlled clinical studies carried out in elderly populations are very scarce. Very recently, a double-blind, placebo-controlled study was carried out in elderly patients with esophagitis aged 65 years and over [56]. After 12 months of treatment with pantoprazole 20 mg daily, the per protocol and intention-to-treat healing rates of esophagitis were, respectively, 95% [95% confidence interval (CI) 88.5–100%] and 80% (95% CI 68.3–90.9%) in the treatment group versus 33% (95% CI 19.9–45.4%) and 30% (95% CI 18.3–42.4%) in the placebo group (fig. 3). The 'absolute risk reduction' of relapse with pantoprazole 20 mg daily versus placebo was 49.2%. Two patients required treatment to decrease esophagitis relapses by one (number needed to treat = 2.03). These findings are in agreement with previous data indicating that elderly patients had higher healing rates of esophagitis than adult or young patients during maintenance therapy with PPIs [46]. Moreover, pantoprazole at the low dose of 20 mg maintained the largest percentage of elderly patients with esophagitis (95% by per protocol analysis) in long-term remission. This is in agreement with the recent report of a comparable clinical efficacy of 20 mg of pantoprazole and 20 mg of omeprazole in patients with grade 1 reflux esophagitis [57].

Treatment of GERD and Quality of Life

Quality of life is an important therapeutic parameter in patients with GERD. Several studies have reported that treatment with PPIs caused a significant improvement not just in reflux symptoms, but in several physical and mental aspects of quality of life, regardless of whether or not the esophagitis was healed [58]. Indeed, PPI treatment may significantly improve quality of life in patients with GERD symptoms but without esophagitis [59]. Evaluating quality of life is a difficult task in old age, principally due to the variability of the physical, psychological and social conditions that determine the overall well-being of the elderly subject. Very recently, a study was carried out in elderly subjects with esophagitis with the aim of evaluating the effect of PPI treatment on both GERD symptoms and depression state [60]. The patients were initially treated with pantoprazole 40 mg a day for 2 months. Those patients with healed esophagitis were included in maintenance treatment with pantoprazole 20 mg a day for 6 months. As expected, the PPI treatment significantly reduced GERD symptoms (acid regurgitation, dysphagia, heartburn, chest pain and epigastric pain). Moreover, the treatment induced a significant improvement in the mental depression score (evaluated by the Zung Self Depression Scale) after both 2 months (37.2 ± 7.9 vs. 34.8 ± 8.3, $p = 0.008$) and 6 months of therapy (33.2 ± 9.5, $p < 0.0001$) [60]. Further studies need to evaluate the role of antisecretory treatment in other aspects of the quality of life in elderly people.

Safety of Long-Term Medical Treatment

Because of their profound acid inhibition, there has been concern about the long-term safety of PPIs. Recent studies suggest that this fear may be unjustified. A study of long-term omeprazole treatment (up to 11 years) of 230 patients with refractory reflux esophagitis (mean age 63 years, 36% were over 70 years) reported that the annual incidence of gastric corpus mucosal atrophy was 4.7 and 0.7% in *H. pylori*-positive and -negative patients, respectively. This was primarily observed in elderly patients who had moderate or severe gastritis at entry into the study. Corpus intestinal metaplasia was rare and no dysplasia or neoplasms were observed [61]. More recently, a study carried out in 150 patients aged

19–78 years and refractory to H_2 blockers reported that maintenance treatment with pantoprazole 40 mg daily for 3 years was associated with a modest elevation in serum gastrin and no significant changes in gastric endocrine cells, while the number of enterochromaffin-like cells tended to decrease [62]. As regards the effect of gastric acid inhibition on absorption and digestion, current evidence suggests that long-term PPI treatment does not significantly modify protein and carbohydrate digestion nor iron and calcium absorption [29]. However, because the clinical effect of long-term PPI therapy on vitamin B_{12} absorption is controversial [63], it may be prudent to periodically monitor vitamin B_{12} levels in elderly patients receiving long-term PPI therapy, especially in frail patients or those with poor diets.

The Role of Surgery

The role of surgery in the treatment of GERD is controversial. While medical treatment is successful in patients with mild to moderate disease, the threshold of severity above which an operation should be considered remains a matter of debate. Laparoscopic fundoplication has greatly reduced the morbidity and mortality of antireflux surgery, also in the elderly [64]. Thus, the indications for surgery seem to be evolving. Traditionally, surgery has been advocated for patients who are medical treatment failures, patients with severe aspiration, dysphagia or pulmonary symptoms or patients who did not want or could not afford long-term medical therapy. However, recently it has been suggested that the elderly patient should not be refused curative antireflux surgery solely on the basis of age [29]. Indeed, analysis of data from 35,735 patients with erosive esophagitis extracted from the database of the US Department of Veterans Affairs suggests that fundoplication improved the clinical outcome of erosive esophagitis with concomitant esophageal ulcers or strictures, but did not improve the outcome of patients without such complications. Furthermore, fundoplication did not reduce the consumption of health care resources [65]. Similar efficacy between antireflux surgery and omeprazole treatment (if the dose of the PPI was adjusted in the case of relapse) has also been reported in Europe [66]. Moreover, because it has been shown that greater experience of the surgical team significantly improves the long-term results of surgery [67], it is possible that the results obtained in specialized units may be superior to those in other clinical series [68].

In conclusion, randomized clinical studies are needed to compare the outcome of antireflux surgery with that of medical therapy in the elderly. Evidence suggests that surgery may be indicated in elderly patients who (1) are medical treatment failures (with full-dose effective drugs), (2) have severe complications, i.e. strictures not treatable by endoscopy, (3) have severe dysphagia, aspiration or atypical symptoms, such as noncardiac chest pain or respiratory symptoms, (4) have an associated large hiatal hernia, and/or (5) have preneo-plastic lesions analogous to Barrett's esophagus. Furthermore, especially for the elderly patient, surgery for GERD should be centralized to units specialized in these techniques.

Long-Term Treatment Strategies and Costs

There is still some disagreement regarding the most appropriate long-term treatment strategy. A cost-utility analysis comparing laparoscopic Nissen fundo-plication versus omeprazole demonstrated that medical therapy was the preferred treatment strategy for most patients with severe erosive esophagitis, particularly elderly subjects [69]. As regards medical treatment of GERD, there are two main clinical strategies. The step-up approach starts with low acid inhibition (antacids, prokinetics or H_2 blockers) and switches to more effective drugs (PPIs) until adequate symptom control is obtained. In contrast, the step-down approach involves the use of PPIs first, eventually switching to less effective drugs if patients have no symptomatic or endoscopic relapse. An economic analysis from the United States suggests that a step-wise utilization of increasingly more potent and more expensive medications to treat GERD would result in appreciable cost savings [70]. Indeed, the step-up strategy was the most commonly used for elderly patients with GERD by primary care physicians from Alabama, USA [71]. In contrast, two economic analyses from Europe (UK and Sweden) suggested that the step-down approach was probably more cost effective [72, 73]. A very recent analysis of alternative management strategies for GERD reported that initial PPI therapy followed by a step-down approach may result in improved symptom relief and quality of life over 1 year of follow-up, with more appropriate utilization of invasive diagnostic testing with a small marginal increase in total costs [74]. These findings warrant prospective trials comparing these two strategies in elderly patients with GERD. Nevertheless, since in the geriatric patient GERD symptoms are an unreliable index of clinical outcome, the disease is more severe than in adult or young patients and the response to medical treatment is excellent, a step-down strategy may be more appropriate in elderly patients with GERD.

References

1   Mold JW, Reed LE, Davis AB, Allen ML, Decktor DL, Robinson M: Prevalence of gastro-esophageal reflux in elderly patients in a primary care setting. Am J Gastroenterol 1991;86: 965–970.
2   Kennedy T, Jones R: The prevalence of gastro-oesophageal reflux symptoms in a UK population and the consultation behaviour of patients with these symptoms. Aliment Pharmacol Ther 2000; 14:1589–1594.

3   El-Serag H, Sonnenberg A: Associations between different forms of gastro-oesophageal reflux disease. Gut 1997;41:594–599.

4   Xie P, Ren J, Bardan E, Mittal RK, Sui Z, Shaker R: Frequency of gastroesophageal reflux events induced by pharyngeal water stimulation in young and elderly subjects. Am J Physiol 1997;272: G233–G237.

5   Ren J, Shaker R, Kusano M, Podvrsan B, Metwally N, Dua KS, Sui Z: Effect of aging on the secondary esophageal peristalsis: Presbyesophagus revisited. Am J Physiol 1995;268: G772–G779.

6   Grishaw EK, Ott DJ, Frederick MG, Gelfand DW, Chen MY: Functional abnormalities of the esophagus: A prospective analysis of radiographic findings relative to age and symptoms. AJR Am J Roentgenol 1996;167:719–723.

7   Nishimura N, Hongo M, Yamada M, Kawakami H, Ueno M, Okuno Y, Toyota T: Effect of aging on the esophageal motor functions. J Smooth Muscle Res 1996;32:43–50.

8   Grande L, Lacima G, Ros E, Pera M, Ascaso C, Visa J, Pera C: Deterioration of esophageal motility with age: A manometric study of 79 healthy subjects. Am J Gastroenterol 1999;94: 1795–1801.

9   Ferriolli E, Dantas RO, Oliveira RB, Braga FJ: The influence of ageing on oesophageal motility after ingestion of liquids with different viscosities. Eur J Gastroenterol Hepatol 1996;8:793–798.

10 Ferriolli E, Oliveira RB, Matsuda NM, Braga FJ, Dantas RO: Aging, esophageal motility, and gastroesophageal reflux. J Am Geriatr Soc 1998;46:1534–1537.

11 Eckardt VF, Le Compte PM: Esophageal ganglia and smooth muscle in the elderly. Dig Dis Sci 1978;23:849–856.

12 Meciano-Filho J, Carvalho VC, De Souza RR: Nerve cell loss in the myenteric plexus of the human esophagus in relation to age: A preliminary investigation. Gerontology 1995;41:18–21.

13 Tack J, Van Trappen G: The aging esophagus. Gut 1997;41:422–424.

14 Pilotto A, Vianello F, Di Mario F, Plebani M, Farinati F, Azzini CF: Effect of age on gastric acid, pepsin, pepsinogen group A and gastrin in peptic ulcer patients. Gerontology 1994;40:253–259.

15 Haruma K, Kamada T, Kawaguchi H, Okamoto S, Yoshihara M, Sumii K, Inoue M, Kishimoto S, Kajiyama G, Miyoshi A: Effect of age and *Helicobacter pylori* infection on gastric acid secretion. J Gastroenterol Hepatol 2000;15:277–283.

16 Amano K, Adachi K, Katsube T, Watanabe M, Kinoshita Y: Role of hiatus hernia and gastric mucosal atrophy in the development of reflux esophagitis in the elderly. J Gastroenterol Hepatol 2001;16:132–136.

17 Cameron AJ: Barrett's esophagus: Prevalence and size of hiatal hernia. Am J Gastroenterol 1999; 94:2054–2059.

18 Perkins AC, Wilson CG, Blackshaw PE, Vincent RM, Dansereau RJ, Juhlin KD, Bekker PJ, Spiller RC: Impaired oesophageal transit of capsule versus tablet formulations in the elderly. Gut 1994;35:1363–1367.

19 Denman SJ: Esophagitis associated with the use of alendronate. J Am Geriatr Soc 1997;45:662.

20 Avidan B, Sonnenberg A, Schnell TG, Sontag SJ: Risk factors for erosive esophagitis: A case-control study. Am J Gastroenterol 2001;96:41–46.

21 Raiha I, Hietanen E, Sourander L: Symptoms of gastro-oesophageal reflux disease in elderly people. Age Ageing 1991;20:365–370.

22 Raiha I, Ivaska K, Sourander L: Pulmonary function in gastro-oesophageal reflux disease of elderly people. Age Ageing 1992;21:368–373.

23 Franceschi M, Leandro G, Novello R, et al: Elderly subjects with esophagitis have different symptomatology and more severe disease than adult and young patients. Gut 2001;49(suppl 3): A2335.

24 Zimmerman J, Shohat V, Tsvang E, Arnon R, Safadi R, Wengrower D: Esophagitis is a major cause of upper gastrointestinal hemorrhage in the elderly. Scand J Gastroenterol 1997;32:906–909.

25 Maekawa T, Kinoshita Y, Okada A, Fukui H, Waki S, Hassan S, Matsushima Y, Kawanami C, Kishi K, Chiba T: Relationship between severity and symptoms of reflux oesophagitis in elderly patients in Japan. J Gastroenterol Hepatol 1998;13:927–930.

26 Lasch H, Castell DO, Castell JA: Evidence for diminished visceral pain with aging: Studies using graded intraesophageal balloon distension. Am J Physiol 1997;272:G1–G3.

27 Fass R, Pulliam G, Johnson C, Garewal HS, Sampliner RE: Symptom severity and oesophageal chemosensitivity to acid in older and young patients with gastro-oesophageal reflux. Age Ageing 2000;29:125–130.

28 Collen MJ, Abdullian JD, Chen YK: Gastroesophageal reflux disease in the elderly: More severe disease that requires aggressive therapy. Am J Gastroenterol 1995;90:1053–1057.

29 Richter JE: Gastroesophageal reflux disease in the older patient: Presentation, treatment and complications. Am J Gastroenterol 2000;95:368–373.

30 Ekberg O, Feinberg MJ: Altered swallowing function in elderly patients without dysphagia: Radiologic findings in 56 cases. Am J Roentgenol 1991;156:1181–1184.

31 Fass R, Sampliner RE, Mackel C, McGee D, Rappaport W: Age- and gender-related differences in 24-hour esophageal pH monitoring of normal subjects. Dig Dis Sci 1993;38:1926–1928.

32 Schenk BE, Kuipers EJ, Klinkenberg-Knol EC, Festen HP, Jansen EH, Tuynman HA, Schrijver M, Dieleman LA, Meuwissen SG: Omeprazole as a diagnostic tool in gastroesophageal reflux disease. Am J Gastroenterol 1997;92:1997–2000.

33 Fass R, Fennerty MB, Ofman JJ, Gralnek IM, Johnson C, Camargo E, Sampliner RE: The clinical and economic value of a short course of omeprazole in patients with noncardiac chest pain. Gastroenterology 1998;115:42–49.

34 Fass R, Ofman JJ, Sampliner RE, Camargo L, Wendel C, Fennerty MB: The omeprazole test is as sensitive as 24-h oesophageal pH monitoring in diagnosing gastro-oesophageal reflux disease in symptomatic patients with erosive oesophagitis. Aliment Pharmacol Ther 2000;14:389–396.

35 Pilotto A, Franceschi M, Costa MC, Di Mario F, Valerio G: Helicobacter pylori test and eradication strategy. Lancet 2000;356:1683–1684.

36 Hamilton JW, Boisen RJ, Yamamoto DT, Wagner JL, Reichelderfer M: Sleeping on a wedge diminishes exposure of the esophagus to refluxed acid. Dig Dis Sci 1988;31:581–586.

37 Avidan B, Sonnenberg A, Schnell TG, Sontag SJ: Walking and chewing reduce postprandial acid reflux. Aliment Pharmacol Ther 2001;15:151–155.

38 Flockhart DA, Desta Z, Mahal SK: Selection of drugs to treat gastro-oesophageal reflux disease: The role of drug interactions. Clin Pharmacokinet 2000;39:295–309.

39 James OFW, Parry-Billings KS: Comparison of omeprazole and histamine H2-receptor antagonists in the treatment of elderly and young patients with reflux oesophagitis. Age Ageing 1994;23:121–126.

40 Chiba N, De Gara CJ, Wilkinson JM, Hunt RH: Speed of healing and symptom relief in grade II to IV gastroesophageal reflux disease: A meta-analysis. Gastroenterology 1997;112:1798–1810.

41 Pilotto A, Franceschi M, Leandro G, Di Mario F, Valerio G: Comparison of omeprazole, lansoprazole and pantoprazole in the treatment of elderly patients with esophagitis. Gastroenterology 1999;116(suppl):A283.

42 Pilotto A on behalf of the Aging and Acid-Related Diseases Study Group: Efficacy of pantoprazole in the short and long-term treatment of elderly patients with esophagitis: A multicenter study. Gut 2001;49(suppl 3):A2217.

43 Klotz U: Pharmacokinetic considerations in the eradication of Helicobacter pylori. Clin Pharmacokinet 2000;38:243–270.

44 Laurent AL, Merritt GJ, Setoyama T, et al: Rabeprazole: Pharmacokinetics and safety in the elderly. Clin Geriatr 1999;7:27–33.

45 Hasselgren G, Hassan-Alin M, Andersson T, Claar-Nilsson C, Rohss K: Pharmacokinetic study of esomeprazole in the elderly. Clin Pharmacokinet 2001;40:145–150.

46 Carlsson R, Galmiche JP, Dent J, Lundell L, Frison L: Prognostic factors influencing relapse of oesophagitis during maintenance therapy with antisecretory drugs: A meta-analysis of long-term omeprazole trials. Aliment Pharmacol Ther 1997;11:473–482.

47 McDougall NI, Johnston BT, Kee F, Collins JS, McFarland RJ, Love AH: Natural history of reflux oesophagitis: A 10 year follow-up of its effect on patient symptomatology and quality of life. Gut 1996;38:481–486.

48 Pilotto A, Franceschi M, Leandro G, Novello R, Di Mario F, Valerio G: Long-term clinical outcome of elderly patients with reflux esophagitis: A six-month to three-year follow-up study. Am J Ther 2002;9:295–300.

49   Vigneri S, Termini R, Leandro G, Badalamenti S, Pantalena M, Savarino V, Di Mario F, Battaglia G, Mela GS, Pilotto A, Plebani M, Davi G: A comparison of five maintenance therapies for reflux esophagitis. N Engl J Med 1995;333:1106–1110.
50   Birbara C, Breiter J, Perdomo C, Hahne W: Rabeprazole for the prevention of recurrent erosive or ulcerative gastro-oesophageal reflux disease. Eur J Gastroenterol Hepatol 2000;12:889–897.
51   Robinson M, Lanza F, Avner D, Haber M: Effective maintenance treatment of reflux erosive esophagitis with low-dose lansoprazole: A randomized, double-blind, placebo-controlled trial. Ann Intern Med 1996;124:859–867.
52   Lauritsen K, Jaup B, Carling L, Raptis S, Aadland E, Färkkilä M, Elawant A, Krejs G, Altorfer J: Comparable efficacy of pantoprazole and omeprazole to prevent relapse in patients with GERD. Gut 2000;47(suppl 3):A60.
53   Vakil NB, Shaker R, Johnson DA, Kovacs T, Baerg RD, Hwang C, D'Amico D, Hamelin B: The new proton pump inhibitor esomeprazole is effective as a maintenance therapy in GERD patients with healed erosive oesophagitis: A 6-month, randomized, double-blind, placebo-controlled study of efficacy and safety. Aliment Pharmacol Ther 2001;15:927–935.
54   Escourrou J, Deprez P, Saggioro A, Geldof H, Fischer R, Maier C: Maintenance therapy with pantoprazole 20 mg prevents relapse of reflux oesophagitis. Aliment Pharmacol Ther 1999;13:1482–1491.
55   Hatlebakk JG, Berstad A: Lansoprazole 15 and 30 mg daily in maintaining healing and symptom relief in patients with reflux oesophagitis. Aliment Pharmacol Ther 1997;11:365–372.
56   Pilotto A on behalf of the Aging and Acid-Related Diseases Study Group: Maintenance therapy of reflux esophagitis with pantoprazole 20 mg daily in elderly patients: A double-blind, placebo-controlled study. Dig Liver Dis 2002;34(suppl 1):A7.
57   Bardhan KD, Van Rensburg C: Comparable clinical efficacy and tolerability of 20 mg pantoprazole and 20 mg omeprazole in patients with grade I reflux oesophagitis. Aliment Pharmacol Ther 2001;15:1585–1591.
58   McDougall NI, Collins JS, McFarland RJ, Watson RG, Love AH: The effect of treating reflux oesophagitis with omeprazole on quality of life. Eur J Gastroenterol Hepatol 1998;10:459–464.
59   Havelund T, Lind T, Wiklund I, Glise H, Hernqvist H, Lauritsen K, Lundell L, Pedersen SA, Carlsson R, Junghard O, Stubberod A, Anker-Hansen O: Quality of life in patients with heartburn but without esophagitis: Effects of treatment with omeprazole. Am J Gastroenterol 1999;94:1782–1789.
60   Pilotto A on behalf of the Aging and Acid-Related Diseases Study Group: The cure of esophagitis improves gastrointestinal symptoms and depression state in elderly patients. Gut 2001;49(suppl 3):A2707.
61   Klinkenberg-Knol EC, Nelis F, Dent J, Snel P, Mitchell B, Prichard P, Lloyd D, Havu N, Frame MH, Roman J, Walan A, Group LT: Long-term omeprazole treatment in resistant gastroesophageal reflux disease: Efficacy, safety, and influence on gastric mucosa. Gastroenterology 2000;118:661–669.
62   Bardhan KD, Cherian P, Bishop AE, Polak JM, Romanska H, Perry MJ, Rowland A, Thompson M, Morris P, Schneider A, Fischer R, Ng W, Luhmann R, McCaldin B: Pantoprazole therapy in the long-term management of severe acid peptic disease. Clinical efficacy, safety, serum gastrin, gastric histology and endocrine cell studies. Am J Gastroenterol 2001;96:1767–1776.
63   Marcuard SP, Albernaz L, Khazamie PG: Omeprazole therapy causes malabsorption of cyanocobalamin (vitamin B12). Ann Intern Med 1994;12:211–215.
64   Trus TL, Laycock WS, Wo JM, Waring JP, Branum GD, Mauren SJ, Katz EM, Hunter JG: Laparoscopic antireflux surgery in the elderly. Am J Gastroenterol 1998;93:351–353.
65   El-Serag HB, Sonnenberg A: Outcome of erosive reflux esophagitis after Nissen fundoplication. Am J Gastroenterol 1999;94:1771–1776.
66   Lundell L, Miettinen P, Myrvold HE, Pedersen SA, Liedman B, Hatlebakk JG, Julkonen R, Levander K, Carlsson J, Lamm M, Wiklund I: Continued (5-year) followup of a randomized clinical study comparing antireflux surgery and omeprazole in gastroesophageal reflux disease. J Am Coll Surg 2001;192:172–181.
67   Luostarinen ME, Isolauri JO: Surgical experience improves the long-term results of Nissen fundoplication. Scand J Gastroenterol 1999;34:117–120.

68   Rantanen TK, Halme TV, Luostarinen ME, Karhumaki LM, Kononen EO, Isolauri JO: The long term results of open antireflux surgery in a community-based health care center. Am J Gastroenterol 1999;94:1777–1781.

69   Heudebert GR, Marks R, Wilcox CM, Centor RM: Choice of long-term strategy for the management of patients with severe esophagitis: A cost-utility analysis. Gastroenterology 1997;112:1078–1086.

70   Sonnenberg A, Inadomi JM, Becker LA: Economic analysis of step-wise treatment of gastro-oesophageal reflux disease. Aliment Pharmacol Ther 1999;13:1003–1013.

71   Wilcox CM, Heudebert G, Klapow J, Shewchuk R, Casebeer L: Survey of primary care physicians' approach to gastroesophageal reflux disease in elderly patients. J Gerontol A Biol Sci Med Sci 2001;56:M514–M517.

72   Bate CM, Richardson PDI: A one year model for the cost-effectiveness of treating reflux oesophagitis. Br J Med Econ 1992;2:5–12.

73   Jonsson B, Stalhammar NO: The cost effectiveness of omeprazole and ranitidine in intermittent and maintenance treatment of reflux oesophagitis: The case of Sweden. Br J Med Econ 1993;6: 111–119.

74   Ofman JJ, Dorn GH, Fennerty MB, Fass R: The clinical and economic impact of competing management strategies for gastro-oesophageal reflux disease. Aliment Pharmacol Ther 2002; 16:261–273.

Alberto Pilotto, Unità Operativa di Geriatria,
Ospedale 'Casa Sollievo della Sofferenza', IRCCS, I–71013 San Giovanni Rotondo (FG) (Italy)
Tel. +39 0882 410271, E-Mail alberto.pilotto@libero.it

Pilotto A, Malfertheiner P, Holt PR (eds): Aging and the Gastrointestinal Tract.
Interdiscipl Top Gerontol. Basel, Karger, 2003, vol 32, pp 118–127

....

Non-Steroidal Anti-Inflammatory Drug-Related Gastroduodenal Damage in the Elderly

Francesco Di Mario, Giulia Martina Cavestro,
Anna Virginia Ingegnoli

Gastroenterology Department, University of Parma, Parma, Italy

Epidemiology of Non-Steroidal Anti-Inflammatory Drug Consumption in the Elderly

The linear increase in life expectancy observed in the last century and the discovery that more than 70% of subjects over 65 years of age suffer from rheumatic diseases certainly account at least in part for the epidemiological and clinical importance of non-steroidal anti-inflammatory drug (NSAID) therapy in old age. Similarly, it is well known that NSAID prescriptions increase with age and that self-prescription of NSAIDs is widely practised in elderly populations. In 1995, the total number of prescriptions per year was approximately 485 million, and it was calculated that more than 30 million people took NSAIDs daily; over 40% of these patients were over 65 years of age.

Several epidemiological studies have reported that serious complications associated with the use of NSAIDs may occur, especially in the elderly [1]. In the USA, 103,000 hospitalizations occur each year, with approximately 16,000 deaths related to adverse events associated with NSAID use [2]. Approximately 34–46% of patients on NSAID therapy are expected to have some manifestation of adverse gastrointestinal events, and the overall risk of developing a serious gastrointestinal complication is three times greater in NSAID users than non-users [3]. A recent study of over 3,000 elderly subjects in Italy reported that 96.4% of subjects over 65 years old were taking drugs and 30.4% were taking an NSAID [4].

Several epidemiological studies have demonstrated that aging is an independent risk factor for severe gastroduodenal injuries. This risk tends to

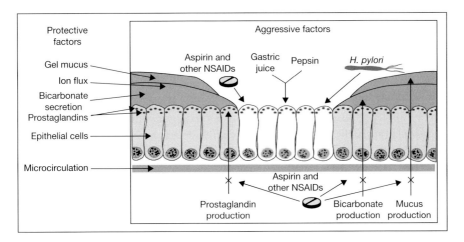

Fig. 1. NSAIDs and gastroduodenal damage.

increase linearly with aging and becomes particularly high in the presence of disability [5], co-morbidity (congestive heart failure, hypertension, renal or hepatic insufficiency and volume depletion) [2], co-medication and concomitant intake of corticosteroids [6], anticoagulants [7] or other NSAIDs, especially at high dosages. Furthermore, the risk of damage is high when a history of ulcer is present, as well as gastroduodenal symptoms, previous haemorrhagic events or anti-ulcer drug use [2]. Interestingly, associations with education level, smoking habit, alcohol consumption and *Helicobacter pylori* infection are still uncertain [2].

Mechanisms of NSAID-Related Gastrointestinal Damage

Gastrointestinal damage associated with NSAID use has been recognized as the most damaging of side effects from any class of therapeutic agents [8]. The most frequent adverse event is peptic ulcer and its complications, i.e. haemorrhage and perforation. Other side effects, including epithelial damage in the small intestine, large bowel haemorrhage and acute liver failure, are also common, but occur with lower incidence and severity. NSAID-related gastroduodenal damage results from a critical disequilibrium between protective and aggressive factors in the gastric and duodenal mucosa (fig. 1). The gastroduodenal mucosa functions as a barrier maintaining tissue integrity, the protective apparatus of which could be classified as pre-epithelial, epithelial and post-epithelial [9].

The first level of protection is offered by the mucus layers, bicarbonate secretion and phospholipids present on the luminal surface of the epithelium. The second line of protection is constituted by the epithelial cells, which are able to maintain an electrical resistance that prevents the back-diffusion of hydrogen ion into the mucosa from the gastric lumen. The third protective mechanism is the capacity of mucosal cells to rapidly migrate to the affected site, promptly restoring the potentially damaged epithelium. This mechanism is dependent on mucosal blood flow, while all three mechanisms are dependent on prostaglandin concentrations in the mucosa.

Two distinct processes have been described for acute and chronic NSAID injury. The first mechanism, commencing within 90 min of ingestion, is a direct effect and is dependent on gastric acid secretion. In fact, in the presence of high gastric acid content, the non-ionized lipophilic NSAIDs may diffuse into epithelial cells, where they are converted into their ionized form, trapping H^+ ions within the cells. This toxic event leads to alterations in the membrane's permeability, reduction of the hydrophobicity of the gastric mucosa, hydrogen ion back-diffusion, inhibition of oxidative phosphorylation and reduction of cell turnover. These local events may induce superficial, acute injury, such as gastric erosions. A recent study demonstrated that the progression from erosion to ulcer is mediated by acid, supporting the hypothesis that NSAID-related acute and occasional damage is caused principally by a high acid environment [10].

The chronic mechanism of NSAID injury consists mainly in the inhibition of prostaglandin synthesis, subsequently leading to alterations in the mucous barrier and possibly ulcer [11]. The cytoprotective action of prostaglandins is mediated mainly by endogenous prostacyclin and prostaglandin E_2, which act by preventing gastric erosions and ulceration. Prostaglandins act by reducing gastric acid secretion and exerting a direct vasodilatory action on the vessels of the gastric mucosa. They are also known to stimulate mucus secretion, gastric fluids and duodenal bicarbonate ions. Some data suggest that prostaglandin physiology may change with age.

Prostaglandins are synthesized through the activity of the cyclooxygenase (COX) enzyme. It has recently been demonstrated that COX exists in at least two isoforms: COX-1 and COX-2. These two isoforms can be distinguished as constitutive (COX-1) and inducible (COX-2), and are encoded by different genes. COX-1 is found under basal conditions in most cells/tissues, including platelets, gastric mucosa and the kidney. COX-1-derived prostanoids regulate platelet aggregation, the integrity and function of the gut and the kidney mucosa. In contrast, COX-2 is not usually present in cells under basal conditions, but its expression is induced during inflammatory processes that involve various cell types such as monocytes, fibroblasts and synovial cells. All NSAIDs act by inhibiting COX enzymes, accounting for both their therapeutic and toxic effects. Recent drugs showing a high potency against COX-2 and a low COX-2/COX-1 activity ratio seem to exert a powerful anti-inflammatory activity with potentially few side effects on both the stomach and kidney [12].

Under NSAID therapy, the gastric mucosa develops the so-called phenomenon of 'gastric adaption'. Indeed, the probability that a gastroduodenal lesion will occur is higher in the first 3 months of treatment, with a peak in the first 3–4 weeks. This has been attributed to the cells' capacity for quick repair under the influence of epidermal growth factor and nitric oxide.

Clinical Aspects of NSAID-Related Gastroduodenal Damage

Nearly 10–20% of patients taking NSAIDs present symptoms related to the first digestive tract [13]. Nevertheless, these symptoms do not always correlate with endoscopic evidence of gastric or duodenal damage, and 40% of patients, in particular the elderly, affected by NSAID-related erosive gastritis have been reported to be asymptomatic [14]. One study reported that only 17% of patients over 65 years of age and affected by an NSAID-related peptic ulcer presented with dyspeptic symptoms, while 65% of patients with peptic ulcers unrelated to NSAID use presented with dyspepsia [15].

In one study of 128 elderly symptomatic patients taking NSAIDs and who had undergone an endoscopic examination [16], epigastric pain was reported by 50% of patients, and a relevant number of patients had anaemia (30%), melaena (17%), vomiting (12%) and anorexia or weight loss (6.2%). Overall, 83% of patients showed endoscopic lesions of the upper gastrointestinal tract and almost 39% of these were haemorrhagic lesions [16]. These findings confirm that in the elderly, the clinical picture of NSAID-related gastroduodenal damage may be non-specific and sometimes misleading, and that the first manifestation might be quite severe, such as haemorrhage and stenosis [17]. A reduction of visceral sensibility and/or the analgesic activity of the NSAID itself may account for these findings.

Indeed, patients over 65 years old have a higher risk of haemorrhagic complications, a risk that escalates even further with increasing aging. Current clinical evidence suggests that even in the elderly, *H. pylori* infection increases the risk of ulcer in patients who take NSAIDs [18]. Two studies carried out in elderly subjects reported that NSAID use and *H. pylori* infection were independent risk factors for upper gastrointestinal bleeding [19, 20].

In conclusion, the main features of NSAID gastroduodenal damage in the elderly are: (1) absence of or mild (and non-specific) abdominal symptoms; (2) poor correlation of symptoms with endoscopic signs, and (3) severe

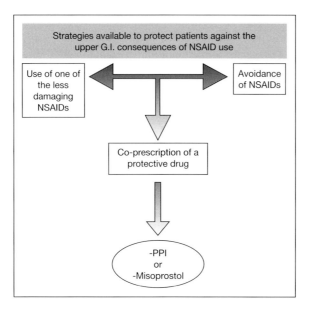

┌───┐
│ Strategies available to protect patients against the │
│ upper G.I. consequences of NSAID use   │
└───┘

Fig. 2. Strategies available for gastroduodenal protection. G.I. = Gastrointestinal.

complications like haemorrhage as the initial event. Direct or indirect consequences of these clinical characteristics can cause a critical delay in diagnosis and therapy.

Strategies for the Prevention of NSAID-Related Gastroduodenal Damage

Several strategies have been suggested to prevent NSAID-related gastroduodenal complications in the elderly (fig. 2), as discussed below.

Discontinuation of NSAID Therapy
The first strategy is the discontinuation of NSAID therapy. A study from the UK reported that the number of NSAID prescriptions in general practice was significantly related to the number of hospitalizations for bleeding ulcer in the elderly [21]. Another study from Canada reported an estimated rate of unnecessary NSAID prescriptions of 37% in elderly patients with osteoarthritis [22]. Recently, an interesting study from the USA reported a significant reduction in re-hospitalization rates for peptic ulcer within 1 year, as well as mortality rates of elderly subjects who participated in a quality improvement project that involved counselling about NSAID toxicity [23].

Table 1. Estimated RRs of upper gastrointestinal complications associated with the use of individual NSAIDs

NSAID	Study			
	Langman et al. 1994 [24] (UK)		Garcia Rodriguez et al. 1998 [25] (Italy)	
	odds ratio	95% CI	odds ratio	95% CI
Ibuprofen	2.0	1.4–2.8	2.9	1.78–5.0
Diclofenac	4.2	2.6–6.8	3.9	2.3–6.5
Naproxen	9.1	5.5–15.1	3.1	1.7–5.9
Ketoprofen	23.7	7.6–74.1	5.4	2.6–11.3
Indomethacin	11.3	6.3–20.3	6.3	3.3–12.2
Piroxicam	13.7	7.1–26.3	18.0	8.3–39.6
Azopropazone	31.5	10.3–96.9	23.4	6.9–79.5

CI = Confidence interval.

Selection of Less Damaging NSAIDs

Several studies have attempted in recent years to rank NSAIDs according to their relative risk (RR) for upper gastrointestinal adverse events. Data indicated a relatively lower risk of upper gastrointestinal complications, particularly bleeding, with ibuprofen (RR 2.0–2.9), diclofenac (RR 3.9–4.2) and naproxen (RR 3.1–9.1) compared to indomethacin (RR 4.9–11.3), piroxicam (RR 9.5–19.1) and azapropazone (RR 23.4–31.5) [24, 25] (table 1).

Furthermore, the risk of complications appears to be directly related to the dose of the given NSAID and inversely related to the duration of therapy. Indeed, as discussed previously, the greatest risk of adverse events tends to occur in the early stages of exposure due to the gastric adaptation mechanism that emerges with chronic use. Moreover, the pharmacodynamics of NSAIDs may influence side effects; a study in elderly subjects with osteoarthritis reported higher faecal blood loss using NSAIDs with a long plasma half-life such as naproxen (2.76 ml) and piroxicam (1.16 ml) compared to NSAIDs with shorter half-lives such as diclofenac (0.53 ml) [26].

COX-2 Inhibitors

In the year 2000, two specific inhibitors of COX-2, celecoxib and rofecoxib, were approved for human use. It is claimed that these COX-2-specific inhibitors are as effective in relieving pain and symptoms in patients with osteoarthritis as traditional NSAIDs such as ibuprofen, diclofenac and naproxen [27, 28]. More recently, celecoxib has been shown to effectively improve the quality of life of patients over 70 years of age [29], and rofecoxib has been successfully used in patients over 80 years of age [30]. Most recent studies demonstrated that COX-2-selective inhibitors have significant safety advantages with regards to gastrointestinal side effects [31]. However, the selective inhibition of COX-2 may induce both cardiac and renal adverse events, especially in the elderly [32]. A comparative study between celecoxib and rofecoxib in 810 elderly patients over 65 years old affected by both hypertension and arthritis reported oedema in 10 and 5%, respectively, with rofecoxib and celecoxib (p < 0.01), while systolic blood pressure was significantly modified in 17% of patients treated with rofecoxib and in 11% of patients treated with celecoxib [33]. These results suggest that selective COX-2 inhibitors need to be carefully evaluated before greater diffusion occurs, particularly in the elderly population.

Co-Treatment with Misoprostol

Prostanoids are synthetic prostaglandins that function by enhancing mucosal defensive properties and, at higher doses, by inhibiting gastric acid secretion. Graham et al. [34] showed that misoprostol at doses of 200 μg four times daily was effective in the prevention of gastric and duodenal ulcer but did not appear to improve dyspeptic symptoms. Indeed, at these doses, adverse effects such as diarrhoea, abdominal complaints and uterine contractions [34] occurred. Lower doses of misoprostol have been shown to be better tolerated. However, the only study carried out in elderly patients demonstrated that misoprostol 200 μg twice daily was effective in treating acute (10 days) NSAID-induced gastric ulcer (25 vs. 43%), but not duodenal ulcer. Furthermore, in this study, adverse events were reported in 28% of patients [35].

Co-Treatment with Anti-Secretory Drugs

One 6-month study reported a beneficial effect of high-dose famotidine, 40 mg twice a day (but not 20 mg twice a day), in preventing both gastric and duodenal ulcers in a sample of 285 patients affected by rheumatoid arthritis and treated with NSAIDs. However, after 6 months of treatment with famotidine 40 mg twice a day, a relapse of gastric or duodenal ulcer occurred in 26% of these NSAID users versus 53% of those treated with placebo [36].

A meta-analysis of 21 controlled trials in healthy volunteers and NSAID users with osteoarthritis co-treated with misoprostol, H_2 antagonists or proton pump inhibitors (PPIs) reported that 68% of placebo-treated subjects presented with acute, severe gastric damage versus 14% of subjects treated with anti-secretory drugs. Severe duodenal damage was found in 22% of placebo-treated subjects versus 2.3% of those treated with gastro-protective NSAIDs. Gastroduodenal protection was found to be significantly higher with misoprostol and PPI than with H_2 antagonists [37].

The preventative role of PPIs against NSAID injury was recently reported in elderly users. One month of therapy with pantoprazole at a dose of 40 mg a day associated with diclofenac 50–100 mg daily was highly effective in preventing gastric and duodenal injuries; not one patient presented a peptic ulcer or severe erosion at endoscopy after 1 month of therapy/follow-up [38]. This PPI treatment was more effective than 1 week of *H. pylori* eradication therapy, confirming that although *H. pylori* eradication may be a useful strategy [39], it is not sufficient to prevent severe gastroduodenal damage in elderly *H. pylori*-positive NSAID users [40].

References

1   Gabriel SE, Jaakkimainen L, Bombardier C: Risk for serious gastrointestinal complications related to use of nonsteroidal anti-inflammatory drugs: A meta-analysis. Ann Intern Med 1991;115:787–796.
2   Wolfe MM, Lichtenstein DR, Singh G: Gastrointestinal toxicity of nonsteroidal antiinflammatory drugs. N Engl J Med 1999;340:1888–1899.
3   Gutthann SP, Garcia Rodriguez LA, Raiford DS: Individual nonsteroidal antiinflammatory drugs and other risk factors for upper gastrointestinal bleeding and perforation. Epidemiology 1997;8:18–24.
4   Pilotto A, Di Mario F, Franceschi M, Dal Bò N on behalf of the Geriatric Gastroenterology Study Group of The Italian Gerontological and Geriatric Society: Drug use and upper gastrointestinal tract in the elderly: An epidemiological survey of general practitioners. Gastroenterology 2000;118(suppl):A1293.
5   Pahor M, Guralnik JM, Salive ME, Chrischilles EA, Manto A, Wallace RB: Disability and severe gastrointestinal hemorrhage. A prospective study of community-dwelling older persons. J Am Geriatr Soc 1994;42:816–825.
6   Piper JM, Ray WA, Daugherty JR, Griffin MR: Corticosteroid use and peptic ulcer disease: Role of nonsteroidal anti-inflammatory drugs. Ann Intern Med 1991;114:735–740.
7   Shorr RI, Ray WA, Daugherty JR, Griffin MR: Concurrent use of nonsteroidal anti-inflammatory drugs and oral anticoagulants places elderly persons at high risk for hemorrhagic peptic ulcer disease. Arch Intern Med 1993;153:1665–1670.
8   Singh G, Rosen Ramey D: NSAID-induced gastrointestinal complications: The ARAMIS perspective – 1997. Arthritis, Rheumatism, and Aging Medical Information System. J Rheumatol Suppl 1998;51:8–16.
9   Davenport HW: Fluid protection by the gastric mucosa during damage by acetic and salicylic acids. Gastroenterology 1966;50:487–499.
10 Clayton NM, Oakley I, Williams LV, Trevethick MA: The role of acid in the pathogenesis of indomethacin-induced gastric antral ulcers in the rat. Aliment Pharmacol Ther 1996;10:339–345.
11 Vane JR: Inhibition of prostaglandin synthesis as a mechanism of action for aspirin-like drugs. Nature 1971;231:232–235.
12 Vane JR, Bakhle YS, Botting RM: Cyclooxygenases 1 and 2. Annu Rev Pharmacol Toxicol 1998;38:97–120.
13 Larkai EN, Smith JL, Lidsky MD, Graham DY: Gastroduodenal mucosa and dyspeptic symptoms in arthritic patients during chronic non-steroidal anti-inflammatory drug use. Am J Gastroenterol 1987;82:1153–1158.

14   Pounder R: Silent peptic ulceration: Deadly silence or golden silence? Gastroenterology 1989;96:626–631.

15   Skander MP, Ryan FP: Non-steroidal anti-inflammatory drugs and pain-free peptic ulceration in the elderly. BMJ 1988;297:833–834.

16   Pilotto A, Franceschi M, Leandro G, Di Mario F, Valerio G: The effect of *Helicobacter pylori* infection on NSAID-related gastroduodenal damage in the elderly. Eur J Gastroenterol Hepatol 1997;9:951–956.

17   Kemppainen H, Raiha I, Sourander L: Clinical presentation of bleeding peptic ulcer in the elderly. Aging (Milano) 1996;8:184–188.

18   Pilotto A: *Helicobacter pylori*-associated peptic ulcer disease in older patients. Current management strategies. Drugs Aging 2001;18:487–494.

19   Pilotto A, Leandro G, Di Mario F, Franceschi M, Bozzola L, Valerio G: Role of *Helicobacter pylori* infection on upper gastrointestinal bleeding in the elderly. A case-control study. Dig Dis Sci 1997;42:586–591.

20   Cullen DJ, Hawkey GM, Greenwood DC, Humphreys H, Shepherd V, Logan RF, Hawkey CJ: Peptic ulcer bleeding in the elderly: Relative roles of *Helicobacter pylori* and non-steroidal anti-inflammatory drugs. Gut 1997;41:459–462.

21   Hawkey CJ, Cullen DJE, Greenwood DC, Wilson JV, Logan RF: Prescribing of nonsteroidal anti-inflammatory drugs in general practice: Determinants and consequences. Aliment Pharmacol Ther 1997;11:293–298.

22   Tamblyn R, Berkson L, Dauphinee WD, Gayton D, Grad R, Huang A, Isaac L, McLeod P, Snell L: Unnecessary prescribing of NSAIDs and the management of NSAID-related gastropathy in medical practice. Ann Intern Med 1997;127:429–438.

23   Brock J, Sauaia A, Ahnen D, Marine W, Schluter W, Stevens BR, Scinto JD, Karp H, Bratzler D: Process of care and outcomes for elderly patients hospitalized with peptic ulcer disease: Results from a quality improvement project. JAMA 2001;286:1985–1993.

24   Langman MJS, Weil J, Wainwright P, Lawson DH, Rawlins MD, Logan RF, Murphy M, Vessey MP, Colin-Jones DG: Risks of bleeding peptic ulcer associated with individual non-steroidal anti-inflammatory drugs. Lancet 1994;343:1075–1078.

25   Garcia Rodriguez LA, Cattaruzzi C, Troncon MG, Agostinis L: Risk of hospitalization for upper gastrointestinal tract bleeding associated with ketorolac, other nonsteroidal anti-inflammatory drugs, calcium antagonists, and other antihypertensive drugs. Arch Intern Med 1998;158:33–39.

26   Scharf S, Kwiatek R, Ugoni A, Christophidis N: NSAIDs and faecal blood loss in elderly patients with osteoarthritis: Is plasma half-life relevant? Aust NZ J Med 1998;28:436–439.

27   Silverstein FE, Faich G, Goldstein JL, Simon LS, Pincus T, Whelton A, Makuch R, Eisen G, Agrawal NM, Stenson WF, Burr AM, Zhao WW, Kent JD, Lefkowith JB, Verburg KM, Geis GS: Gastrointestinal toxicity with celecoxib vs nonsteroidal anti-inflammatory drugs for osteoarthritis and rheumatoid arthritis: The CLASS study. A randomized controlled trial. Celecoxib Long-term Arthritis Safety Study. JAMA 2000;284:1247–1255.

28   Bombardier C, Laine L, Reicin A, Shapiro D, Burgos-Vargas R, Davis B, Day R, Ferraz MB, Hawkey CJ, Hochberg MC, Kvien TK, Schnitzer TJ: Comparison of upper gastrointestinal toxicity of rofecoxib and naproxen in patients with rheumatoid arthritis. VIGOR Study Group. N Engl J Med 2000;343:1520–1528.

29   Lisse J, Espinoza L, Zhao SZ, Dedhiya SD, Osterhaus JT: Functional status and health-related quality of life of elderly osteoarthritic patients treated with celecoxib. J Gerontol A Biol Med Sci 2001;56:167–175.

30   Truitt KE, Sperling RS, Ettinger WH Jr, Greenwald M, De Tora L, Zeng Q, Bolognese J, Ehrich E: A multicentre, randomized, controlled trial to evaluate the safety profile, tolerability, and efficacy of rofecoxib in advanced elderly patients with osteoarthritis. Aging (Milano). 2001;13:112–121.

31   Fitzgerald GA, Patrono C: The coxibs, selective inhibitors of cyclooxygenase-2. N Engl J Med 2001;345:433–442.

32   Swan SK, Rudy DW, Lasseter KC, Ryan CF, Buechel KL, Lambrecht LJ, Pinto MB, Dilzer SC, Obrda O, Sundblad KJ, Gumbs CP, Ebel DL, Quan H, Larson PJ, Schwartz JI, Musliner TA, Gertz BJ, Brater DC, Yao SL: Effect of cyclooxygenase-2 inhibition on renal function in elderly persons receiving a low-salt diet. A randomized controlled trial. Ann Intern Med 2000;133:1–9.

33   Whelton A, Fort JG, Puma JA, Normandin D, Bello AE, Verburg KM: Cyclooxygenase-2-specific inhibitors and cardiorenal function: A randomized, controlled trial of celecoxib and rofecoxib in older hypertensive osteoarthritis patients. Am J Ther 2001;8:85–95.

34   Graham DY, White RH, Moreland LW, Schubert TT, Katz R, Jaszewski R, Tindall E, Triadafilopoulos G, Stromatt SC, Teoh LS: Duodenal and gastric ulcer prevention with misoprostol in arthritis patients taking NSAIDs. Misoprostol Study Group. Ann Intern Med 1993;119:257–262.

35   Piette F, Teillet L, Naudin R, Boichut D, Capron MH: Efficacy of misoprostol in the prophylaxis of gastroduodenal lesions induced by short-term nonsteroidal antiinflammatory drug therapy in elderly patients. A multicenter double-blind, placebo-controlled trial. Rev Rhum Engl Ed 1997;64:259–266.

36   Taha AS, Hudson N, Hawkey CJ, Swannell AJ, Trye PN, Cottrell J, Mann SG, Simon TJ, Sturrock RD, Russell RI: Famotidine for the prevention of gastric and duodenal ulcers caused by nonsteroidal antiinflammatory drugs. N Engl J Med 1996;334:1435–1439.

37   Leandro G, Pilotto A, Franceschi M, Bertin T, Lichino E, Di Mario F: Prevention of acute NSAID-related gastroduodenal damage: A meta-analysis of controlled clinical trials. Dig Dis Sci 2001;46:1924–1936.

38   Pilotto A, Di Mario F, Franceschi M, Leandro G, Battaglia G, Germana B, Marin R, Valerio G: Pantoprazole versus one-week *Helicobacter pylori* eradication therapy for the prevention of acute NSAID-related gastroduodenal damage in elderly subjects. Aliment Pharmacol Ther 2000;14:1077–1082.

39   Chan FK, Chung SC, Sue BY, Lee YT, Leung WK, Leung VK, Wu JC, Lau JY, Hui Y, Lai MS, Chan HL, Sung JJ: Preventing recurrent upper gastrointestinal bleeding in patients with *Helicobacter pylori* infection who are taking low-dose aspirin or naproxen. N Engl J Med 2001; 344:967–973.

40   Pilotto A, Malfertheiner P: Review article: An approach to *Helicobacter pylori* infection in the elderly. Aliment Pharmacol Ther 2002;16:683–691.

Francesco Di Mario
Chairman, Gastroenterology Department, University of Parma,
Ospedale Maggiore, Via Gramsci, 14, I–43100 Parma (Italy)
Tel. +39 0521 991772, E-Mail francesco.dimario@unipr.it

Pilotto A, Malfertheiner P, Holt PR (eds): Aging and the Gastrointestinal Tract.
Interdiscipl Top Gerontol. Basel, Karger, 2003, vol 32, pp 128–144

....

Helicobacter pylori Infection
in the Elderly

Alberto Pilotto[a], *Peter Malfertheiner*[b]

[a] Geriatric Unit, 'Casa Sollievo della Sofferenza' Hospital, IRCCS,
   San Giovanni Rotondo, Italy;
[b] Department of Gastroenterology, Hepatology and Infectious Diseases,
   Otto-von-Guericke University of Magdeburg, Magdeburg, Germany

The prevalence of *Helicobacter pylori* infection increases with age world-wide, reaching levels of 40–60% in asymptomatic elderly subjects and over 70% in elderly patients with gastroduodenal diseases [1]. In reality, however, the percentage of elderly patients who are treated for their *H. pylori* infection remains very low. A recent study of 2,267 Medicare beneficiaries hospitalized for peptic ulcer disease in 80 hospitals located in five American states reported that the rate of diagnostic screening or treatment for *H. pylori* infection was only 55.6% [2]. In agreement with these results, an additional two studies from the US [3, 4] demonstrated that only 40–56% of patients 65 years and older who were hospitalized for ulcer disease were tested for *H. pylori* infection. Subsequently, only 50–73% of patients who had a positive test were treated with antibiotics. The reasons for such a low rate of diagnosis and therapy in elderly people are not clear; however, these data indicate a substantial opportunity to improve the medical care of elderly patients with *H. pylori*-associated diseases.

Indications for Treatment in the Elderly

Peptic Ulcer Disease

The incidence of gastric and duodenal ulcers and their severe complications, such as bleeding or perforation, is increasing in old-aged populations worldwide [5–7] despite improvements in the quality of healthcare and the recent widespread use of new very effective antiulcer drugs, such as H_2 blockers and proton pump inhibitors (PPIs). Two factors that might explain these observed changes in the incidence of peptic ulcer in elderly patients are the increasing use of damaging drugs, i.e. nonsteroidal antiinflammatory drugs (NSAIDs), low-dose aspirin and warfarin, and *H. pylori* infection.

A recent cohort study of 4,292 Medicare beneficiaries 65 years and older hospitalized in 1995 and 1997 at acute care hospitals in the United States with a diagnosis of peptic ulcer disease reported that only 26% of patients who were tested for the infection were *H. pylori* positive, while recent use of NSAIDs was documented in 82% of patients [8]. The low prevalence of *H. pylori* detected in this population explains why a quality improvement program consisting of screening for and treating *H. pylori* infection did not influence rehospitalization and mortality of these elderly subjects with peptic ulcer, while counseling about NSAID use was associated with a decrease both in the risk of 1-year rehospitalization for ulcer and mortality rates [8].

In contrast, many clinical studies have reported that approximately 50–70% of elderly peptic ulcer patients are *H. pylori* positive [9–11]. Indeed, we now have data that demonstrate the benefit of curing the infection in elderly patients with *H. pylori*-associated peptic ulcer disease. Some controlled, short-term studies performed on elderly patients reported that the treatment of *H. pylori* infection healed ulcers in over 95% of patients [12] and improved symptomatology in over 85% of patients [13]. Moreover, a 1-year follow-up study performed in elderly patients with peptic ulcer demonstrated that the eradication of *H. pylori* infection significantly improved clinical outcome, reducing ulcer recurrences, symptomatology and gastritis activity [14].

Nonulcer Dyspepsia

The clinical efficacy of anti-*H. pylori* treatment in patients with nonulcer dyspepsia is still under debate [15]. A study in elderly patients documented an improvement of dyspeptic symptoms in 70% of patients with nonulcer chronic gastritis 2 months after treatment [13]. Another study performed on subjects over 60 years old reported a significant reduction in the symptoms of functional dyspepsia in patients in whom *H. pylori* was eradicated versus *H. pylori*-positive patients 2 months after therapy [16]. As yet, no studies have evaluated the efficacy of *H. pylori* therapy on symptomatology after longer periods of follow-up. However, an important aspect of the clinical management of dyspepsia in elderly subjects is the diagnostic approach. A recent study carried out in 445 elderly patients with dyspepsia reported that 238 (53.5%) were *H. pylori* positive and 207 (46.5%) were *H. pylori* negative [17]. Of these *H. pylori*-negative patients, 53 were NSAID users and 45 had reflux symptoms; thus, 109 subjects (24.5% of the overall dyspeptic elderly population) were non-NSAID users and had no reflux symptoms. In this last group, a high prevalence of peptic ulcer (15.6%),

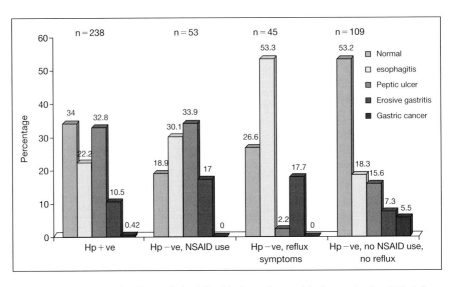

Fig. 1. Endoscopic diagnosis in 445 elderly patients with dyspepsia (modified from Pilotto et al. [17]). Hp = *H. pylori.*

esophagitis (18.3%), erosive gastritis (7.3%) and even gastric cancers (5.5%) was found (fig. 1). These findings suggested that for elderly patients with dyspepsia, it is mandatory to adopt a full diagnostic approach by endoscopy and that the test-and-treatment strategy could be misleading and possibly dangerous [17].

Chronic Atrophic Gastritis

Chronic atrophic gastritis and *H. pylori* infection are commonly found together in elderly subjects; yet, it is not clear whether *H. pylori* infection and age act as co-risk factors. A study in healthy volunteers reported that advancing age was independently related to chronic atrophic gastritis [18], while other studies suggested that atrophic changes of the gastric mucosa were associated with *H. pylori* infection rather than with aging [19–21]. In agreement with these data, a study reported that advanced age per se had no influence on gastric acid secretion in *H. pylori*-negative subjects, whereas gastric acid secretion decreased with age in *H. pylori*-positive subjects because of the increasing prevalence of fundic atrophic gastritis [22]. Another report suggested that elevated serum gastrin concentrations that were observed with increasing age were due to the greater incidence of *H. pylori* infection or gastric autoantibodies, and not to advancing age [23].

A randomized 1-year follow-up study reported that *H. pylori* eradication was beneficial in preventing progression of atrophy and intestinal metaplasia of the gastric mucosa [24]. By stratifying patients according to age, the study demonstrated that, with persistent infection, the intensity of mononuclear infiltration of chronic gastritis as well as the increase in intestinal metaplasia were significantly higher in subjects older than 45 years compared to younger patients.

Another study of 132 adult volunteers from Columbia with a baseline diagnosis of gastric atrophy reported a significant improvement in antral atrophy 6 years after they had received anti-*H. pylori* treatment [25]. Moreover, a recent study carried out in 22 elderly patients from Finland with *H. pylori* infection and moderate or severe atrophic corpus gastritis reported a significant improvement in the histological scores of inflammation, atrophy and intestinal metaplasia in the corpus mucosa 2.5 years after *H. pylori* eradication therapy [26].

Since the response to treatment was similar in patients of different ages, we may assume that the cure of *H. pylori* infection in elderly patients with gastric mucosal modifications is the same as that for young and adult patients.

Use of NSAIDs

The relation between *H. pylori* infection and the use of NSAIDs in the pathogenesis of peptic ulcer disease is controversial. A recent meta-analysis of 25 studies carried out in adult NSAID takers [27] confirmed that both *H. pylori* infection and NSAID use independently and significantly increase the risk of peptic ulcer and ulcer bleeding. *H. pylori* infection increased the risk of peptic ulcer in NSAID takers 3.5-fold in addition to the risk associated with NSAID use; similarly, in the presence of the risk of peptic ulcer associated with *H. pylori* infection, use of NSAIDs increased the risk of peptic ulcer 3.55-fold. Indeed, both factors, NSAID use and *H. pylori* infection, were shown to be independent and unrelated risk factors for peptic ulcer [28] and gastroduodenal bleeding even in elderly subjects [29, 30].

These findings are in agreement with recent pathophysiological studies that demonstrated that age and *H. pylori* infection may decrease gastric mucosal hydrophobicity [31] and the gastric mucus gel layer [32] independently.

Eradication of *H. pylori* before NSAID therapy reduced the occurrence of NSAID-related peptic ulcers in acute (2 months) NSAID users [33]. Moreover, a recent randomized trial carried out in patients who were starting long-term treatment with an NSAID (diclofenac slow release 100 mg daily) reported that the cure of *H. pylori* infection significantly reduced the 6-month risk of peptic ulcer [34].

However, a study performed in elderly patients reported that the use of PPIs, concomitantly with the NSAID diclofenac, 50 or 100 mg daily, reduced the occurrence of acute (1-month) NSAID-related gastroduodenal damage more effectively than the eradication of *H. pylori* infection [35]. Similarly, a prospective study carried out in patients who needed chronic treatment with NSAIDs reported that continuous PPI treatment for 6 months in association with naproxen 500 mg twice daily might prevent rebleeding significantly more than eradication of *H. pylori* [36]. No differences between the two strategies were observed for subjects who were treated with low-dose aspirin (80 mg daily) as a vascular antiplatelet prevention therapy. The study was not carried out specifically in elderly subjects; however, the mean age was almost 70 years in both the groups [36].

All these findings suggest that, in elderly subjects, eradication therapy alone is not sufficient to prevent peptic ulcer or rebleeding related to acute or chronic NSAID use. More studies are needed to suggest the most effective prevention strategy for those elderly patients who need to be treated with low-dose aspirin.

Gastroesophageal Reflux Disease

In the elderly, the prevalence of both *H. pylori* infection and gastro-esophageal reflux disease (GERD) are higher than in adult and young populations. However, the relationship between *H. pylori* infection and the clinical behavior of GERD has not yet been clarified, particularly in old age. A study carried out in elderly patients failed to find any significant association between the presence of *H. pylori* and reflux esophagitis [37]. More recently, a significantly lower prevalence of *H. pylori* infection was found in patients over 60 years of age with reflux esophagitis in comparison with sex- and age-matched controls [38]. Controversy also exists with regard to the influence of *H. pylori* on the clinical response to antisecretory therapy. A randomized clinical trial carried out in 971 patients with grade 2–3 reflux esophagitis reported that *H. pylori*-positive patients with reflux esophagitis responded significantly better to short-term treatment with the PPI pantoprazole than *H. pylori*-negative patients [39]. Conversely, a recent study carried out in 271 elderly patients (mean age 79.2 years) with esophagitis reported that healing of esophagitis after a 2-month treatment with PPIs was similar in *H. pylori*-positive and -negative patients [40]. Moreover, in this elderly population, the eradication therapy did not influence the clinical response to short-term PPI therapy. This finding was in agreement with the results of a pH-metric study that found no consistent change in gastroesophageal acid reflux in patients with grade 1 or 2 esophagitis 12 weeks after *H. pylori* eradication [41]. Recently, a double-blind, placebo-controlled study in 58 nonelderly patients (mean age 54 years, range 18–75 years) with GERD reported that *H. pylori*-positive patients relapsed earlier (54 days) than did those in whom *H. pylori* was eradicated (100 days, $p < 0.05$). As expected, time to relapse was also affected by esophagitis grade.

However, when the results were corrected for the effect of esophagitis grade, *H. pylori*-positive patients relapsed earlier than *H. pylori*-eradicated patients (p = 0.086) and *H. pylori*-negative controls (p = 0.001). This suggests that *H. pylori* infection affected the relapse rate of GERD and that eradication of *H. pylori* could help to prolong the disease-free interval in patients with GERD [42]. In contrast, a recent prospective study carried out in 52 *H. pylori*-positive elderly patients (mean age 72.3 years) with esophagitis reported that the eradication of *H. pylori* did not influence the short- (2 months) and long-term (8 months) healing rates of esophagitis, nor the symptomatology of reflux disease [43]. It is unknown whether such discrepancies are due to an age-sensitive pathophysiological characteristic such as gastric acid secretion in response to *H. pylori* infection and/or to antisecretory therapy.

Extradigestive Diseases

A scientific debate has arisen about the possible association of *H. pylori* infection with extradigestive diseases, principally cardiovascular diseases, but also liver and biliary tract diseases, skin diseases, iron deficiency and pernicious anemia [44]. The few studies performed in elderly populations failed to find any association between *H. pylori* infection and coronary heart disease [45, 46] or extracardiac atherosclerosis [47]. To date, the presence of extradigestive diseases is not an indication for the testing or treatment of *H. pylori*.

Subjects Living in Nursing Homes

For many people, advanced age coincides with institutional living and, thus, with an increased risk of infection. The seroprevalence of *H. pylori* infection in asymptomatic elderly people living in a nursing home for at least 5 years was reported to be 86% [48]. A study carried out in elderly patients aged 70 years or more living in nursing homes showed that the prevalence of *H. pylori* was significantly higher in subjects who stayed in nursing homes for more than 15 months compared to subjects with a shorter duration of institutionalization (84 vs. 63%, p < 0.05) [49]. Another study reported that employees of institutions for the intellectually disabled, especially those with a long duration of employment and who have close physical contact with patients, were at high risk of developing *H. pylori* infection [50]. However, no significant correlation was found between seropositivity and cognitive status, the grade of disability [51], nutritional status [48, 51] or gastric function parameters [48] in elderly subjects.

To date, no specific hygienic or behavioral measures are currently recommended for minimizing *H. pylori* transmission among elderly and professional people in nursing homes.

The Diagnosis of *H. pylori* Infection in the Elderly

Upper gastrointestinal endoscopy is always indicated for elderly subjects with new abdominal symptoms because of the high prevalence of serious gastric diseases in this age group [17]. *H. pylori* infection may be easily diagnosed by means of either histology evaluation, rapid urease test or culture performed on gastric biopsies taken during endoscopy [52]. However, the biopsy site needs to be selected with care since *H. pylori* may only be found in the fundus or body and not in the antral mucosa of elderly patients who are taking antisecretory drugs [53]. Moreover, the prevalence of chronic atrophic gastritis associated with past colonization of *H. pylori* is higher in elderly than in adult or young patients [54, 55]. Supporting this is the finding that the prevalence of *H. pylori* infection detected by a positive antibody titer was significantly higher than the prevalence of *H. pylori* as documented by gastric mucosal histology [56]. For the same reasons, the rapid urease test performed on antral biopsies had lower sensitivity in subjects 60 years and older compared with patients less than 60 years of age (57 vs. 75%) [57].

These findings may suggest that in the elderly (1) it is advisable to perform gastric biopsies at the least both from the antrum and the body of the stomach, and (2) a second test for *H. pylori* should be performed in this age group if a urease-based or histological test is negative.

Posttreatment Evaluation of Patients

The recent European guidelines on the management of *H. pylori* infection published by the European *H. pylori* Study Group reported that successful eradication should always be confirmed by a noninvasive or endoscopy-based test if endoscopy is clinically indicated [58]. Elderly patients with a diagnosis of peptic ulcer (especially gastric ulcer), gastric mucosa-associated lymphoid tissue, lymphoma or severe gastritis should be evaluated by endoscopy and gastric mucosal histology after completion of anti-*H. pylori* therapy. Most experts agree that this evaluation must be carried out at least 1 month after completion of therapy in order to minimize false-negative results.

Elderly patients with mild or moderate forms of chronic gastritis may be evaluated after therapy by a noninvasive test. Recently, the ^{13}C-urea breath test demonstrated significantly higher sensitivity (100%), specificity (95.7%) and diagnostic accuracy (98%) in elderly subjects than serology (IgG anti-*H. pylori* antibodies). Furthermore, the ^{13}C-urea breath test was shown to be unaffected by potential covariables such as cognitive function, disability, comorbidity and cotreatments [59]. This is in agreement with a previous study that demonstrated the low sensitivity (62%) and specificity (56%) of serology in monitoring *H. pylori* treatment in elderly people [60]. Thus, the routine use of serum IgG antibodies for the monitoring of *H. pylori* infection should not be a recommended clinical practice since it does not accurately reflect the elderly patient's true gastric *H. pylori* status [61, 62]. Recently, a stool antigen test for the detection of *H. pylori* was suggested as a new valuable option with a high potential role in the first diagnosis [63] as well as after eradication therapy [64]. A very recent study of geriatric subjects reported that the stool antigen test had a posttreatment diagnostic accuracy comparable to the ^{13}C-urea breath test (91 vs. 92%); furthermore, cognitive status, disability, concomitant diseases and cotreatments did not influence the feasibility and accuracy of the test [65]. Other new noninvasive diagnostic tests have been developed involving the detection of antibodies in saliva and whole blood [66]. All these methods, however, have not yet been evaluated sufficiently in older populations.

Treatment

Regimens

The recommended first-line anti-*H. pylori* therapy of the recent European *H. pylori* Study Group Maastricht 2-2000 Consensus Meeting is a triple therapy using a PPI or ranitidine bismuth citrate combined with clarithromycin and amoxicillin or metronidazole [58].

Studies performed in elderly subjects demonstrated that PPI-based triple therapies for 1 week were highly effective in old-aged patients [67]. One controlled study carried out in 134 patients greater than 60 years of age treated for the first time with omeprazole 20 mg twice daily plus clarithromycin 250 mg and tinidazole 500 mg twice daily reported a 92.9% cure rate [95% confidence interval (CI) 88.2–97.6%] [68]. Excellent cure rates were also obtained with a 1-week treatment with 30 mg of lansoprazole twice daily in combination with (1) 250 mg of clarithromycin twice daily and 250 mg of metronidazole four times a day (86% eradication rate, 95% CI 76–96%), or (2) 1 g of amoxicillin twice daily plus clarithromycin 250 mg twice daily (82% eradication rate, 95% CI 71–93%), or (3) 1 g of amoxicillin twice daily plus metronidazole 250 mg four times daily (80% eradication rate, 95% CI 69–91%) [13].

In elderly patients, a reduction of the dosage of omeprazole from 40 to 20 mg daily did not influence the cure rates of a triple therapy consisting of the PPI plus clarithromycin 250 mg twice daily and metronidazole 250 mg four times a day [83.3 versus 85.5% intention to treat (ITT) cure rates, respectively, with omeprazole 40 and 20 mg daily] [69]. Pantoprazole also demonstrated high efficacy when it was used at the dosage of 40 mg once daily in combination

Table 1. Cumulative results of nine clinical trials [12, 13, 16, 35, 68–71, 73] evaluating 1-week PPI-based double or triple anti-*H. pylori* therapies in elderly patients

	Number of patients	ITT eradication, %	PP eradication, %	Dropouts, %	Side effects, %
Double therapies					
PPI + C	37	43.2	47.0	8.1	8.1
PPI + A1 or A2	83	59.0	61.2	3.6	3.6
Triple therapies					
PPI + C + M or T	296	88.2	90.9	3.0	3.4
PPI + A1 + C	253	84.2	89.1	5.5	7.1
PPI + A1 + M	154	79.8	83.7	4.5	7.1

PPIs used were omeprazole 20 mg daily or twice daily, lansoprazole 30 mg twice daily or pantoprazole 40 mg daily. PP = Per protocol analysis; C = clarithromycin 250 mg twice daily; M = metronidazole 250 mg four times a day or 500 mg twice daily; T = tinidazole 500 mg twice daily; A1 = amoxicillin 1 g twice daily; A2 = amoxicillin 500 mg three times a day.

with (1) amoxicillin 1 g and clarithromycin 250 mg twice daily (85% ITT cure rate, 95% CI 74–96%), or (2) clarithromycin 250 mg and metronidazole 500 mg twice daily (82% ITT cure rate, 95% CI 69–94%), or (3) amoxicillin 1 g and metronidazole 500 mg twice daily (79% ITT cure rate, 95% CI 66–92%) [70]. Excellent eradication rates were recently reported also with rabeprazole at the low dosage of 20 mg once daily in combination with clarithromycin 250 mg and tinidazole 500 mg twice daily (88.5% ITT cure rate) or clarithromycin 250 mg and amoxicillin 1 g twice daily (86.3% ITT cure rate) for 1 week [71]. All these data demonstrate that 1-week PPI-based triple therapies are very effective in elderly patients; moreover, low doses of PPIs are sufficient to obtain excellent cure rates in elderly subjects (table 1).

Side Effects and Dosages of Drugs
Triple PPI-based therapies have been shown to be well tolerated. Adverse event rates of less than 13% were reported in controlled studies performed in the elderly, with less than 6% of patients discontinuing therapy due to these effects [72]. Such a low rate of side effects and high rate of compliance are probably due to the short (1-week) duration and the low dosage of both PPIs and antibiotics used. Pertinent information has been culled from a recent study demonstrating that the reduction of clarithromycin dose from 500 to 250 mg twice daily in combination with amoxicillin 1 g twice daily and pantoprazole 40 mg once daily resulted in no significant differences in cure rates and tolerability in elderly subjects [73]. These results are in disagreement with data

reported in nonelderly populations, in whom 500 mg twice daily of clarithromycin (in combination with a standard dose of PPI and amoxicillin 1 g twice daily) was more effective than lower dosages [74]. A possible explanation for the varying drug response in subjects of different ages is that aging per se has little influence on the pharmacokinetics of amoxicillin and metronidazole, whereas a direct effect of age on clarithromycin disposition is observed and is known to be independent of renal function [75]. These findings suggest that, for the elderly, PPI-based triple therapies may include clarithromycin at a low dose of 250 mg twice daily when combined in a triple regimen with a PPI and amoxicillin (at the standard dosage of 1 g twice daily) or metronidazole (at the dosage of 400 or 500 mg twice daily).

Risk Factors for Treatment Failure

To date, only a few studies have concentrated on the risk factors for treatment failure specifically in elderly patients. Relevant for clinical practice was the finding that concomitant diseases and concomitant treatments did not influence the efficacy of anti-*H. pylori* therapy [60].

A study from Italy reported that age higher than 45 years was an independent predictor of eradication failure with a 1-week PPI-based triple therapy [76]. In contrast, a study carried out in 234 *H. pylori*-positive subjects reported that age higher than 55 years was significantly associated with treatment success, while smoking, history of peptic ulcer and metronidazole resistance were associated with eradication failure [77]. Two independent studies reported that a 1-week PPI-based eradication therapy was more effective in peptic ulcer patients than in subjects with nonulcer dyspepsia [78, 79], while in another study, the only variable significantly associated with the result of this therapy outcome was daily alcohol consumption, with a higher probability of success in consumers than in nonconsumers [80].

Resistance of *H. pylori* to antibiotics (especially to clarithromycin and metronidazole) is one of the major reasons for treatment failure also in old age. In the presence of nitroimidazole resistance, a drop in efficacy by 15–50% was found for bismuth-based and PPI-based triple therapies containing a nitroimidazole [81]. Clarithromycin resistance is still low in most communities; however, when present, it has a higher negative impact on treatment outcome than metronidazole resistance [82]. Only a few studies have concentrated on this topic in old age. A recent study from northeastern Italy, carried out in subjects 25–90 years old, documented that resistance to metronidazole was 15% and resistance to clarithromycin was 1.8% [83]. These percentages were very similar to those observed in a group of elderly subjects aged 60–96 years living in the same geographical area: 21 and 5%, respectively, for resistance to metronidazole and macrolides [84].

Table 2. Clinical characteristics of *H. pylori* infection in elderly subjects compared to young or adult subjects

Prevalence of infection	1. increases with age worldwide in asymptomatic subjects 2. decreases in elderly subjects with peptic ulcer disease (50–70 vs. 80–90% of adult peptic ulcer patients) 3. is higher in elderly subjects who are living in nursing homes for longer periods of time 4. no significant correlations between *H. pylori* infection and cognitive status, disability, nutritional status and extracardiac atherosclerosis
Indications for treatment of infection	1. similar benefit of curing *H. pylori* infection in young and elderly patients with peptic ulcer, gastric MALT lymphoma, nonulcer dyspepsia and chronic atrophic gastritis 2. in elderly subjects, eradication therapy alone is not sufficient to prevent peptic ulcer or rebleeding related to acute or chronic NSAID use 3. no definite role of *H. pylori* eradication in elderly users of low-dose aspirin nor in elderly patients with GERD
Diagnosis of infection	1. test and treatment strategies are not useful and possibly unsafe in elderly subjects 2. rapid urease test and histology may have lower sensitivity in the elderly than in adults 3. in the elderly, a second test for *H. pylori* should be performed if a urease-based or histological test is negative
Posttreatment evaluation	1. ^{13}C-urea breath test has higher sensitivity and specificity than serology and it is unaffected by cognitive function, disability, comorbidity and cotreatments 2. the potential role of the stool antigen test remains to be explored in old age
Treatment	1. 1-week, PPI-based triple therapies are very effective also in elderly patients 2. low doses of both PPIs and clarithromycin (in combination with amoxicillin or nitroimidazoles) are sufficient to obtain excellent cure rates 3. concomitant diseases and concomitant treatments did not influence the efficacy of anti-*H. pylori* therapy 4. similarly to young and adult patients, low compliance and antibiotic resistance are the main factors related to treatment failure

MALT = Mucosa-associated lymphoid tissue.

A recent study including 1,064 patients from the UK reported an overall resistance to clarithromycin of 4.4% and to metronidazole of 40.3%. Metronidazole resistance decreased with age (odds ratio for patients over 60 years 0.63, 95% CI 0.48–0.80) [85]. A meta-analysis of 20 trials including 3,624 men and women in the United States reported that overall resistance to clarithromycin, metronidazole and amoxicillin was 10.1, 36.9 and 1.4%, respectively. Clarithromycin resistance was significantly associated with geographic region, older age and female sex, while no influence of age was documented for metronidazole and amoxicillin resistances [86].

Antibiotic resistances may change with time even within the same population, principally due to the emergence of secondary resistances [87]. Indeed, an increased resistance to recommended antibiotics, especially clarithromycin, has been reported all over the world [88, 89]. Since the ideal way to prevent secondary resistance is probably to obtain the highest possible eradication rate with first-line regimens, a continuous surveillance of *H. pylori* susceptibility to antibiotics would be needed to establish the most effective primary treatment in a specific geographic area [90].

A recent review article confirmed that the most common reason for treatment failure was poor compliance with eradication guidelines [91]. Indeed, a study from Germany reported that only a fraction of *H. pylori* infections were actually eradicated, principally due to the gap existing between 'state-of-the-art' recommendations and what is actually being carried out in daily clinical practice [92]. In agreement with these findings, a study reported that the use of enhanced compliance programs [93] consisting of medication counseling (written and oral) from a pharmacist, along with a medication calendar and a minipillbox, as well as a telephone call after initiation of therapy, significantly improved the compliance of patients with *H. pylori* eradication therapy. More recently, another study reported that structured patient counseling and follow-up may have a significant effect on *H. pylori* eradication rates [94]. These results suggest a new approach to anti-*H. pylori* treatment and encourage further studies, especially in elderly patients [95].

Table 2 summarizes the characteristics of *H. pylori* infection in elderly subjects compared to young or adult subjects.

References

1   Pilotto A: Aging and the gastrointestinal tract. Ital J Gastroenterol Hepatol 1999;31:137–153.
2   Hood HM, Wark C, Burgess PA, Nicewander D, Scott MW: Screening for *Helicobacter pylori* and nonsteroidal anti-inflammatory drug use in Medicare patients hospitalized with peptic ulcer disease. Arch Intern Med 1999;159:149–154.
3   Roll J, Weng A, Newman J: Diagnosis and treatment of *Helicobacter pylori* infection among California Medicare patients. Arch Intern Med 1997;157:994–998.

4 Ofman JJ, Etchason J, Alexander W, Stevens BR, Herrin J, Cangialose C, Ballard DJ, Bratzler D, Elward KS, FitzGerald D, Culpepper-Morgan J, Marshall B: The quality of care for Medicare patients with peptic ulcer disease. Am J Gastroenterol 2000;95:106–113.

5 Fock KM: Peptic ulcer disease in the 1990s: An Asian perspective. J Gastroenterol Hepatol 1997;12:S23–S28.

6 Dominitz JA, Provenzale D: Prevalence of dyspepsia, heartburn and peptic ulcer disease in veterans. Am J Gastroenterol 1999;94:2086–2093.

7 Higham J, Kang JY, Majeed A: Recent trends in admissions and mortality due to peptic ulcer in England: Increasing frequency of haemorrhage among older subjects. Gut 2002;50:460–464.

8 Brock J, Sauaia A, Ahnen D, Marine W, Schluter W, Stevens BR, Scinto JD, Karp H, Bratzler D: Process of care and outcomes for elderly patients hospitalized with peptic ulcer disease: Results from a quality improvement project. JAMA 2001;286:1985–1993.

9 Safe AF, Warren B, Corfield A, McNulty CA, Watson B, Mountford RA, Read A: *Helicobacter pylori* infection in elderly people: Correlation between histology and serology. Age Ageing 1993; 22:215–220.

10 Kemppainen H, Raiha I, Sourander L: Clinical presentation of peptic ulcer in the elderly. Gerontology 1997;43:283–288.

11 Pilotto A, Franceschi M, Di Mario F: *Helicobacter pylori*-associated peptic ulcer disease in elderly patients. Clin Geriatr 2000;8:49–58.

12 Murakami M, Saita H, Takahashi Y, et al: Therapeutic effects of lansoprazole on peptic ulcers in elderly patients. J Clin Gastroenterol 1995;20(suppl 2):S79–S82.

13 Pilotto A, Franceschi M, Leandro G, Bozzola L, Fortunato A, Rassu M, Meli S, Soffiati G, Scagnelli M, Di Mario F, Valerio G: Efficacy of 7 day lansoprazole-based triple therapy for *Helicobacter pylori* infection in elderly patients. J Gastroenterol Hepatol 1999;14:468–475.

14 Pilotto A, Franceschi M, Di Mario F, Leandro G, Bozzola L, Valerio G: The long-term clinical outcome of elderly patients with *Helicobacter pylori*-associated peptic ulcer disease. Gerontology 1998;44:153–158.

15 McColl K, Malfertheiner P: *Helicobacter pylori* and functional dyspepsia. Curr Opin Gastroenterol 2000;16(suppl 1):S29–S32.

16 Catalano F, Branciforte G, Brogna A, Bentivegna C, Luca S, Terranova R, Michalos A, Dawson BK, Chodash HB: *Helicobacter pylori*-positive functional dyspepsia in elderly patients. Comparison of two treatments. Dig Dis Sci 1999;44:863–867.

17 Pilotto A, Franceschi M, Costa MC, Di Mario F, Valerio G: *Helicobacter pylori* test-and-eradication strategy. Lancet 2000;356:1683–1684.

18 Feldman M, Cryer B, McArthur KE, Huet BA, Lee E: Effects of aging and gastritis on gastric acid and pepsin secretion in humans: A prospective study. Gastroenterology 1996;110: 1043–1052.

19 Asaka M, Kato M, Kudo M, Katagiri M, Nishikawa K, Koshiyama H, Takeda H, Yoshida J, Graham DY: Atrophic changes of gastric mucosa are caused by *Helicobacter pylori* infection rather than aging: Studies in asymptomatic Japanese adults. Helicobacter 1996;1:52–56.

20 Kawaguchi H, Haruma K, Komoto K, Yoshihara M, Sumii K, Kajiyama G: *Helicobacter pylori* is the major risk factor for atrophic gastritis. Am J Gastroenterol 1996;91:959–962.

21 Pilotto A, Rassu M, Bozzola L, Leandro G, Franceschi M, Furlan F, Meli S, Scagnelli M, Di Mario F, Valerio G: Cytotoxin-associated gene A-positive *Helicobacter pylori* infection in the elderly. Association with gastric atrophy and intestinal metaplasia. J Clin Gastroenterol 1998;26: 18–22.

22 Haruma K, Kamada T, Kawaguchi H, Okamoto S, Yoshihara M, Sumii K, Inoue M, Kishimoto S, Kajiyama G, Miyoshi A: Effect of age and *Helicobacter pylori* infection on gastric acid secretion. J Gastroenterol Hepatol 2000;15:277–283.

23 Jassel SV, Ardill JES, Fillmore D, Bamford KB, O'Connor FA, Buchanan KD: The rise in circulating gastrin with age is due to increases in gastric autoimmunity and *Helicobacter pylori* infection. Q J Med 1999;92:373–377.

24 Sung JJ, Lin SR, Ching JY, Zhou LY, To KF, Wang RT, Leung WK, Ng EK, Lau JY, Lee YT, Yeung CK, Chao W, Chung SC: Atrophy and intestinal metaplasia one year after cure of *H. pylori* infection: A prospective, randomized study. Gastroenterology 2000;119:7–14.

25   Ruiz B, Garay J, Correa P, Fontham ET, Bravo JC, Bravo LE, Realpe JL, Mera R: Morphometric evaluation of gastric antral atrophy: Improvement after cure of *Helicobacter pylori* infection. Am J Gastroenterol 2001;96:3281–3287.

26   Kokkola A, Sipponen P, Rautelin H, Harkonen M, Kosunen TU, Haapiainen R, Puolakkainen P: The effect of *Helicobacter pylori* eradication on the natural course of atrophic gastritis with dysplasia. Aliment Pharmacol Ther 2002;16:515–520.

27   Huang JQ, Sridhar S, Hunt RH: Role of *Helicobacter pylori* infection and non-steroidal anti-inflammatory drugs in peptic ulcer disease: A meta-analysis. Lancet 2002;359:14–22.

28   Pilotto A, Franceschi M, Leandro G, Di Mario F, Valerio G: The effect of *Helicobacter pylori* infection on NSAID-related gastroduodenal damage in the elderly. Eur J Gastroenterol Hepatol 1997;9:951–956.

29   Cullen DJ, Hawkey GM, Greenwood DC, Humphreys H, Shepherd V, Logan RF, Hawkey CJ: Peptic ulcer bleeding in the elderly: Relative roles of *Helicobacter pylori* and non-steroidal anti-inflammatory drugs. Gut 1997;41:586–591.

30   Pilotto A, Leandro G, Di Mario F, Franceschi M, Bozzola L, Valerio G: Role of *Helicobacter pylori* infection on upper gastrointestinal bleeding in the elderly. A case-control study. Dig Dis Sci 1997;42:586–591.

31   Hackelsberger A, Platzer U, Nilius M, Schulze V, Gunther T, Dominguez-Munoz JE, Malfertheiner P: Age and *Helicobacter pylori* decrease gastric mucosal surface hydrophobicity independently. Gut 1998;43:465–469.

32   Newton JL, Jordan N, Pearson J, Williams GV, Allen A, James OFW: The adherent gastric antral and duodenal mucus gel layer thins with advancing age in subjects infected with *Helicobacter pylori*. Gerontology 2000;46:153–157.

33   Chan FKL, Sung JJ, Chung SC, To KF, Yung MY, Leung VK, Lee YT, Chan CS, Li EK, Woo J: Randomised trial of eradication of *Helicobacter pylori* before non-steroidal anti-inflammatory drug therapy to prevent peptic ulcers. Lancet 1997;350:975–979.

34   Chan FKL, To KF, Wu JCY, Yung MY, Leung WK, Kwok T, Hui Y, Chan HL, Chan CS, Hui E, Woo J, Sung JJ: Eradication of *Helicobacter pylori* and risk of peptic ulcers in patients starting long-term treatment with nonsteroidal anti-inflammatory drugs: A randomised trial. Lancet 2002;359:9–13.

35   Pilotto A, Di Mario F, Franceschi M, Leandro G, Battaglia G, Germanà B, Marin R, Valerio G: Pantoprazole versus one-week *Helicobacter pylori* eradication therapy for the prevention of acute NSAID-related gastroduodenal damage in elderly subjects. Aliment Pharmacol Ther 2000;14:1077–1082.

36   Chan FKL, Chung SCS, Suen BY, Lee YT, Leung WK, Leung VKS, Wu JC, Lau JY, Hui Y, Lai MS, Chan HL, Sung JJ: Preventing recurrent upper gastrointestinal bleeding in patients with *Helicobacter pylori* infection who are taking low-dose aspirin or naproxen. N Engl J Med 2001;344:967–973.

37   Liston R, Pitt MA, Banarjee AK: Reflux oesophagitis and *Helicobacter pylori* infection in elderly patients. Postgrad Med J 1996;72:221–223.

38   Haruma K, Hamada H, Mihara M, Kamada T, Yoshihara M, Sumii K, Kajiyama G, Kawanishi M: Negative association between *Helicobacter pylori* infection and reflux esophagitis in older patients: Case-control study in Japan. Helicobacter 2000;5:24–29.

39   Holtmann G, Cain C, Malfertheiner P: Gastric *Helicobacter pylori* infection accelerates healing of reflux esophagitis during treatment with the proton pump inhibitor pantoprazole. Gastroenterology 1999;117:11–16.

40   Pilotto A, Franceschi M, Leandro G, Rassu M, Bozzola L, Valerio G, Di Mario F: Influence of *Helicobacter pylori* infection on severity of oesophagitis and response to therapy in the elderly. Dig Liver Dis 2002;34:328–331.

41   Tefera S, Hatlebakk JG, Berstad A: The effect of *Helicobacter pylori* eradication on gastro-oesophageal reflux. Aliment Pharmacol Ther 1999;13:915–920.

42   Schwizer W, Thumshirn M, Dent J, Guldenschuh I, Menne D, Cathomas G, Fries M: Helicobacter pylori and symptomatic relapse of gastro-oesophageal reflux disease: A randomised controlled trial. Lancet 2001;357:1738–1742.

43   Pilotto A on behalf of the Study Group 'Aging and Acid Related Diseases': Effect of *H. pylori* eradication on long-term outcome of esophagitis in elderly subjects. A randomized, prospective study. Gut 2001;49(suppl 2):A65.

44 De Koster E, De Bruyne I, Langlet P, Deltenre M: Evidence based medicine and extradigestive manifestations of *Helicobacter pylori*. Acta Gastroenterol Belg 2000;63:388–392.

45 Strandberg TE, Tilvis RS, Vuoristo M, Lindroos M, Kosunen TU: Prospective study of *Helicobacter pylori* seropositivity and cardiovascular diseases in a general elderly population. BMJ 1997;314: 1317–1318.

46 Ossewaarde JM, Feskens EJ, De Vries A, Vallinga CE, Kromhout D: *Chlamydia pneumoniae* is a risk factor for coronary heart disease in symptom-free elderly men, but *Helicobacter pylori* and cytomegalovirus are not. Epidemiol Infect 1998;120:93–99.

47 Pilotto A, Rumor F, Franceschi M, Leandro G, Novello R, Soffiati G, Scagnelli M, Di Mario F, Valerio G: Lack of association between *Helicobacter pylori* infection and extracardiac atherosclerosis in dyspeptic elderly subjects. Age Ageing 1999;28:367–371.

48 Pilotto A, Fabrello R, Franceschi M, Scagnelli M, Soffiati F, Di Mario F, Fortunato A, Valerio G: *Helicobacter pylori* infection in asymptomatic elderly subjects living at home or in a nursing home: Effects on gastric function and nutritional status. Age Ageing 1996;25:245–249.

49 Regev A, Fraser GM, Braun M, Maoz E, Laibovici L, Niv Y: Seroprevalence of *Helicobacter pylori* and length of stay in a nursing home. Helicobacter 1999;4:89–93.

50 Bohmer CJ, Klinkenberg-Knol EC, Kuipers EJ, Niezen-de Boer MC, Schreuder H, Schuckink-Kool F, Meuwissen SG: The prevalence of *Helicobacter pylori* infection among employees of institutes for the intellectually disabled. Am J Gastroenterol 1997;92:1000–1004.

51 Neri MC, Lai L, Bonetti P, Baldassarri AR, Monti M, De Luca P, Cunietti E, Quatrini M: Prevalence of *Helicobacter pylori* infection in elderly inpatients and institutionalized old people: Correlation with nutritional status. Age Ageing 1996;25:17–21.

52 Peura DA: *Helicobacter pylori:* A diagnostic dilemma and a dilemma of diagnosis. Gastroenterology 1995;109:313–315.

53 Malfertheiner P, Leodolter A, Gerards C: Pitfalls in *Helicobacter pylori* diagnosis; in Hunt RH, Tytgat GNJ (eds): *Helicobacter pylori*. Basic Mechanisms to Clinical Cure 2000. Boston, Kluwer Academic, 2000, pp 123–133.

54 Faisal MA, Warren B, Samloff IM, Holt PR: *Helicobacter pylori* infection and atrophic gastritis in the elderly. Gastroenterology 1990;99:1543–1544.

55 Hackelsberger A, Gunther T, Schultze V, Peitz U, Malfertheiner P: Role of aging in the expression of *Helicobacter pylori* gastritis in the antrum, corpus and cardia. Scand J Gastroenterol 1999;34: 138–143.

56 Pilotto A: Helicobacter pylori infection in the elderly. Clin Geriatr 1996;4:53–70.

57 Abdalla AM, Sordillo EM, Hanzely Z, Perez-Perez GI, Blaser MJ, Holt PR, Moss SF: Insensitivity of the CLO test for *H. pylori*, especially in the elderly. Gastroenterology 1998;115: 243–244.

58 Malfertheiner P, Megraud F, O'Morain C, Hungin APS, Jones R, Axon A, Graham DY, Tytgat G: Current concepts in the management of *Helicobacter pylori* infection. The Maastricht 2-2000 Consensus Report. Aliment Pharmacol Ther 2002;16:167–180.

59 Pilotto A, Franceschi M, Leandro G, Rassu M, Zagari RM, Bozzola L, Furlan F, Bazzoli F, Di Mario F, Valerio G: Noninvasive diagnosis of *Helicobacter pylori* infection in older subjects: Comparison of the ^{13}C-urea breath test with serology. J Gerontol A Biol Sci Med Sci 2000;55: M163–M167.

60 Pilotto A, Franceschi M, Leandro G, Di Mario F, Soffiati G, Scagnelli M, Bozzola L, Fabrello R, Valerio G: The clinical usefulness of serum pepsinogens, specific IgG anti-Hp antibodies and gastrin for monitoring *Helicobacter pylori* treatment in older people. J Am Geriatr Soc 1996;44: 665–670.

61 Tsai CJ: *Helicobacter pylori* infection in elderly people. Does quantitative serological testing predict gastroduodenal ulcer disease? Dig Dis Sci 1999;44:96–101.

62 Shirin H, Bruck R, Kenet G, Krepel Z, Wardi Y, Reif S, Zaidel L, Geva D, Avni Y, Halpern Z: Evaluation of a new immunochromatographic test for *Helicobacter pylori* IgG antibodies in elderly symptomatic patients. J Gastroenterol 1999;34:7–10.

63 Vaira D, Malfertheiner P, Megraud F, Axon AT, Deltenre M, Hirschl AM, Gasbarrini G, O'Morain C, Garcia JM, Quina M, Tytgat GN: Diagnosis of *Helicobacter pylori* infection with a new noninvasive antigen-based assay. HpSA European study group. Lancet 1999;354:30–33.

64 Leodolter A, Agha-Amiri K, Peitz U, Gerards C, Ebert MP, Malfertheiner P: Validity of a *Helicobacter pylori* stool antigen assay for the assessment of *H. pylori* status following eradication therapy. Eur J Gastroenterol Hepatol 2001;13:673–676.

65 Pilotto A, Franceschi M, Furlan F, Bozzola L, Fucito L, Rassu M, Peron A, Valerio G, Scognelli M, Leandro G: The noninvasive diagnosis of *H. pylori* infection in geriatric subjects by the ^{13}C-urea breath test and the stool antigen test: The role of disability and cognitive status. Gut 2002;51(suppl 2):A108.

66 Reilly T, Poxon V, Sanders DSA, Elliott TSJ, Walt RP: Comparison of serum, salivary, and rapid whole blood test diagnostic tests for *Helicobacter pylori* and their validation against endoscopy based tests. Gut 1997;40:454–458.

67 Pilotto A, Di Mario F, Franceschi M: Treatment of *Helicobacter pylori* infection in elderly subjects. Age Ageing 2000;29:103–109.

68 Moshkowitz M, Brill S, Konikoff FM, Reif S, Arber N, Halpern Z: The efficacy of omeprazole-based short-term triple therapy in *Helicobacter pylori*-positive patients with dyspepsia. J Am Geriatr Soc 1999;47:720–722.

69 Pilotto A, Di Mario F, Franceschi M, Leandro G, Soffiati G, Scagnelli M, Bozzola L, Valerio G: Cure of *Helicobacter pylori* infection in the elderly: Effects of eradication on gastritis and serological markers. Aliment Pharmacol Ther 1996;10:1021–1027.

70 Pilotto A, Leandro G, Franceschi M, Rassu M, Bozzola L, Furlan F, Di Mario F, Valerio G: The effect of antibiotic resistance on the outcome of three 1-week triple therapies against *Helicobacter pylori*. Aliment Pharmacol Ther 1999;13:667–673.

71 Pilotto A, Di Mario F, Franceschi M, Dal Bò N, Bozzola L, Rassu M, Novello R: Efficacy of one-week triple therapies with low-dose rabeprazole and clarithromycin plus standard-dose amoxicillin or tinidazole for the cure of *H. pylori* infection in elderly patients. Gut 2001;49(suppl 2):A95.

72 Pilotto A: Helicobacter pylori-associated peptic ulcer disease in older patients: Current management strategies. Drugs Aging 2001;18:487–494.

73 Pilotto A, Franceschi M, Leandro G, Bozzola L, Rassu M, Soffiati G, Di Mario F, Valerio G: Cure of *Helicobacter pylori* infection in elderly patients: Comparison of low versus high doses of clarithromycin in combination with amoxicillin and pantoprazole. Aliment Pharmacol Ther 2001;15:1031–1036.

74 Huang JQ, Hunt RH: The importance of clarithromycin dose in the management of *Helicobacter pylori* infection: A meta-analysis of triple therapies with a proton pump inhibitor, clarithromycin and amoxycillin or metronidazole. Aliment Pharmacol Ther 1999;13:719–729.

75 Ammon S, Treiber G, Kes F, Klotz U: Influence of age on the steady state disposition of drugs commonly used for the eradication of *Helicobacter pylori*. Aliment Pharmacol Ther 2000;14:759–766.

76 Perri F, Villani MR, Festa V, Quitadamo M, Andriulli A: Predictors of failure of *Helicobacter pylori* eradication with the standard 'Maastricht triple therapy'. Aliment Pharmacol Ther 2001;15:1023–1029.

77 Treiber G, Wittig J, Ammon S, Walker S, van Doorn LJ, Klotz U: Clinical outcome and influencing factors of a new short-term quadruple therapy for *Helicobacter pylori* eradication: A randomized controlled trial (MACLOR study). Arch Intern Med 2002;162:153–160.

78 Gisbert JP, Marcos S, Gisbert JL, Pajares JM: *Helicobacter pylori* eradication therapy is more effective in peptic ulcer than in non-ulcer dyspepsia. Eur J Gastroenterol Hepatol 2001;13:1303–1307.

79 Rudi J, Reuther S, Sieg A, Hoerner M, Stremmel W: Relevance of underlying disease and bacterial vacA and cagA status on the efficacy of *Helicobacter pylori* eradication. Digestion 2002;65:11–15.

80 Baena JM, Lopez C, Hidalgo A, Rams F, Jimenez S, Garcia M, Hernandez MR: Relation between alcohol consumption and the success of *Helicobacter pylori* eradication therapy using omeprazole, clarithromycin and amoxicillin for 1 week. Eur J Gastroenterol Hepatol 2002;14:291–296.

81 Dorè MP, Leandro G, Realdi G, Sepulveda AR, Graham DY: Effect of pretreatment antibiotic resistance to metronidazole and clarithromycin on outcome of *Helicobacter pylori* therapy: A meta-analytical approach. Dig Dis Sci 2000;45:68–76.

82 Megraud F: Resistance of *Helicobacter pylori* to antibiotics: The main limitation of current proton pump inhibitor triple therapy. Eur J Gastroenterol Hepatol 1999;11(suppl 2):S35–S37.

---

83   Pilotto A, Rassu M, Leandro G, Franceschi M, Di Mario F: Prevalence of *Helicobacter pylori* resistance to antibiotics in Northeast Italy: A multicentre study. GISU. Interdisciplinary Group for the Study of Ulcer. Dig Liver Dis 2000;32:763–768.

84   Pilotto A, Di Mario F, Malfertheiner P, Valerio G, Naccarato R: Upper gastrointestinal diseases in the elderly: Report of a meeting held at Vicenza, Italy, on 20 March 1998. Eur J Gastroenterol Hepatol 1999;11:801–808.

85   Parsons HK, Carter MJ, Sanders DS, Winstanley T, Lobo AJ: *Helicobacter pylori* antimicrobial resistance in the United Kingdom: The effect of age, sex and socio-economic status. Aliment Pharmacol Ther 2001;15:1473–1478.

86   Meyer JM, Silliman NP, Wang W, Siepman NY, Sugg JE, Morris D, Zhang J, Bhattacharyya H, King EC, Hopkins RJ: Risk factors for *Helicobacter pylori* resistance in the United States: The surveillance of *H. pylori* antimicrobial resistance partnership (SHARP) study, 1993–1999. Ann Intern Med 2002;136:13–24.

87   Pilotto A, Franceschi M, Rassu M, Leandro G, Bozzola L, Furlan F, Di Mario F: Incidence of secondary *Helicobacter pylori* resistance to antibiotics in treatment failures after 1-week proton pump inhibitor-based triple therapies: A prospective study. Dig Liver Dis 2000;32:667–672.

88   Grove DI, Koutsouridis G: Increasing resistance of *Helicobacter pylori* to clarithromycin: Is the horse bolting? Pathology 2002;34:71–73.

89   Ecclissato C, Marchioretto MA, Mendonca S, Godoy AP, Guersoni RA, Deguer M, Piovesan H, Ferraz JG, Pedrazzoli J: Increased primary resistance to recommended antibiotics negatively affects *Helicobacter pylori* eradication. Helicobacter 2002;7:53–59.

90   Megraud F, Doerman HP: Clinical relevance of resistant strains of *Helicobacter pylori:* A review of current data. Gut 1998;43:S61–S65.

91   Qasim A, O'Morain C: Treatment of *Helicobacter pylori* infection and factors influencing eradication. Aliment Pharmacol Ther 2002;16(suppl 1):24–30.

92   Perez E, Schroder-Bernhardi D, Dietlein G: Treatment behaviour of doctors regarding *Helicobacter pylori* infections. Int J Clin Pharmacol Ther 2002;40:126–129.

93   Lee M, Kemp JA, Canning A, Enag C, Tataronis G, Farraye FA: A randomized controlled trial of an enhanced patient compliance program for *Helicobacter pylori* therapy. Arch Intern Med 1999;159:2312–2319.

94   Al-Eidan FA, McElnay JC, Scott MG, McConnell JB: Management of *Helicobacter pylori* eradication: The influence of structured counselling and follow-up. Br J Clin Pharmacol 2002;53:163–171.

95   Pilotto A, Malfertheiner P: An approach to *Helicobacter pylori* infection in the elderly. Aliment Pharmacol Ther 2002;16:683–691.

Alberto Pilotto, Unità Operativa di Geriatria,
Ospedale 'Casa Sollievo della Sofferenza', IRCCS, I–71013 San Giovanni Rotondo (FG) (Italy)
Tel. +39 0882 410271, E-Mail alberto.pilotto@libero.it

Pilotto A, Malfertheiner P, Holt PR (eds): Aging and the Gastrointestinal Tract.
Interdiscipl Top Gerontol. Basel, Karger, 2003, vol 32, pp 145–156

······················

Gastric Cancer in the Elderly

Alastair McKinlay[a,b]*, Ken Park*[c]*, Rohan Gunasekera*[d]*,
Emad M. El-Omar*[a,b]

[a]Gastrointestinal Unit and Departments of [b]Medicine and Therapeutics and
[c]Surgery, Aberdeen University and Aberdeen Royal Infirmary, Aberdeen,
Scotland, and [d]Academic Unit of Surgery, University of Liverpool,
Clinical Sciences Centre, University Hospital, Liverpool, UK

Introduction

Gastric cancer remains a major health problem, with an estimated 21,700 new diagnoses in the US in 2001 and 12,800 patients expected to die in the same year [1]. On a global scale, gastric cancer remains the world's second commonest malignancy, having only been overtaken by lung cancer in the late 1980s [2]. The risk of gastric cancer is strongly related to age. The median age of patients presenting with this cancer is around 72 years, and since the early 1990s, one quarter of newly diagnosed gastric cancer patients are over 80 years of age [3]. A high proportion of these patients present with co-morbid disease that limits their treatment options. Despite significant advances in the understanding of the aetiology and pathogenesis of gastric cancer, the mortality rate remains depressingly high and no more than 10% of patients will be alive at 5 years [4].

Epidemiology

The incidence of gastric cancer shows marked worldwide variation. Cancer death rates of <10 per 100,000 are found in northern European countries, North America, Australia and New Zealand. Moreover, the incidence has shown a substantial and continuing decline since the 1940s. Intermediate death rates of 10–20 per 100,000 are found in southern Europe and the Middle East.

Age-adjusted death rates of 20–30 per 100,000 have been reported from South America, India and Eastern Europe whilst the highest rates of >30 per 100,000 are found in Russia, China and Japan [5]. The situation in Japan is particularly interesting because whilst the incidence is falling, it remains much higher than in other Western economies, suggesting that particular genetic or environmental factors must be involved.

Classification

Adenocarcinoma makes up 90% of malignant gastric tumours, with lymphoma accounting for a further 5% [6]. The Lauren classification is traditionally used to divide adenocarcinoma into an intestinal form, where the malignant cells form a glandular-like structure, and a diffuse form, where the cells infiltrate through the wall of the stomach with relatively little disturbance of the mucosa itself, making endoscopic diagnosis more difficult. It may, however, be more relevant to classify tumours on the basis of their location within the upper gastrointestinal tract, as tumours in different locations display a remarkable divergence in their incidence and epidemiologic features. Thus, distal gastric adenocarcinoma is commoner in Afro-Asian populations and seems to be declining in incidence worldwide, but particularly in Western countries, while carcinoma of the cardia and fundus (proximal cancers) are more common in Caucasians and their incidence is rising at an alarming rate [7].

Presentation

The introduction of mass screening programs in Japan in the 1960s has allowed the detection of very early lesions in which the tumour is limited to the mucosa and submucosa. Eighty percent of patients with early gastric cancer are asymptomatic. Ten percent have peptic ulcer symptoms and there are a number of other non-specific features such as nausea, anorexia or early satiety. A symptomatic presentation is almost by definition indicative of advanced stage, and unfortunately this is the usual mode of presentation in the West. In Western countries, the commonest presenting symptoms are weight loss followed by abdominal pain, nausea and vomiting, anorexia and dysphagia. Most of these symptoms are non-specific and are very common in elderly patients for other reasons. As a result, late presentation is a particular problem in older patients, and detection requires a high level of suspicion.

In some studies, 40% of patients will have had symptoms for <3 months but 60% will have been symptomatic for 3 months or longer and up to 20% for over 1 year. The late presentation of the disease probably explains why its prognosis remains so dismal, with only 10% of patients still alive at 5 years.

The clinical manifestations also depend critically on the anatomical location of the tumour. Large tumours in the fundus and body may simply manifest with occult blood loss. In contrast, tumours of the antrum will delay gastric emptying and lead to early satiety, anorexia and eventually the features of gastric outlet obstruction. Tumours of the proximal stomach may involve the distal oesophagus and present with dysphagia. What is often more surprising, however, is the considerable size gastric tumours may reach before becoming symptomatic.

As might be anticipated, presentation with local or distant metastatic disease is frequent. Local spread is usually to local and regional nodes, but occasionally lymphatic spread will involve more distant nodes such as the supraclavicular (Virchow's) node or the rare umbilical (Sister Mary Joseph) node. More advanced local spread may involve the omentum, pancreas and even the transverse colon. In advanced gastric cancer, up to 90% of patients have local spread, and this can make radical resection a formidable undertaking, particularly in elderly malnourished patients. Distant spread to the liver, lungs and bone is very common, but peritoneal spread and malignant ascites can also occur.

Aetiology

Although many of the known associations have been described for years, a clear understanding of their interaction has been lacking until recently. Pernicious anaemia with its hallmark of atrophic gastritis has long been known to confer an increased risk of gastric cancer. Similarly, it is well established that benign ulcer surgery, such as partial gastrectomy, is also associated with gastric cancer, with a lead-in time of 15–30 years [8, 9]. Following gastric surgery, inflammation of the gastric remnant is common and usually associated with the reflux of bile. Some authors recognise this 'chemical' gastritis as an entity distinct from the autoimmune atrophic gastritis of pernicious anaemia. Although the histological appearances are different, both pernicious anaemia and the surgical stomach share a common pathophysiological abnormality, namely hypochlorhydria.

The discovery of *Helicobacter pylori* by Marshall and Warren in 1983 was a turning point in gastroenterology. Its causative role in peptic ulcer disease was soon recognised and extensively studied, but the link with gastric cancer lagged almost a decade behind. The main reason for this was the fact that unlike the situation in benign ulcer disease, the organism was often absent from pathological specimens of neoplastic tissue. It is now clear that *H. pylori* infection induces, in genetically predisposed hosts [10, 11], a cascade of events that could ultimately lead to gastric neoplasia. The key pathophysiological events include the onset of gastric atrophy and hypochlorhydria. The increased proliferation induced by inflammation creates a genetically unstable gastric mucosa, which is further compromised by the presence of genotoxic substances generated by inflammatory and bacterial products. The hypochlorhydria contributes to bacterial overgrowth, which further exacerbates the inflammation and leads to the generation of carcinogenic nitrogenous products. Diets that are high in salt content and lacking in fresh fruits and vegetables are likely to contribute to the malignant transformation. Elderly patients have a much higher prevalence of *H. pylori* infection, and those who are infected develop a gradual decline in gastric acid secretory function, which is induced by the chronic gastritis and atrophy. In the presence of other environmental factors such as poor diet and smoking, the neoplastic process is accelerated.

Diagnosis

Diagnosis of gastric cancer is frequently straightforward, particularly in advanced cases, but may require a high index of suspicion, and a careful history and examination are therefore essential. Whilst the presence of weight loss, a sucussion splash or a mass in the epigastrium are clearly suggestive of gastric cancer, no single presentation is unique to the disease. More typically, the history may be non-specific, with loss of appetite, weight loss, abdominal pain and other vague symptoms. Physical examination is frequently unrewarding even in advanced gastric cancer.

A hypochromic, microcytic anaemia is a common finding, and the faecal occult blood test may be positive, although again this does not localise the source of blood loss and is rarely diagnostic on its own. The liver function tests may be deranged in advanced disease, and both the C-reactive protein and erythrocyte sedimentation rate may be elevated, but all of these findings can occur in other contexts, particularly in elderly patients. For these reasons, some form of examination of the upper gastrointestinal tract is indicated if gastric carcinoma is suspected.

Endoscopy
Upper gastrointestinal endoscopy has been shown to be more accurate than barium radiology in the diagnosis of gastric cancer. The procedure is generally well tolerated in the elderly, although complications can occur, particularly in patients with co-morbid disease [12]. The results from retrospective studies

typically quote a significant complication rate of 1 in 1,000 procedures, with a mortality rate of 1 in 10,000 [13].

The principle advantage of endoscopy is its ability to allow close inspection of the mucosa, which is generally the only circumstance under which early gastric carcinoma is found, but more importantly to allow biopsy and a firm histological diagnosis to be made. Gastric carcinoma is usually obvious at endoscopy, either due to gross distortion of the stomach or the presence of an obvious polypoid mass. Certain presentations are more difficult. Firstly, it is well recognised that gastric cancer can present as a typical gastric ulcer. For this reason, gastric ulcers should always be biopsied unless there are obvious contra-indications. It is also good practice to follow gastric ulceration to healing, with repeated biopsy if required, as acid-suppressing drugs such as H_2 blockers or proton pump inhibitors can produce temporary healing of malignant ulcers. Finally, non-steroidal anti-inflammatory drugs, which are frequently prescribed in the elderly, can produce large malignant-looking ulcers.

Diffuse gastric carcinoma presenting as a 'leather bottle' stomach may also be difficult to diagnose at endoscopy. The gastric mucosa itself may not appear particularly abnormal, but an experienced endoscopist may become aware of a different 'feel' to the stomach or a failure to produce normal inflation. Mucosal biopsies may not be diagnostic because the carcinoma is infiltrative. Under these circumstances, a double-contrast barium meal demonstrating abnormal motility or CT scanning confirming a thickened wall may be helpful.

Finally, examination of the post-operative stomach may present particular difficulties. As previously indicated, surgery for benign ulcer disease was a common operation until the late 1960s, when H_2 blockers became available. The cohort of patients who received surgery has now aged, and with the typical lead-in time for gastric carcinoma being 30 years, malignancy may not appear until the 7th or 8th decade.

A variety of procedures were in common use, including antrectomy and gastroenterostomy (Polya gastrectomy), antrectomy and primary anastomosis (Billroth I partial gastrectomy), vagotomy and pyloroplasty, and vagotomy and gastroenterostomy. Achieving adequate inflation of the stomach in patients with a gastroenterostomy may be difficult. In addition, bile reflux gastritis is common and may produce a fragile and mottled mucosa. The appearance of cancer around the margins of a gastroenterostomy may, therefore, be difficult to determine and requires particular vigilance.

Multiple biopsies are essential for diagnosis. As mentioned previously, gastric atrophy and intestinal metaplasia are common findings in elderly patients. The presence of high-grade dysplasia, however, should always be regarded as significant because it may indicate a high risk of malignant transformation or it may reflect the presence of adjacent malignancy.

Radiology
Barium Studies
The double-contrast barium meal was for many years the mainstay of diagnosis in gastric cancer. Typically, the patient ingests barium with a 'gassing' agent to produce distension of the stomach. The procedure is usually well tolerated and can be useful in older patients who are felt to be unfit for endoscopy. It should, however, be borne in mind that a patient who is unfit for endoscopy is unlikely to be fit for major surgery, and in the very frail, even the diagnosis of gastric cancer may be academic.

Some patients find it difficult to retain gas and double-contrast barium meals can be difficult to interpret without adequate inflation of the stomach. Similarly, an abnormality detected on barium examination usually requires endoscopic examination to confirm the presence of gastric cancer. Thus, whilst a barium meal may seem an attractive alternative in a very frail patient, it may not always provide a definitive answer.

The barium meal can be a useful alternative to endoscopy if there is no ready access to endoscopy. It may also help to define the extent of a tumour, although this can also be determined by endoscopy, and most patients being considered for surgery will undergo more advanced staging techniques such as CT scanning. The role of the barium meal has, therefore, become less important in the diagnosis of gastric carcinoma, particularly with the wide availability of upper gastrointestinal endoscopy.

Techniques for Staging and Pre-Operative Assessment
Gastric cancer is sometimes diagnosed at routine abdominal ultrasound scan if a thickened gastric wall is noted. Typically, however, the stomach is not distended at the time of ultrasonography, and gastric wall thickness may not be easy to determine. Ultrasonography is useful for assessing the spread of gastric carcinoma. It may detect evidence of lymphadenopathy but can be particularly valuable in detecting metastases within the liver.

Ready availability of CT scanning now makes its use almost routine in the assessment of patients with gastric carcinoma, particularly if surgery is being considered. CT scanning is particularly useful for picking up pulmonary and hepatic metastases, although it cannot detect lesions less than 5 mm in size. Most gastric tumours produce wall thickening that is usually readily apparent on CT examination. It may also help to determine the presence of lymph nodes, although distinguishing reactive nodes from local spread can be difficult. CT scanning may also detect peritoneal seeding, omental involvement and spread to the ovaries and rectal shelf. Some studies have suggested 90% accuracy of CT in detecting distant metastases. However, up to 50% of gastric tumours are under-staged and a further 15% may be over-staged by CT scanning.

More recent technical advances have allowed ultrasound probes to be mounted directly onto the tip of endoscopes. Both radial and linear rays are available, and whilst radial scanning is more commonly available, linear rays allow targeted biopsy, which can be useful [14]. A number of studies suggest that endoscopic ultrasound has an accuracy of 90% in defining the depth of invasion within the stomach itself. It is also sensitive to wall thickening and will pick up diffuse carcinomas, and it may allow the identification of regional lymph nodes [15]. In many areas, however, the availability of endoscopic ultrasound is still limited.

In patients where a radical surgical resection is contemplated, some surgeons will use laparoscopic visualisation and even laparoscopic ultrasonography to search for local and peritoneal spread. Once again, however, the use of advanced techniques to stage gastric carcinoma should be considered in the light of the patient's overall fitness. Whilst it may be clinically relevant to produce a definitive diagnosis of gastric cancer in a frail elderly patient because of its important implications for life expectancy and the need for palliative care, detailed staging techniques should probably be reserved for patients where definitive surgery seems a real prospect. It may, therefore, be equally valid to carry out pulmonary function and cardiac tests to determine the patient's fitness for surgery before initiating invasive and potentially uncomfortable staging tests. Similarly, in elderly patients where it is clear that only palliative therapy will be possible, it is advisable to move directly to the appropriate surgery with minimum delay rather than put the patient through extensive staging investigations.

Management of Gastric Cancer

Surgery

Patients with early gastric tumours may be cured by appropriate treatment, whereas patients with more advanced disease will have a limited life expectancy and treatment must be aimed at providing good-quality symptom relief. Although surgical resection remains the only proven method of providing long-term survival in patients with gastric cancer, it is only likely to be effective if a complete macro- and microscopic clearance of the tumour is possible (R_0 resection).

In patients with very early tumours of the stomach, alternatives to resection have been proposed, including laser ablation, photodynamic therapy and endoscopic mucosal resection (EMR) [16]. Clearly, such treatments avoid both the immediate and long-term morbidity associated with surgery but can only be recommended if they are effective in disease control. For tumours limited to the gastric mucosa, it would appear that the incidence of lymphatic spread is minimal; accordingly, mucosal techniques are likely to be effective. As tumours invade into the submucosa, the incidence of lymphatic spread increases and mucosal ablative techniques are unlikely to achieve clearance of the disease. Unfortunately, currently available imaging techniques are unable to differentiate between mucosal and submucosal tumours, and we have thus adopted diagnostic EMR; i.e., in patients with endoscopic early tumours, an EMR is performed and the pathologist is asked to comment specifically on the depth of invasion and the lateral excision margins. If there is evidence of submucosal invasion, a formal resection is performed, whereas in patients with mucosal disease, a policy of regular endoscopic surveillance is undertaken and this is often combined with ablation of the surrounding mucosa. Care must be taken to ensure that the specimen is correctly orientated for the pathologist and that excess diathermy is avoided as this may make histological interpretation difficult. Lesions that are ulcerated pose particular problems with infiltration and may also be difficult for the pathologist to interpret; furthermore, some reports have indicated that such lesions may metastasise early to regional lymph nodes. Accordingly, we would tend not to recommend EMR in such tumours.

In Western countries, the majority of stomach tumours coming to surgery are not suitable for EMR. In such cases, perhaps the area of greatest controversy for surgeons is the extent of lymphadenectomy that is required to obtain tumour clearance: local (D1) versus extended systemic dissection (D2). The advocates of D2 dissection argue that such an approach provides better local control and allows a more accurate determination of the tumour stage and therefore prognosis, whereas those opposed to this approach argue that the excess morbidity associated with a longer and more involved operation is not justified by any tangible benefit to the individual patient [17, 18].

Outcome of Gastric Cancer Surgery in the Elderly in the UK:
The ASCOT Project

The ASCOT project is a multicentre prospective database for gastro-oesophageal cancer surgery [19]. It was initiated in 1999 and aims to collect detailed prospective data on co-morbidity, surgery, stage and outcome in a large cohort of patients from a wide variety of hospitals in the UK. It was designed to audit the practice of 32 centres in the UK and to allow comparison of performance by appropriate risk stratification. The accumulation of a large representative data set permits detailed study of particular subgroups; we took the opportunity to examine the outcome of gastric cancer surgery in elderly patients compared to the rest and present some interesting preliminary data. The patients were aged between 34 and 94 years (median 65.5 years). The overall mortality rate was 15.5%. Table 1 shows the number of patients in the

Table 1. Mortality rates from gastric cancer surgery in the different age groups

Age, years	Number of patients	Mortality rate, %
<70	109 (41.3)	12.8
70–79	111 (42.0)	17.1
>80	44 (16.7)	18.2

Figures in parentheses represent percentages.

Table 2. Mortality rates from gastric cancer surgery stratified on the basis of ASA status

Age, years	Mortality rate, %	
	ASA I and II	ASA III and IV
<70	10.5	20.8
70–79	10.6	25.6
>80	15.8	45.5

Overall ASA distribution was as follows: ASA I = 17%; ASA II = 49%; ASA III = 31%; ASA IV = 3%.

age categories <70, 70–79 and >80 years and the overall mortality rates by age. Table 2 shows the mortality rates for the different age groups stratified on the basis of their pre-operative American Society of Anesthesiology (ASA) status. As might be expected, the mortality rate associated with gastric cancer surgery is heavily dependent on the pre-operative condition of patients of all ages, and this is particularly the case in patients aged over 80 years. These results echo findings in other elderly populations [20, 21].

Chemotherapy

The low survival associated with gastric cancer has prompted investigation into post-operative (adjuvant) chemotherapy and pre-operative (neo-adjuvant) treatment. In patients with gastric cancer, there is no evidence that either adjuvant or neo-adjuvant chemotherapy is of value in patients in whom a complete surgical resection is possible. The consensus seems to be that the use of either pre-operative or post-operative chemotherapy in gastric cancer, even in young patients, cannot be justified outside the context of trials. In the case of elderly patients, even greater caution should be exercised. The elderly are more likely to have cardiac and renal disease and are therefore less likely to tolerate chemotherapy well and have a greater risk of side effects. Adjuvant chemotherapy would therefore have to show significant survival benefit to offset days lost due to toxicity or time in hospital, and in reality, chemotherapy is rarely a viable option in patients over the age of 75.

Palliative Therapy

The majority of elderly patients present with late gastric cancer at an advanced stage. Most will not be amenable to curative surgical resection and the issue of palliation is therefore very important. The principal complications of late gastric cancer can be divided into local and distant problems. Distal tumours involving the antrum frequently progress to outlet obstruction. In some patients, this will be due to physical stenosis of the pylorus, while in others, gradual infiltration of the antrum leads to loss of functionality and the failure of gastric emptying. Medical treatment of outlet obstruction with prokinetics is usually unhelpful. The symptoms are usually unpleasant, with vomiting, regurgitation and reflux and rapid nutritional failure. Because of this, palliative surgical therapy is often justified and options include antrectomy or, more usually, the formation of a gastroenterostomy to relieve obstruction. Alternative approaches may include laser of more localised lesions or, under certain circumstances, the placement of a venting gastrostomy to allow gastric contents to be drained externally. Patients with large tumours may also develop dysphagia if the distal oesophagus is involved. This complication is usually amenable to stenting or sometimes to laser therapy.

Large tumours frequently bleed and result in chronic blood loss. Patients with advanced gastric carcinoma may therefore develop chronic iron deficiency anaemia. This may on occasion again warrant consideration of surgery, although the difficulties of performing surgery in frail elderly patients should not be underestimated. Another alternative is to try to shrink the tumour using a neodymium YAG laser, but in the authors' experience, laser therapy purely to reduce blood loss is usually disappointing.

Most patients with advanced gastric cancer develop nutritional problems and weight loss is almost invariable. Extensive infiltration alters the compliance of the stomach and frequently leads to sensations of early satiety and loss of appetite. In addition, advanced gastric cancer frequently leads to profound metabolic effects such as cachexia and loss of muscle bulk. Some patients may be amenable to naso-gastric feeding, but this is unusual because infiltration of the stomach usually prevents it from emptying normally and enteral support may be less well tolerated. Parenteral support is frequently required post-operatively, but is rarely used long-term in the United Kingdom. There is no evidence, however, that parenteral feeding improves survival. It is possible that it might improve quality of life, but there are no good data to support this. Finally, the difficulty of home parenteral feeding in the elderly should not be underestimated.

Local spread of gastric cancer is usually via the lymph nodes, but can occur by direct infiltration into all the surrounding organs. Many patients will experience pain. Some patients may benefit from radiotherapy, but adenocarcinoma is frequently not radiosensitive. The role of hospices and organised palliative care and pain teams is extremely important in improving the comfort of patients. Finally, distant metastases to the liver and lung are usually associated with short survival times. In elderly patients with distant spread, very little direct treatment is usually available and the prognosis is usually measured in months.

Conclusions

Gastric cancer is an important disease in elderly patients. The incidence of gastric cancer in industrialised countries is falling, but it remains a common cancer and despite improved surgery and the use of adjuvant therapies there has been virtually no improvement in survival. In many less developed countries, gastric cancer remains extremely common and often affects younger people. In developed countries, however, changes in the epidemiology of *H. pylori* infection and an ageing cohort of patients with previous gastric surgery mean that the disease is increasingly found in the elderly. Diagnosis requires a high index of clinical suspicion. In Europe and North America, unlike Japan, early gastric cancer is usually a chance finding, presentation is frequently late and the symptoms and signs are non-specific.

In terms of treating elderly patients with gastric cancer, it is clear that age in itself is not a contraindication to aggressive treatment, including curative surgery, provided the operative risk defined by the co-morbid assessment is favourable. While aggressive treatment such as surgery may not improve survival, it may provide good palliation and a better quality of life at the risk of considerable operative mortality. Less aggressive palliative therapy may avoid unpleasant surgery and chemotherapy, but runs the risk of leaving the patient with unpleasant complications and the final stages of the disease that may be difficult to treat.

References

1   Greenlee RT, Murray T, Bolden S, Wingo PA: Cancer statistics, 2000. CA Cancer J Clin 2000;50: 7–33.
2   Parkin DM, Pisani P, Ferlay J: Estimates of the worldwide incidence of 25 major cancers in 1990. Int J Cancer 1999;80:827–841.

3   Kranenbarg EK, van de Velde CJ: Gastric cancer in the elderly. Eur J Surg Oncol 1998;24: 384–390.
4   Bray F, Sankila R, Ferlay J, Parkin DM: Estimates of cancer incidence and mortality in Europe in 1995. Eur J Cancer 2002;38:99–166.
5   Parkin DM, Bray F, Ferlay J, Pisani P: Estimating the world cancer burden: Globocan 2000. Int J Cancer 2001;94:153–156.
6   Koh TJ, Wang TC: Tumors of the stomach; in Feldman M, Friedman LS, Sleisenger MF (eds): Sleisenger and Fordtran's Gastrointestinal and Liver Disease. Philadelphia, WB Saunders, 2002, pp 829–855.
7   El Serag HB, Mason AC, Petersen N, Key CR: Epidemiological differences between adenocarcinoma of the oesophagus and adenocarcinoma of the gastric cardia in the USA. Gut 2002;50: 368–372.
8   Safatle-Ribeiro AV, Ribeiro U Jr, Reynolds JC: Gastric stump cancer: What is the risk? Dig Dis 1998;16:159–168.
9   Tersmette AC, Giardiello FM, Tytgat GN, Offerhaus GJ: Carcinogenesis after remote peptic ulcer surgery: The long-term prognosis of partial gastrectomy. Scand J Gastroenterol Suppl 1995;212: 96–99.
10   El-Omar EM, Carrington M, Chow WH, McColl KE, Bream JH, Young HA, Herrera J, Lissowska J, Yuan CC, Rothman N, Lanyon G, Martin M, Fraumeni JF Jr, Rabkin CS: Interleukin-1 polymorphisms associated with increased risk of gastric cancer. Nature 2000;404:398–402.
11   El Omar EM, Chow WH, Rabkin CS: Gastric cancer and H. pylori: Host genetics open the way. Gastroenterology 2001;121:1002–1004.
12   Lockhart SP, Schofield PM, Gribble RJ, Baron JH: Upper gastrointestinal endoscopy in the elderly. Br Med J (Clin Res Ed) 1985;290:283.
13   Cotton PB, Williams CB: Practical Gastrointestinal Endoscopy. Oxford, Blackwell Scientific, 1996.
14   Ziegler K, Sanft C, Zimmer T, Zeitz M, Felsenberg D, Stein H, Germer C, Deutschmann C, Riecken EO: Comparison of computed tomography, endosonography, and intraoperative assessment in TN staging of gastric carcinoma. Gut 1993;34:604–610.
15   Kelly S, Harris KM, Berry E, Hutton J, Roderick P, Cullingworth J, Gathercole L, Smith MA: A systematic review of the staging performance of endoscopic ultrasound in gastro-oesophageal carcinoma. Gut 2001;49:534–539.
16   Ono H, Kondo H, Gotoda T, Shirao K, Yamaguchi H, Saito D, Hosokawa K, Shimoda T, Yoshida S: Endoscopic mucosal resection for treatment of early gastric cancer. Gut 2001;48:225–229.
17   Bonenkamp JJ, Hermans J, Sasako M, van de Velde CJ: Extended lymph-node dissection for gastric cancer. Dutch Gastric Cancer Group. N Engl J Med 1999;340:908–914.
18   Cuschieri A, Weeden S, Fielding J, Bancewicz J, Craven J, Joypaul V, Sydes M, Fayers P: Patient survival after D1 and D2 resections for gastric cancer: Long-term results of the MRC randomized surgical trial. Surgical Co-operative Group. Br J Cancer 1999;79:1522–1530.
19   Cummins J, McCulloch P: ASCOT: A comprehensive clinical database for gastro-oesophageal cancer surgery. Eur J Surg Oncol 2001;27:709–713.
20   Kitamura K, Sugimachi K, Saku M: Evaluation of surgical treatment for patients with gastric cancer who are over 80 years of age. Hepatogastroenterology 1999;46:2074–2080.
21   Roviello F, Marrelli D, De Stefano A, Messano A, Pinto E, Carli A: Complications after surgery for gastric cancer in patients aged 80 years and over. Jpn J Clin Oncol 1998;28:116–122.

Professor Emad M. El-Omar
Department of Medicine and Therapeutics,
Polwarth Building, Foresterhill, Aberdeen AB25 2ZD, Scotland (UK)
Tel. +44 1224 553021/554578, Fax +44 1224 554761, E-Mail e.el-omar@abdn.ac.uk

Pilotto A, Malfertheiner P, Holt PR (eds): Aging and the Gastrointestinal Tract.
Interdiscipl Top Gerontol. Basel, Karger, 2003, vol 32, pp 157–166

· ·

The Pancreas and Aging

Gianpiero Manes[a], *Peter Malfertheiner*[b]

[a] Department of Gastroenterology, Ospedale A. Cardarelli, Naples, Italy;
[b] Department of Gastroenterology, Hepatology and Infectious Disease,
Otto-von-Guericke University of Magdeburg, Magdeburg, Germany

Introduction

With improvement in health care, living standards and socioeconomic status, more adults are living to old age. As the population ages, it is increasingly important to identify the factors which might impact on the nutritional status and thus the health status of the elderly. To guarantee an adequate nutritional status, it is important to understand how aging affects the digestive system in order to allow appropriate interventions in the case of digestive functional impairment.

The pancreas has a central role in the digestive process due to the production of essential digestive enzymes and bicarbonate. Astonishingly, the gastrointestinal tract, and the pancreas as well, undergo few clinically apparent changes with aging. The relative preservation of the complex gastrointestinal functions with aging is likely due to the large reserve capacity of this organ system.

This article will evaluate the structural, morphological and functional changes of the exocrine pancreas occurring in the elderly, as well as the peculiarities of exocrine pancreatic diseases, i.e. acute and chronic pancreatitis and pancreatic cancer, in aging adults.

Structural Changes of the Pancreas

Investigations conducted in animals showed us that with advancing age, the pancreas undergoes alterations, such as atrophy, fibrosis and fatty infiltration [1]. Similarly, in 112 unselected autopsies of adults without clinical manifestation of pancreatic disease, an increase in lipomatosis, fibrosis and both ductal and ductal epithelial alterations was observed in old age [2]; these morphological alterations were accompanied by a steady decrease in the mean weight of the gland, starting at the age of about 40 years. A further finding of this study was that severe generalized atherosclerosis was correlated with the presence of lipomatosis and fibrosis [2]. Other changes reported in the elderly are a pancreas of smaller size and an increase in the duct diameter [3]. At the microscopic level, the pancreatic ducts may show epithelial hyperplasia, periductular fibrosis and cystic widening [4]. All these changes increase with age, both in frequency and intensity, and usually appear after the age of 50 [4].

Several studies based on imaging, i.e. computed tomography (CT) [5], ERCP [6] and ultrasonography (US) [7, 8], have identified a series of structural alterations. Of particular note is a Japanese study that evaluated the parenchymal perfusion of the normal pancreas using dynamic CT in correlation with the patients' demographic characteristics [9]. The authors reported that the pancreas perfusion, ranging from 0.554 to 1.698 ml $\cdot$ min^{-1} $\cdot$ ml^{-1}, decreased with the patients' age. They attributed this to the increasing atrophy of the exocrine pancreas. Conversely, an increase in the fatty tissue with age was unlikely to be the cause of the reduced perfusion, as pancreatic parenchymal density measured before the injection of contrast material did not correlate with the perfusion measured by dynamic CT nor with age [9].

Changes in Pancreatic Function

Over the years, gastroenterologists have assumed that gastrointestinal function declines with age. However, this assumption did not stand the test of a rigorous scientific investigation [10].

In animal studies, it was shown that pancreatic function was diminished in older rats as compared with younger animals [11]. In particular, in the basal condition, enzymes and protein concentrations in pancreatic tissue were not significantly different in the two age groups. Interestingly, after 7 days of a diet enriched with fat or starch, lipase and amylase concentrations increased by about 25% in young, but not in aging rats. The authors concluded that aging induces modest changes in pancreatic digestive enzymes which are unlikely to be physiologically important, but the pancreas of aging rats does not adapt to changes in dietary intake as well as that of young rats [11]. The same conclusion is drawn from studies conducted in humans. In older humans, pancreatic secretion is not diminished upon initial stimulation with either secretin or cholecystokinin [12, 13]. This was demonstrated by Gullo et al. using either a secretin-cerulein test [12] or a tubeless, noninvasive pancreatic function test such as the pancreolauryl test [13]. However, upon repeated stimulation, pancreatic secretion drops significantly in older persons as compared with younger control individuals [14]. Thus, it appears that in the elderly, the pancreas might be able to function well under unstressed conditions. This was confirmed in a more recent study by Arora et al. [10] which showed that fat malabsorption did not occur in elderly humans up to the age of 91 years; 24-hour fecal fat excretion on a diet of 100 g fat/day was found to be 2.8 g for both age groups of 19–44 and 70–91 years. However, in a Swedish study, it was found that elderly volunteers developed mild steatorrhea when the dietary fat content was increased to rather uncharacteristically high levels of 115–120 g/day [15].

With regards to carbohydrate digestion and/or absorption, a study was conducted by Feibusch and Holt [16], which was interpreted as showing decreased carbohydrate digestive or absorptive capacity with aging. Mixed carbohydrate meals containing about 200 g of carbohydrate were fed to elderly individuals and young control subjects. Breath hydrogen tests were subsequently carried out, and in the elderly group, the prevalence of positive tests was about 60%. In the control group there were no positive breath hydrogen tests, even in subjects on the 200-gram carbohydrate meal. Interpreting findings of carbohydrate maldigestion/malabsorption with age as a sign of pancreatic insufficiency is complicated by the increased numbers of bacteria that can overgrow in the intestine of elderly adults as a result of hypochlorhydria of aging [17]. Hypochlorhydria comes about in advanced age as a result of a high prevalence of atrophic gastritis, which affects as many as 10–30% of elderly persons over the age of 60 [18]. We know today that *Helicobacter pylori* infection is the main cause of atrophic gastritis. The decreased acid secretion in persons with atrophic gastritis results in increased survivability of swallowed bacteria in the stomach and small intestine, which in younger, normochlorhydric persons would be killed by stomach acid. Thus, an abnormal result on a breath test in an elderly person might not reflect carbohydrate malabsorption, but rather simply exposure of the carbohydrate load to the bacteria residing in the small intestine.

The demonstration that pancreatic function is well preserved with aging has the following practical consequence: encountering true pancreatic insufficiency in an elderly person should raise concern as to whether a significant disease process is under way in the pancreas.

Imaging of the Pancreas in the Elderly

The anatomical and microscopic alterations of the pancreas occurring in aged patients may influence the appearance of the organ in common imaging procedures such as US, CT and ERCP. Studies which correlate imaging of the pancreas with different anatomical findings in the elderly are, however, lacking, due to the difficulty of obtaining histological specimens of the pancreas.

An increased, sometimes heterogeneous echogenicity of the pancreas, with multiple tiny hyperechoic spots, is usually considered a typical sign of chronic pancreatitis, occurring in about 53–74% of patients [19, 20]. In advanced disease, the pancreatic duct becomes dilated, usually irregularly, with increased echogenicity of the wall [19, 20]. These signs are likely to be nonspecific for chronic pancreatitis in the elderly. In fact, the aging pancreas shows atrophy, fibrosis and fatty infiltration, which are likely to increase the echogenicity of the gland on US [8, 21]. A moderate dilation of the main pancreatic duct is also revealed by US in the elderly [8]. Comparing the echogenicity of the pancreas with that of the liver, Glaser and Stienecker [8] found that while the majority of patients younger than 40 have a pancreatic echogenicity lower or similar to that of the liver, from 50 years, most individuals show a pancreatic echogenicity distinctly higher than that of the liver. All patients over 80 have a higher pancreatic echogenicity compared to that of the liver. In the same study, the diameter of the main pancreatic duct was demonstrated to increase from a mean of 1.5 mm in the group aged 18–29 years to 2.3 mm in patients over 80, but never exceeded 3 mm.

The US-secretin test has been introduced in an attempt to improve the diagnostic value of US. In one study, US pancreatic duct measurements were performed before and after secretin stimulation in two groups of patients with distinctly different mean ages (30 vs. 68 years) [22]. It was observed that no difference between the two groups existed concerning the extent and temporal development of secretin-induced pancreatic duct dilation [22]. According to these data, diagnosis of chronic pancreatitis in the elderly, especially in the early stage of disease, cannot be based only on the use of US, since false-positive results may occur if too much confidence is placed in single nonspecific signs like echogenicity and duct enlargement.

The considerations reported above for US regarding the evaluation of the parenchyma and duct system in the elderly may also be applied to CT [23]. The size of the aging pancreas may also be reduced [5], similarly to what happens in advanced chronic pancreatitis with atrophy of the gland. However, in this stage of the disease, the CT diagnosis of chronic pancreatitis is usually easy due to the presence of other typical features such as calcifications, irregular duct dilations and pseudocysts; conversely, in the early phase of chronic pancreatitis, especially in the elderly, recognition of single alterations such as increased parenchymal density and duct dilation could lead to false-positive results.

Increased diameter of the main pancreatic duct in the elderly can also be demonstrated by ERCP [6]. This dilation is homogeneous in the whole organ

Table 1. Morphologic changes of the pancreas in common imaging procedures in comparison to chronic pancreatitis and pancreatic cancer

	Pancreas in the elderly	Differential diagnosis	
		chronic pancreatitis	pancreatic cancer
Parenchyma	increased homogeneous echogenicity, sometimes with tiny spots (US) increased homogeneous density, sometimes inhomogeneous patchy structures (lipomatosis) (CT) reduced pancreatic perfusion (contrast-enhanced CT)	increased heterogeneous echogenicity with multiple spots, intraparenchymal calcifications, pseudocysts (US) increased, inhomogeneous density, intraparenchymal calcifications, pseudocysts (CT)	focal tumor mass with surrounding normal parenchyma (US and CT)
Duct system	diffuse homogeneous smooth enlargement of the duct system (US, CT, ERCP)	multiple irregular dilatations and strictures in the whole gland, irregular side branches, calcifications, cystic structures with regular contours (US, CT, ERCP)	singular, irregular stenosis or obstruction, regular dilation of the upstream tract, normal aspect of the downstream tract, irregular cavities and extravasation (US, CT, ERCP)
Size and shape	homogeneous reduction in size with preserved shape (US and CT)	increase in size and sometimes pseudotumor mass, decrease in size in advanced stages (US and CT)	focal enlargement due to the tumor mass; otherwise preserved size and shape

and usually does not represent a problem in the diagnosis of chronic pancreatitis and pancreatic cancer.

Table 1 summarizes the morphologic changes of the pancreas of elderly persons seen with common imaging procedures (US, CT and ERCP) in comparison to chronic pancreatitis and pancreatic cancer.

Acute Pancreatitis in the Elderly

Acute pancreatitis may be seen in patients of every age, but most often the disease is seen in adults between the age of 30 and 70 years [24]. In 1972, Parkash [25] related the incidence of pancreatitis in various age groups to the number of individuals in the corresponding age groups in the general population. In this way, he calculated a 'corrected' age distribution for the risk of morbidity of acute pancreatitis and found a sudden significant increase in persons over the age of 50 years [25]. Acute pancreatitis is therefore a disease which occurs frequently in old adults and may present some peculiarities in this age group. According to some authors [26], the rate of biliary pancreatitis increases significantly with age, while that of alcoholic pancreatitis decreases. This would fit well with the age distribution of alcoholism and biliary tract disease in the Western population. Other causes of pancreatitis in the elderly are rare. A variety of benign and malignant conditions of the main pancreatic duct have been reported to cause acute pancreatitis by obstructing the duct. They represent rare causes of pancreatitis; however, due to the higher incidence of pancreatic cancer in the elderly, they should be taken into account when acute pancreatitis occurs in an old adult without any other recognizable cause. Also, periampullary duodenal diverticula, which occur more frequently in the elderly, may represent a possible cause of acute pancreatitis [27].

The clinical course of acute pancreatitis is not different between young and old adults in terms of severity of disease (i.e. rate of edematous and necrotizing acute pancreatitis) and development of local and systemic complications [26]. In the series of Cataldi et al. [26], age did not represent a factor determining the outcome of the disease. In several reports [28, 29], however, age did represent a prognostic factor in acute pancreatitis, due to the higher morbidity of aging patients related to associated preexisting diseases. The factor 'age' is, moreover, included in several multifactorial scoring systems in the prognostic assessment of acute pancreatitis [28, 29].

Diagnosis and treatment of acute pancreatitis in the elderly is not different from that in younger patients. Old patients may safely undergo ERCP and sphincterotomy without significantly increased morbidity and mortality [26]. A recent study has demonstrated that in old patients with gallstones, endoscopic sphincterotomy, performed after a first episode of acute pancreatitis, significantly reduces the recurrence rate of disease if these patients cannot be cholecystectomized because they are considered unfit for surgery [30].

Table 2 summarizes the clinical characteristics of acute pancreatitis in the elderly.

Chronic Pancreatitis in the Elderly

Chronic pancreatitis is a dynamic, evolving disease in which a progressive destruction of the pancreatic parenchyma due to inflammation and consequent biosynthesis of large amounts of fibrotic tissue lead to complete changes in the architecture of the gland and impairment of its function [31]. The typical clinical picture of chronic pancreatitis in the elderly is that of a patient who, after years of alcohol abuse and a history of recurrent abdominal pain, develops

Table 2. Clinical characteristics of acute and chronic pancreatitis in the elderly

Acute pancreatitis	Chronic pancreatitis
Occurs frequently in the elderly	The onset is usually in young adulthood
The rate of biliary etiology is increased, while the rate of alcoholic pancreatitis decreases	In the elderly, we usually observe the terminal stage of disease
Pancreatic cancer is a possible cause of pancreatitis	Steatorrhea, diabetes mellitus and malnutrition are the typical clinical features, while pain has usually subsided
The rate of edematous/necrotizing pancreatitis is not different than in younger patients	Diagnosis may involve some problems due to the morphological changes of the pancreas related to age
Possible higher morbidity is due to age and associated diseases	Functional tests maintain their accuracy
Diagnosis and treatment is not different than in younger patients	Treatment is mainly oriented at compensation of exocrine pancreatic insufficiency and diabetes mellitus

steatorrhea, diabetes mellitus and general malnutrition. However, this is only the late aspect of a disease which has developed years before. Chronic pancreatitis is usually diagnosed in young adults who suffer from recurrent attacks of abdominal pain with still normal exocrine and endocrine pancreatic function. The evolution of the disease leads to progressive alteration of the pancreatic architecture with the development of ductal strictures and occasionally pseudocysts. In this phase, pain tends to occur more frequently or even to be continuous, and pancreatic function becomes abnormal. In the terminal stage of chronic pancreatitis, which usually characterizes the disease of elderly patients, the pancreatic gland appears to be totally fibrotic and calcifications and pseudocysts are usually present. Exocrine (steatorrhea, malnutrition) and endocrine (diabetes mellitus) insufficiencies develop, whereas pain tends to disappear (burning out pancreas) [31].

The vast majority of patients with chronic pancreatitis is likely to live to old age. In one study, only 13% of patients died from a condition directly related to chronic pancreatitis [32]. However, alcohol consumption seems to be the most important determinant of prognosis in chronic pancreatitis patients since it may determine the evolution of the disease and development of complications as well as the need for surgery. The mean life expectancy from the onset of symptoms is 37 years for alcoholics and 39 years for nonalcoholics [32]. In that study, 10 years after the onset of symptoms, 80% of nonalcoholics and only 65% of alcoholics were still alive [32].

Diagnosis of chronic pancreatitis in the elderly may involve some problems related to the morphological changes in the pancreatic gland related to age (see above). Conversely, since the pancreatic function is preserved with age, current tests of pancreatic function maintain their accuracy. However, a first diagnosis of chronic pancreatitis in old age is a rare event. Furthermore, in aging people, the disease is usually at an advanced stage, so that typical morphological and functional features allow an easy diagnosis.

While in young chronic pancreatitis patients, treatment should aim mainly at pain relief, the main problem in older patients is the compensation of exocrine pancreatic insufficiency and the management of diabetes mellitus. Avoidance of alcohol, dietetic management, enzyme supplementation and analgesia as well as endoscopic and surgical procedures may be recommended similarly to old and younger patients with chronic pancreatitis.

The clinical characteristics of chronic pancreatitis in the elderly are shown in table 2.

Pancreatic Cancer in the Elderly

Pancreatic ductal adenocarcinoma is the 4th or 5th leading cause of death from cancer in the Western industrialized countries [33]. Its incidence is still increasing with time in many countries (e.g. in Japan). Its incidence increases markedly with age [33]. In a Swedish epidemiological study, the age-standardized incidence rate in 1988 per 100,000 inhabitants was 15.1 for men and 14.6 for women. Above 55 years of age, these incidence rates were higher, and reached almost 1 per 1,000 at the age of 80 or more [34]. In the same study, the median survival time after diagnosis was strongly correlated with age; younger patients lived longer than older patients. In the older age group, in whom cancer is most common, the median survival was most often only 1 month [34]. These data demonstrate that pancreatic cancer is most of all a disease of the elderly, which is of importance when treatment, quality of life and other factors are considered. It has been suggested that hyperplastic changes of the duct epithelium of the pancreas may give rise to ductal adenocarcinoma. A recent study conducted on 140 postmortem pancreases of patients without pancreatic disease has demonstrated that hyperplastic and dysplastic lesions of the duct system are more common beyond the age of 40 and their frequency increases with age [35].

Diagnosis and treatment of pancreatic cancer in the elderly is not different than in younger patients.

The outcome of major pancreatic surgery in the elderly has been evaluated by a recent German study [36] in a series of 300 pancreatic resections. Both surgical and general complications occurred more frequently in patients over 70 years, but the mortality rate 30 and 90 days after surgery was not different from that in patients of younger age. However, due to age and the diseases frequently associated with old age, most old patients may not be fit for surgery, and thus careful selection of patients eligible for surgery is mandatory to further improve the outcome of pancreatic operation in the elderly.

Acknowledgment

Dr. Gianpiero Manes is the recipient of a grant of the Alexander von Humboldt Foundation in the Department of Gastroenterology, Hepatology and Infectious Disease of the University of Magdeburg, Director Prof. P. Malfertheiner.

References

1   Andrew W: Senile changes in the pancreas of Wistar institute rats and of man with special regard to the similarity of locule and cavity formation. Am J Anat 1944;74:97–127.
2   Stamm BH: Incidence and diagnostic significance of minor pathologic changes in the adult pancreas at autopsy: A systematic study of 112 autopsies in patients without known pancreatic disease. Hum Pathol 1984;15:677–683.
3   Schmitz-Moormann P, Otte CA, Ihm P, Schmidt G: Vergleichende röntgenologische und morphometrische Untersuchungen am menschlichen Pankreas. 3. Z Gastroenterol 1979;17:256–263.
4   Schmitz-Moormann P, Hein J: Changes of the pancreatic duct system associated with aging: Their relations to parenchyma (in German). Virchows Arch A Pathol Anat Histol 1976;371:145–152.
5   Heuck A, Maubach PA, Reiser M, Feuerbach S, Allgayer B, Lukas P, Kahn T: Age-related morphology of the normal pancreas on computed tomography. Gastrointest Radiol 1987;12:18–22.
6   Hastier P, Buckley MJ, Dumas R, Kuhdorf H, Staccini P, Demarquay JF, Caroli-Bosc FX, Delmont JP: A study of the effect of age on pancreatic duct morphology. Gastrointest Endosc 1998;48:53–57.
7   Perret RS, Sloop GD, Borne JA: Common bile duct measurements in an elderly population. J Ultrasound Med 2000;19:727–730.
8   Glaser J, Stienecker K: Pancreas and aging: A study using ultrasonography. Gerontology 2000;46:93–96.
9   Tsushima Y, Kusano S: Age-dependent decline in parenchymal perfusion in the normal human pancreas: Measurement by dynamic computed tomography. Pancreas 1998;17:148–152.
10 Arora S, Kassarjian Z, Krasinski SD, Kaplan MM, Russel RM: Effect of age on tests of intestinal and hepatic function in healthy humans. Gastroenterology 1989;96:1560–1565.
11 Greenberg RE, Holt PR: Influence of aging upon pancreatic digestive enzymes. Dig Dis Sci 1986;31:970–977.
12 Gullo L, Priori P, Daniele C, Ventrucci M, Gasbarrini G, Labo G: Exocrine pancreatic function in the elderly. Gerontology 1983;29:407–411.
13 Gullo L, Ventrucci M, Naldoni P, Pezzilli R: Aging and exocrine pancreatic function. J Am Geriatr Soc 1986;34:790–792.
14 Bartos V, Groh J: The effect of repeated stimulation of the pancreas on the pancreatic secretion in young and aged men. Gerontol Clin (Basel) 1969;11:56–62.
15 Werner I, Hambraeus L: The digestive capacity of elderly people; in Carlson LA (ed): Nutrition in Old Age. Uppsala, Almqvist and Wicksel, 1972, pp 55–60.

16   Feibusch JM, Holt PR: Impaired absorptive capacity for carbohydrate in the aging human. Dig Dis Sci 1982;27:1095–1100.
17   Saltzman JR, Kowdley KV, Pedrosa MC, Sepe T, Golner B, Perrone G, Russell RM: Bacterial overgrowth without clinical malabsorption in elderly hypochlorhydric subjects. Gastroenterology 1994;106:615–623.
18   Hurwitz A, Brady A, Schaal E, Samloff I, Delon J, Ruhl C: Gastric acidity in older adults. JAMA 1997;278:659–662.
19   Otte M: Ultrasound in chronic pancreatitis; in Malfertheiner P, Ditschunheit H (eds): Diagnostic Procedures in Pancreatic Disease. Berlin, Springer, 1986, pp 143–148.
20   Alpern MB, Sandler MA, Kellman GM, Madrazo BL: Chronic pancreatitis: Ultrasonic features. Radiology 1985;155:215–219.
21   Worthen NJ, Beabeau D: Normal pancreatic echogenicity: Relation to age and body fat. AJR Am J Roentgenol 1982;139:1095–1098.
22   Glaser J, Stienecker K: Does aging influence pancreatic response in the ultrasound secretin test by impairing hydrokinetic exocrine function or sphincter of Oddi motor function? Dig Liver Dis 2000;32:25–28.
23   Ferrucci JT, Wittember J, Black EB, Kirkpatrick RH, Hall DA: Computed body tomography in chronic pancreatitis. Radiology 1979;130:175–182.
24   Uomo G, Visconti M, Manes G, Calise F, Laccetti M, Rabitti PG: Nonsurgical treatment of acute necrotizing pancreatitis. Pancreas 1996;12:142–148.
25   Parkash O: On the anomalous age-dependence of acute pancreatitis. Digestion 1972;5:269–274.
26   Cataldi F, Rabitti PG, De Pasquale M, Cavallera A, Esposito P, Manes G, Uomo G, Rengo F: Considerazioni su di una casistica ospedaliera di pancreatiti acute in età geriatrica. G Gerontol 1995;11:651.
27   Uomo G, Manes G, Rabitti PG: Periampullary extraluminal duodenal diverticula and acute pancreatitis: An underestimated etiological association. Am J Gastroenterol 1996;91:1186–1188.
28   Ranson JHC, Rifkind KM, Roses DF, Fink SD, Eng K, Spencer FC: Prognostic signs and the role of operative management in acute pancreatitis. Surg Gynecol Obstet 1974;139:69–81.
29   Ranson JHC: The timing of biliary surgery in acute pancreatitis. Ann Surg 1979;189:654–662.
30   Uomo G, Manes G, Laccetti M, Cavallera A, Rabitti PG: Endoscopic sphincterotomy and recurrence of acute pancreatitis in gallstone patients considered unfit for surgery. Pancreas 1997;14: 28–31.
31   Amman R, Akovbiantz A, Largiader F, Schüler G: Course and outcome of chronic pancreatitis. Gastroenterology 1984;86:820–828.
32   Lankisch PG, Löhr-Happe A, Otto J, Creutzfeld W: Natural course in chronic pancreatitis. Pain, axocrine and endocrine pancreatic insufficiency and prognosis of the disease. Digestion 1993;54: 148–155.
33   Boyle P, Hsieh CC, Maisonneuve , La Vecchia C, McFarlane GJ, Walker AM, Trichopoulos D: Epidemiology of pancreas cancer. Int J Pancreatol 1988;5:327–346.
34   Andren-Sandberg A, Bäckmann PL: Demographics of pancreatic cancer; in Beger HG, Büchler MV, Schoemberg MH (eds): Cancer of the Pancreas. Ulm, Universitätsverlag Ulm, 1996, pp 3–7.
35   Lüttges J, Reinecke-Lüthge A, Möllmann B, Menke MAOH, Clemens A, Klimpfinger M, Sipos B, Kloppel G: Duct changes and K-ras mutations in the disease-free pancreas: Analysis of type, age relation and spatial distribution. Virchows Arch 1999;435:461–468.
36   Bottger TC, Engelmann R, Junginger T: Is age a risk factor for major pancreatic surgery? An analysis of 300 resections. Hepatogastroenterology 1999;46:2589–2598.

Prof. Peter Malfertheiner
Abteilung für Gastroenterologie, Hepatologie und Infektiologie,
Otto-von-Guericke-Universität, Leipzigerstrasse 44, D–39120 Magdeburg (Germany)
Tel. +49 391 6713100, Fax +49 391 6713105,
E-Mail Peter.Malfertheiner@medizin.unimagdeburg.de

Pilotto A, Malfertheiner P, Holt PR (eds): Aging and the Gastrointestinal Tract.
Interdiscipl Top Gerontol. Basel, Karger, 2003, vol 32, pp 167–175

....
Liver Diseases in the Elderly

Annarosa Floreani

Department of Surgical and Gastroenterological Sciences,
University of Padua, Padua, Italy

Introduction

Although there are no specific age-related liver diseases, it is increasingly recognized that it is important to consider special features and differences between old and young persons in relation to clinical liver disease and its management [1]. In particular, chronic hepatitis is an important cause of death and hospitalization in the elderly. In an American study, chronic hepatitis (including cirrhosis) was a common cause of death in the elderly [2]; the mortality rate was highest in patients between 65 and 74 years old. It has also been demonstrated that the trend in mortality for both sexes increases in subjects over 65 years [3].

During the 1970s, several studies examined morphological and functional changes in the elderly liver. With advancing age, liver size diminishes and liver blood flow declines. Histologically, a reduction in the volume of lobules and hepatocytes is observed, as well as changes in the mitochondrial volume of the hepatocytes, in the endoplasmic reticulum and in the deposition of hepatic pigments. Biochemical parameters show substantially normal findings, though a slightly reduced bile acid synthesis and an increase in cholesterol synthesis and secretion are observed. The consequence is an increase in bile saturation with a greater risk of gallstones. Most indicators of dynamic liver function – sulfobromophtalein retention, galactose elimination, aminopyrine demethylation and caffeine clearance – fall due to the reduction in liver volume and hepatic blood flow. Growth factors correlated with hepatic regeneration decrease with advancing age, and a number of studies have demonstrated that old age coincides with a high incidence of acute liver failure after hepatectomy [4]. In this chapter, we describe a few aspects of parenchymal liver disease that have recently been revisited in the elderly.

Viral Hepatitis

Hepatitis A Virus Infection

Thanks to improved sanitation, hepatitis A virus (HAV) infection is becoming progressively less frequent in childhood and adolescence, when it is asymptomatic. We are thus moving towards a situation in which a large proportion of adults and, in the near future, elderly people, will be susceptible to HAV infection. This is more likely in countries with high levels of sanitation and/or among the wealthier classes.

Limited food-related outbreaks of HAV have already been described, also affecting the elderly [5]. This may become an important problem in geriatric medicine because HAV hepatitis can be severe, frequently cholestatic and potentially lethal in old people.

Vaccines against HAV infection are now available. They are based on inactivated virus, attenuated live virus or recombinant subunit proteins, administered by parenteral routes. Antibody response occurs in nearly 100% of adults, providing the full cycle of 3 injections is given. So far, no studies on elderly people have been completed. Good sanitation minimizes the risk of transmission in the community, though outbreaks can also stem occasionally from contaminated foods (such as commercially available frozen fruits). No outbreaks have been reported in institutions for the elderly so far. This possibility should be considered, however, especially in developed countries.

Hepatitis B Virus Infection

Hepatitis B virus (HBV) infection is declining in many countries. This is only partially due to vaccination campaigns, which are generally aimed at children or high-risk groups. In our experience, the decline in HBV infection in old people's homes, as in other closed communities, is due to improvements in hygienic standards and medical care [6]. Infected elderly people often develop a subclinical or oligosymptomatic hepatitis with a low rate of HBV clearance, possibly due to their impaired immunological status. This can produce highly infective chronic hepatitis B surface antigen carriers who are substantially healthy. Chronic hepatitis and/or cirrhosis (due to infection acquired earlier in life) are generally inactive and progress slowly (maybe because patients with more severe disease do not reach old age).

Hepatitis Delta Virus Infection

Hepatitis delta virus (HDV) is a defective virus which requires HBV particles for its transmission. No special infection has been described in the elderly. HDV infection is also declining in high-prevalence countries.

Hepatitis C Virus Infection

This is the most important clinical form in the elderly. From the epidemiological point of view, the prevalence of antibodies against hepatitis C virus (HCV) increases with advancing age. In studies carried out in the Italian general population, the proportion of infected subjects over 65 years old ranged from 4.1 to 33.1% [7–9]. On the other hand, only sporadic cases of new HCV infection have been recorded in the elderly during the last decade. Moreover, closed communities, e.g. old people's homes, do not represent a risk factor for HCV infection [10]. As the natural history of HCV infection is characterized by a high rate of chronicity (>80%), and the severity of the liver disease is determined by a number of cofactors, including coinfection with other hepatotropic viruses (HBV, HIV, HDV), alcohol abuse and several underestimated environmental factors, we can assume that HCV-infected elderly people represent a cohort of subjects whose infection was acquired many years before. Epidemiological figures, in fact, suggest an epidemic spread of HCV infection during the Second World War and in the early postwar years.

Anti-HCV-positive elderly people have detectable HCV RNA in 54.3–62.5% of cases. As far as HCV genotype is concerned, the elderly are more likely to have the 1b genotype, indicating a very long-standing infection. In Italy and France, Nousbaum et al. [11] observed that the 1b genotype represented 30.8% of HCV-infected subjects under 40 years old, while this proportion increased with advancing age to up to 82.3% in subjects over 60. Similarly, in a population of 610 patients with chronic hepatitis, Simmonds et al. [12] observed that genotype 3 was more frequent in young adults, whereas genotypes 1 and 2 increased with advancing age.

At the onset of infection or the diagnosis of chronic hepatitis, old age is associated with more severe histological damage and the presence of cirrhosis [13]. Moreover, most studies including a logistic regression analysis demonstrate that old age is a risk factor for progression to cirrhosis [13]. In an Italian multicenter study on liver cirrhosis considering 1,829 subjects [14], the presence of HCV, alone or in association with other cofactors of liver damage, was reported in 83% of cases. Subjects with HCV-related cirrhosis were a median 60 years old, those with HBV-related cirrhosis were 51 years old and those with HDV-related cirrhosis were 42 years old.

On the strength of these findings, elderly HCV-positive subjects could be divided into three groups: (1) those who were cleared of the virus with no signs of active replication (anti-HCV+/HCV RNA−), estimated to account for 20–30% of the subjects; (2) those with a long history of infection, with active viremia and compensated liver disease, and with normal transaminase levels (liver disease can range from minimal changes to compensated cirrhosis) – this group included the majority of infected subjects, the estimated proportion being

60–70%; (3) elderly subjects with decompensated chronic liver disease, possibly with superimposed hepatocellular carcinoma, estimated to account for <5%.

New Viral Agents

In recent years, at least two new viral agents have been described: hepatitis G virus (HGV) and TT virus. These two viruses do not seem, however, to have a pathogenic role in determining acute or chronic hepatitis. Dawson et al. [15] observed that, in 290 residents in West Africa, the prevalence of HGV RNA-positive subjects increased with advancing age, but this report only included 13 subjects over 40 years of age. In Japan, the prevalence of the viral genome in hemodialyzed subjects was reportedly 3.1% (mean age 56 years) [16]. None of the infected patients had biochemical or clinical evidence of liver damage. In France, a surprisingly high HGV RNA prevalence (57.5%) has been reported [17] in a series of hemodialyzed subjects (mean age 61 years).

A new DNA virus was recently isolated in a serum sample from a Japanese patient with posttransfusion hepatitis of unknown etiology. This agent was named TT virus (TTV) after the initials of the patient concerned. TTV DNA has since been detected in patients with fulminant hepatitis or acute hepatitis of various etiologies, in chronic liver diseases and in considerable proportions (1.9–12%) of blood donors in several countries. We recently carried out an epidemiological survey in an old people's nursing home in northeastern Italy [18]. The overall sample included 285 subjects with a mean age of 83 years. Twenty-seven subjects (9.5%) were found to be TTV DNA positive, whereas anti-HCV positivity was 11.6%; only 2 anti-HCV positive patients were coinfected with TTV. Our study confirmed the lack of association between TTV and overt liver disease.

Drug-Related Liver Damage

The incidence of drug-related liver damage is very high in elderly subjects who are very high consumers of medication. In a recently published review of drug-induced hepatic reactions notified to the spontaneous surveillance system of two Italian regions between 1988 and 1998, a total of 13,118 reports were filed, 388 of them referring to a liver disorder [19]. The majority referred to patients aged 65–74 years, though their age per se does not indicate any age-specific risk for liver reactions.

Drug toxicity is multifactorial and includes: depression of the enzyme system, especially P450 cytochrome and metabolite conjugation; liver changes in the elderly; competition with enzyme systems; renal failure, and a consequent increase in the median life and bioavailability of drugs.

Table 1. Histological changes in drug-induced liver damage

Histological changes	Drugs	Mechanism
Hepatic necrosis	clometacin, nitrofurantoin, methyldopa, thienilic acid, papaverine, dantrolene, iproniazid, isoniazid	immunoallergic
Chronic cholestasis	chlorpromazine, ajmaline, arsenicals, flucloxacillin, amoxicillin, clavulanic acid	unknown
Microvesicular steatosis and steatohepatitis	sex hormones, amiodarone, tetracyclines, perhexiline	inhibition of β-oxidation
Hepatic fibrosis	methotrexate	metabolite-mediated toxicity

Moreover, drug reactions due to immunoallergic mechanisms are more common with advancing age. An example is isoniazid toxicity, which rarely occurs in patients under 20 years old, but is much more frequent in patients over 50 years. Acute drug-related liver damage is usually characterized by an asymptomatic picture, except for a cholestatic reaction. Drug-related liver toxicity sometimes evolves to chronic damage, despite the withdrawal of the medication, e.g. with amiodarone and perhexiline, whose metabolites persist in the liver tissue for several months after suspending the treatment. Table 1 summarizes the most important histological lesions in drug-induced liver damage. As far as the group characterized by hepatic necrosis is concerned, a genetic susceptibility associated with some HLA alleles has been hypothesized for some drugs. Thienilic acid is associated with the development of anti-liver/kidney microsomal type 2 antibodies directed against the P450 isoenzyme, which converts thienilic acid into active metabolite. Non-organ-specific autoantibodies can develop in chronic hepatitis due to methyldopa (50–70% of cases); in addition, iproniazid liver damage can be associated with the development of antimitochondrial antibodies of the M6 subtype.

Chronic cholestatic lesions evolve in vanishing bile duct syndrome. The main lesions involve ductules or ducts and the main clinical manifestations are pruritus and jaundice. Cholestasis is occasionally prolonged, resulting in progressive ductopenia.

Drugs responsible for microvesicular steatosis and steatohepatitis can inhibit β-oxidation by sequestering coenzyme A, and thus inhibiting mitochondrial β-oxidation enzymes, or impairing mitochondrial structure and function. Fatty acids, which are poorly oxidized by mitochondria, are mainly esterified into triglycerides, which accumulate in small vesicles. Histological features include Mallory bodies, microvesicular steatosis and steatohepatitis.

A typical example of fibrosis-inducing medication is methotrexate, an antiblastic drug also used in psoriasis, rheumatoid arthritis and other autoimmune conditions. Liver toxicity is associated with diabetes, obesity and renal failure. The incidence of hepatic damage increases in proportion to the cumulative dose and the risk threshold is above 2 g.

Alcoholic Liver Disease

Signs and symptoms of alcoholic liver disease in old people are no different from the situation in younger subjects and are related to cirrhosis and its complications [20]. However, the prognosis is worse in the elderly (the 1-year mortality risk is 48% in the elderly vs. 20% in young adults) [18]. Risk factors influencing the progression of liver damage include sex, genetic factors, nutritional status, HBV and HCV infection. It has been suggested that the higher susceptibility to alcohol-related liver damage in the elderly is due to a lower gastric alcohol metabolism as a consequence of a decline in gastric alcohol dehydrogenase activity [21].

It has been estimated that 5–15% of elderly people (over 65 years old) have alcohol-related problems. About two thirds of these subjects already had an excessive alcohol intake when younger (early drinkers), whereas one third develop alcohol-related problems in older life, often as a consequence of changing lifestyles (late drinkers) [22]. Drinking habits are influenced by socioeconomic status; overall, late drinkers have a better education and a higher income than early drinkers.

Autoimmune Chronic Liver Disease

Autoimmune Hepatitis
Although it has been thought to be largely a disease of young adults, 17–56% of all patients with autoimmune hepatitis (AIH) are over 65 years old at presentation [23–25]. The most common presenting sign in these subjects is acute icteric hepatitis. The histological picture often shows more severe necroinflammatory and fibrotic changes than in younger adults, but the prognosis is excellent; very few elderly patients with AIH have clinically aggressive disease (overt jaundice, ascites and encephalopathy). AIH should be considered in the older patient, nonetheless, to avoid any delay in starting immunosuppressive therapy.

Primary Biliary Cirrhosis
Primary biliary cirrhosis (PBC) is a chronic cholestatic liver disease with an autoimmune pathogenesis which develops in middle-aged female subjects.

In an epidemiological study in Newcastle, UK, over one third of PBC patients were over 65 years old [1]. Of 111 new cases diagnosed in patients aged over 65, 26% died of liver-related causes. In the elderly, PBC is generally the result of the survival of asymptomatic patients up to geriatric age and the disease is often discovered by chance. The clinical picture at presentation is less severe than in younger adults and the percentage of asymptomatic patients is higher among the elderly. Itching is rarely the most important symptom and the frequency of association with autoimmune conditions is low. A major complication of PBC, which may pose very important problems in terms of morbidity in the elderly, is osteoporosis. As most PBC patients over 65 are asymptomatic or have only minor symptoms, ursodeoxycholic acid (15–20 mg/kg/day) is the only treatment to suggest for such patients. Osteoporosis management includes bisphosphonates. In our experience, alendronate is well tolerated even in elderly patients. Alternatively, clodronate or etidronate might be administered parenterally.

Management of Chronic Hepatitis

Apart from specific treatment (e.g. in cases of AIH), caution is recommended in the management of chronic hepatitis and the complications of cirrhosis in the elderly. As far as viral hepatitis is concerned, elderly patients are not candidates for interferon (IFN) treatment because of the expected low rate of response and high rate of adverse effects. Selected individual cases might be candidates for IFN plus ribavirin treatment in the case of hepatitis C. No experience has been reported with pegylated IFNs in old people. Amantadine, an antiviral antigen active against the influenza A virus, was used for monotherapy in a pilot study including 23 patients over 65 years old with chronic hepatitis C. HCV RNA remained detectable in all patients and no consistent effects on aminotransferase were observed [26]. Colchicine may have an antiviral effect in the case of chronic hepatitis B and could be useful in cases of active replication in elderly subjects [27].

The management of decompensated cirrhosis should be modified if there are coexistent extrahepatic conditions [28]. For instance, the association of decompensated cirrhosis with congestive heart failure requires particular attention.

Strict dietary restrictions, e.g. a low-protein diet, should be avoided in the elderly because they are often undernourished. Caution is also needed with furosemide treatment because of the greater risk of azotemia and electrolyte disturbances. Vasopressin and glypressin should be avoided because these drugs reduce coronary flow and cardiac input, with a high probability of triggering an ischemic event. In cases of portal hypertension, older patients do not tolerate beta-blockers as well as younger individuals. Spontaneous bacterial peritonitis could escape detection in older patients because of the lack of systemic symptoms (fever, abdominal pain).

Liver transplantation is considered an accepted form of therapy for fulminant liver damage and end-stage liver disease. With improvements in surgical techniques and intensive care, the age of recipients on the waiting list has risen. Some centers have reported good results in selected patients over 60 years of age. Experience with liver transplantation in older recipients has recently been published by the Birmingham Liver Unit in the UK [29]; the authors retrospectively evaluated 875 consecutive adult patients undergoing liver transplantation for chronic liver disease, 174 (19.6%) of whom were over 60 years old. The overall actuarial patient survival tended to be better in the younger group. The crude mortality probability showed a stable trend up to 45 years, a gradual increase in mortality between 45 and 60 years and then acceleration of the risk. An adverse effect of older age on outcome was also seen, and this was more marked in more severely diseased patients. In general, it should be stressed that it is not age itself that counts, but rather that age is associated with a worse outcome after surgery. On the other hand, it has been suggested that graft survival is worse with livers from donors over 60 years old [30].

References

1   James OFW: Parenchymal liver disease in the elderly. Gut 1997;41:430–432.
2   NCHS: Advanced Report of Final Mortality Statistics, 1989. Hyattsville, US Department of Health and Human Services, Public Health Service, CDC, 1992 (monthly vital statistics report, vol 40, No. 8, suppl 2).
3   Corrao G, Aricò S, Ascione A: Epidemiology of chronic liver disease in Italy. Ital J Gastroenterol 1994;26:44–49.
4   Fortner JG, Lincer RM: Hepatic resection in the elderly. Ann Surg 1990;211:141–145.
5   Papaevangelou G: Epidemiology of hepatitis A in Mediterranean countries. Vaccine 1992; 10(suppl 1):S63–S66.
6   Floreani A, Bertin T, Soffiati G, Naccarato R, Chiaramonte M: Are homes for the elderly still a risk area for HBV infection? Eur J Epidemiol 1992;8:808–811.
7   Bellentani S, Tiribelli C, Saccoccio G, Sodde M, Fratti N, De Martin C, Cristianini G: Prevalence of chronic liver disease in the general population of Northern Italy: The Dionysus study. Hepatology 1994;20:1442–1449.
8   Stroffolini T, Menchinelli M, Taliani G, et al: High prevalence of hepatitis C virus infection in a small central Italian town: Lack of evidence of parenteral exposure. Ital J Gastroenterol 1995;27: 235–238.
9   Guadagnino V, Stroffolini T, Rapicetta M, Costantino A, Kondili LA, Mennini-Ippolito F, Caroleo B, Costa C, Griffo G, Loiacono P, Pisani V, Foca A, Piazza M: Prevalence, risk factors, and genotype distribution of hepatitis C virus infection in the general population: A community-based survey in Southern Italy. Hepatology 1997;26:1006–1011.
10 Baldo G, Floreani A, Menegon T, Angiolelli G, Trivello R: Prevalence of antibodies against hepatitis C virus in the elderly: A seroepidemiological study in a nursing home and in an open population. Gerontology 2000;46:194–198.

11   Nousbaum J-B, Pol S, Nalpas B, Landais P, Berthelot P, Brechot C: Hepatitis C virus type 1b (II) infection in France and Italy. Ann Int Med 1995;122:161–168.

12   Simmonds P, Mellor J, Craxi A, Sanchez-Tapias JM, Alberti A, Prieto J, Colombo M, Rumi MG, Lo Iacano O, Ampurdances-Mingall S, Forns-Bernhardt X, Chemello L, Civeira MP, Frost C, Dusheiko G: Epidemiological, clinical and therapeutic associations of hepatitis C types in western European patients. J Hepatol 1996;24:517–524.

13   Pagliaro L, Peri V, Linea C, Cammà C, Giunta M, Magrin S: Natural history of chronic hepatitis C. Ital J Gastroenterol Hepatol 1999;31:28–44.

14   De Bac C, Stroffolini T, Gaeta GB, Taliani G, Giusti G: Pathogenic factors in cirrhosis with and without hepatocellular carcinoma: A multicenter Italian study. Hepatology 1994;20:1225–1230.

15   Dawson GJ, Schlauder GG, Pilot-Matias TJ, Thiele D, Leary TP, Murphy P, Rosenblatt JE, Simons JN, Martinson FE, Gutierrez RA, Lentino JR, Pachucki C, Muerhoff AS, Widell A, Tegtmeier G, Desai S, Mushahwar IK: Prevalence studies of GB virus-C infection using reverse transcriptase-polymerase chain reaction. J Med Virol 1996;50:97–103.

16   Masuko K, Mitsui T, Iwano K, Yamazaki C, Okuda K, Meguro T, Murayama N, Inoue T, Tsuda F, Okamoto H, Miyakawa Y, Mayumi M: Infection with hepatitis GB virus C in patients on maintenance hemodialysis. N Engl J Med 1996;334:1485–1490.

17   de Lamballerie X, Charrel RN, Dussol B: Hepatitis GB virus C in patients on hemodialysis. N Engl J Med 1996;334:1549.

18   Floreani A, Baldo V, Buoro S, Mazzariol L, Favarato G, Trivello R: Prevalence of infection with an unenveloped DNA virus (TTV) in elderly subjects. J Am Geriatr Soc 2000;48:1534–1536.

19   Conforti A, Leone R, Ghiotto E, Velo G, Moretti U, Venegoni M, Bissoli F: Spontaneous reporting of drug-related hepatic reactions from two Italian regions (Lombardy and Veneto). Dig Liver Dis 2000;32:718–723.

20   Woodhouse KW, James OFW: Alcoholic liver disease in the elderly: Presentation and outcome. Age Ageing 1985;14:113–118.

21   Seitz HK, Egere G, Simanowski UA, Waldherr R, Eckey R, Agarwal DP, Goedde HW, von Wartburg JP: Human gastric alcohol dehydrogenase activity: Effect of age, sex and alcoholism. Gut 1993;34:1433–1437.

22   Alcoholism in the elderly. Council on Scientific Affairs, American Medical Association. JAMA 1996;275:797–801.

23   Newton JL, Burt AD, Park JB, Matthew J, Bassendine MF, James OFW: Autoimmune hepatitis in older patients. Age Ageing 1997;26:441–444.

24   Parker DR, Kingham JGC: Type I autoimmune hepatitis is primarily a disease of later life. QJM 1997;90:289–296.

25   Schramm C, Kanzler S, zum Buschenfelde KH, Galle PR, Lohse AW: Autoimmune hepatitis in the elderly. Am J Gastroenterol 2001;96:1587–1591.

26   Torre F, Campo N, Giusto R, Ansaldi F, Icardi GC, Picciotto A: Antiviral activity of amantadine in elderly patients with chronic hepatitis C. Gerontology 2001;47:330–333.

27   Floreani A, Lobello S, Brunetto M, Aneloni V, Chiaramonte M: Colchicine in chronic hepatitis B: A pilot study. Aliment Pharmacol Ther 1998;12:653–656.

28   Anand BS: Drug treatment of the complications of cirrhosis in the older adult. Drugs Aging 2001;18:575–585.

29   Garcia CE, Garcia RFL, Mayer AD, Neuberger J: Liver transplantation in patients over sixty years of age. Transplantation 2001;72:679–684.

30   Showstack J, Katz PP, Lake JR, Brown RS Jr, Dudley RA, Belle S, Wiesner RH, Zetterman RK, Everhart J: Resource utilization in liver transplantation: Effects of patient characteristics and clinical practice. NIDDK Liver Transplantation Data Base Group. JAMA 1999;281:1381–1386.

Prof. Annarosa Floreani
Department of Surgical and Gastroenterological Sciences,
Via Giustiniani, 2, I–35128 Padua (Italy)
Tel. +39 049 8212894, Fax +39 049 8760820, E-Mail annarosa.floreani@unipd.it

Pilotto A, Malfertheiner P, Holt PR (eds): Aging and the Gastrointestinal Tract.
Interdiscipl Top Gerontol. Basel, Karger, 2003, vol 32, pp 176–186

······················

Disorders of the Small Intestine in the Elderly

Peter R. Holt

St. Luke's Hospital Center, and Institute for Cancer Prevention,
New York, N.Y., USA

Gastrointestinal symptoms are reported by older patients to their physicians very frequently. One study from the United Kingdom indicated that as many as one third of elderly symptomatic subjects had a history consistent with some sort of functional bowel disorder [1]. In the United States as well, in studies from the Mayo Clinic, about one quarter of elderly individuals reported the presence of frequent abdominal pain, another quarter constipation and 14% chronic diarrhea. Thus, abdominal complaints are very common in the older population and frequently are dismissed as 'due to getting older'. Furthermore, the diagnosis of an acute abdominal emergency is often missed or delayed for a variety of reasons that have been stated before [2]. It is also well known that major abdominal surgery in the emergency environment can present very serious problems in elderly patients who have other concomitant illnesses. Most surgeons believe that age increases mortality and morbidity, but this occurs only as a result of associated cardiovascular and respiratory diseases and not age per se.

In this chapter, we will consider the effect of age upon clinical syndromes associated with diarrhea, intestinal malabsorption, motility disorders, inflammatory bowel disease (IBD) and cancer.

Diarrhea

Diarrhea is usually not considered a major clinical problem when thinking of disorders in the elderly. However, although acute diarrheal disorders usually affect young children, over 50% of deaths occur among individuals aged over 74. The elderly may be at increased risk of dying from diarrhea because of dehydration and electrolyte problems. They also have impaired immunity and frequently are institutionalized. Most deaths from diarrheal disorders occur in the winter and in patients in long-term care facilities. It is likely that defects in both immune and nonimmune defenses may play a role in gastrointestinal infections in the elderly [3].

Physicians must ask specifically about diarrhea since older patients often complain freely of constipation but may not volunteer complaints of diarrhea, since diarrhea in this age group frequently produces incontinence. When considering the causes of diarrhea, as with other clinical problems in the elderly, a disease may start in advanced age or may be caused by disorders that have been present in patients for many years. Diarrhea is defined as an intestinal disorder characterized by abnormal frequency or liquidity of fecal evacuation. Some older patients would use the term diarrhea when they actually mean that they have rectal urgency.

Diarrhea should be divided into acute disease, representing symptoms present for less than 2 weeks, and chronic disease that is longer than 2 weeks' duration. Acute diarrhea is most frequently caused by intestinal infections, many of which are not associated with specifically identified organisms. Acute diarrhea and the diagnosis of 'gastroenteritis' is accompanied with an increased incidence of hospitalization and mortality in older individuals. In the United States, hospitalization data for the elderly suggest that in 78% of patients, the etiology of the acute diarrheal disease is unknown. Amongst infections, viruses are thought to be responsible for approximately 14% of hospital discharges, and in only 9% are specific bacterial organisms detected. Both the length of hospital stays and mortality rates are greater in the elderly than in the young [4].

Specific organisms that are recovered in acute diarrheal episodes include *Shigella*, *Salmonella* and *Campylobacter jejuni*. *Escherichia coli* 0157H7 and enteroadherent *E. coli* are being diagnosed as causing diarrhea more frequently in the elderly. The presence of fecal leukocytes in patients presenting with acute diarrhea suggests the presence of invasive intestinal infections. It should be pointed out that acquired immunodeficiency disease (AIDS) is being diagnosed in the elderly more often than in the past and may be present in individuals who have been treated with effective life-prolonging antiretroviral drug therapy. Whether a patient with AIDS who gets older is more susceptible than younger individuals to intestinal infections has not been determined. Giardiasis and even *Cryptosporidium* have been diagnosed not infrequently in older individuals. Most acute gastrointestinal infections resulting in diarrhea are probably due to viruses for which a specific microbiologic diagnosis cannot be reached [5]. Rotavirus can be recovered if the correct cultures are obtained.

If chronic diarrhea is present, one must first consider whether *Clostridium difficile*-associated colitis is responsible. *C. difficile*-associated colitis occurs commonly in the elderly and may be difficult to diagnose with certainty because *C. difficile* toxin is found in the feces of over 30% of nursing home residents [6]. It is likely that the frequency of *C. difficile* infection is due mainly to the prevalence of antibiotic therapy in the old. The majority of patients who have diarrhea have symptoms which resolve within 2 weeks with appropriate medical treatment. Although classical endoscopic changes are well known, in at least 25% of patients, specific endoscopic changes can only be found if colonoscopy extends to a point proximal to the splenic flexure. The death rate for *C. difficile* toxin-positive patients in nursing homes in some studies has been as high as 40%; in some individuals, it is accompanied by hypoalbuminemia associated with protein-losing enteropathy. Because of the high rate of detection of *C. difficile* infections in patients in chronic care facilities, physicians have attempted to eradicate the infection by treating all toxin-positive patients with metronidazole, implementing isolation procedures and limiting antibiotic use. Such approaches usually tend to be unsuccessful since new patients harboring *C. difficile* are often brought into the facility. The administration of the nonpathogenic yeast *Saccharomyces boulardii* was not found to lower the incidence of the disease in the elderly in one study [7]. The belief that the infection is more serious in the elderly than in the young may not be correct. One explanation for this observation is that the incidence of serum antibodies to *C. difficile* organisms increases with age and the antibodies potentially may modify the clinical disease in a favorable direction [8].

Drug-Induced Diarrhea

Drugs are a common cause of chronic diarrhea in the elderly, principally because they consume so many medications. The mechanism of drug-induced diarrhea for most drugs is poorly understood. The drug may interact with one of the many receptors that are present in the gastrointestinal tract, it may induce mucosal cell toxicity, for example with colchicine or neomycin, it may alter colonic bacterial flora, or occasionally diarrhea may be due to the filler in the medication, such as lactose in a susceptible lactase-deficient individual. Altered intestinal motility or increased sodium or water secretion by the gut may be responsible in some individuals. So many drugs have been incriminated as causing diarrhea in older individuals that it might be advisable to eliminate as many medications as possible in an individual before drug-induced diarrhea is excluded as the cause [6].

What drugs should be considered? Antibiotic-induced diarrhea is common, whether caused by *C. difficile* toxin or in the absence of *C. difficile* infection.

Antineoplastic drugs produce diarrhea principally by direct toxic effects upon epithelial cells. Many cardiovascular drugs that are used by elderly patients are associated with diarrhea, e.g. antiarrhythmic agents such as quinidine, antihypertensive agents including beta-blockers, diuretics including furosemide, cholesterol-lowering agents such as lovastatin and gemfibrosil and central nervous system agents, particularly antiparkinsonian drugs such as L-DOPA, can all induce diarrhea. Gastroenterologists will appreciate that many gastrointestinal drugs such as antiulcer agents, drugs to dissolve gallstones such as ursodeoxycholic acid, some of the 5-aminosalicylic acid compounds used to treat patients with IBD and nonsteroidal antiinflammatory drugs can cause bowel disturbances with diarrhea.

Diabetes mellitus occurs very commonly in persons of advanced age and diarrhea may occur in such patients. Diabetic diarrhea is usually correlated with the presence of neuropathy, but this association does not occur all the time. When very severe, such diarrhea can be treated with alpha-agonists such as clonidine and lidamidine [9]. There are many explanations for causes of diabetic diarrhea, including changes in the autonomic nervous system, intestinal malabsorption and changes in intestinal motility with associated bacterial overgrowth [10].

Intestinal Malabsorption

It is important to recognize that any disease that causes malabsorption in younger patients can also occur in the old. Intestinal malabsorption may be found in an older individual because he or she has had a malabsorptive disorder for many years, such a disease may occur at an advanced age with equal frequency as in the young, or a specific disease might occur much more frequently in the elderly. Reviews of causes of intestinal malabsorption in older individuals have suggested that the prevalence of pancreatic disease, even without pancreatic cancer, was quite high, that celiac sprue was diagnosed commonly and that bacterial overgrowth syndrome, either associated with some alterations in intestinal motility or structure or in the absence of other intestinal disease, was often found [11].

Chronic pancreatitis is well known to occur in the elderly, at times appearing in advanced age without the usual associated etiologies. Idiopathic pancreatic calcification has also been found in some older patients without overt clinical evidence of chronic pancreatitis. Of course, some patients with pancreatic cancer may present with clinical features of pancreatitis, so that this diagnosis must be carefully excluded in any older patient who has not had evidence of pancreatitis before.

Celiac Disease

Previously, celiac disease was believed to be solely a disease of the young, principally of children. Now it is recognized that the incidence of new cases of celiac sprue is bimodal, with a first peak in the fourth decade and a second in the seventh decade. It has been estimated that up to one third of patients now diagnosed with celiac disease are older than 60 years of age, in part because of the availability of specific antibodies for celiac disease such as the endomysial antibody or transglutaminase assays. Studies using serologic tests for celiac disease suggest that the disease may be present in as many as 1 in 200 or 300 individuals.

The clinical presentation of sprue in elderly patients may differ considerably from that seen in the young. Only about 25% of older patients have diarrhea and weight loss as major clinical symptoms and most present clinically with vague symptoms of dyspepsia and ill health [12]. Physicians must be aware that celiac disease in this age group often presents with evidence of vitamin deficiency such as a low serum folate concentration. Increasing numbers of patients are also diagnosed by finding low serum iron levels in the absence of occult gastrointestinal bleeding. Unexpected findings of severe osteopenia by bone densitometry testing also detect sprue in some elderly patients. The frequency of making a diagnosis of clinically significant celiac disease is directly related to how often small intestinal biopsies are performed. It is important to emphasize that an abnormal small bowel biopsy has the same diagnostic accuracy in elderly patients as in the young, and serologic tests for celiac disease have a similar sensitivity and specificity in older and younger individuals. Lymphoma of the small intestine and small intestinal and esophageal cancers occur more often than expected from age-adjusted cancer registries. Splenic atrophy associated with cavitation of lymph nodes or intestinal pseudoobstruction occur with increased frequency. T cell lymphomas may also present as sprue [13].

Once the diagnosis of celiac sprue is made, clinical management is essentially similar to that in younger individuals. However, it must be recognized that elderly patients have difficulty in changing their dietary lifestyle, so that careful and constant evaluation of the gluten-free diet by nutritionists is crucial. Secondary vitamin and micronutrient deficiencies must be treated vigorously, particularly to maintain calcium and vitamin D homeostasis. In this great age group, repeated measurements of bone densitometry are an important component of follow-up.

Bacterial overgrowth syndrome occurs in older patients in the presence of anatomic changes in the proximal small intestine such as small intestinal strictures, postgastrectomy states and upper intestinal diverticulosis resulting in intestinal stasis. There is a unique syndrome of bacterial overgrowth in the absence of anatomic intestinal abnormalities which may be restricted to elderly individuals [14]. Such patients have very few gastrointestinal symptoms; it is the exception rather than the rule for patients with intestinal bacterial overgrowth syndrome to have overt diarrhea and abdominal pain [15]. Most patients have few gastrointestinal symptoms and present clinically with failure to gain weight or malnutrition.

Bacterial overgrowth syndromes are not easy to diagnose and most patients need intubation and collection of intestinal fluid under aerobic and anaerobic conditions. Techniques of breath testing are particularly useful in elderly patients, but their clinical utility for diagnosis has engendered considerable controversy. ^{14}C or ^{13}C cholylglycine breath tests or breath hydrogen analysis following a small glucose load are difficult to interpret. The ^{14}C or ^{13}C xylose breath test is considered the gold standard for this diagnosis, but the test is not generally used. There is also disagreement about the clinical impact of bacterial overgrowth on nutrition in the absence of intestinal structural changes [16, 17]. One hypothesis points to changes in intestinal motility as the major cause of bacterial overgrowth of unknown etiology. If this is the case, then prokinetic agents may be quite useful in management.

Although small bowel diverticulosis is well known to cause bacterial overgrowth syndrome, it is clear that upper intestinal diverticulosis very frequently occurs in the absence of significant bacterial overgrowth or malabsorption [18]. Rather than malabsorption, such diverticula can produce local complications, including perforation, hemorrhage or inflammation, just as in diverticula of other parts of the gastrointestinal tract. Benign duodenal diverticula can also be associated with obstruction of the common bile duct or pancreatic duct.

Cancer

The majority of gastrointestinal cancers occur in individuals older than 65 years of age and most mortality occurs in this age group. Factors that have been suggested to explain the rapid increase in gastrointestinal epithelial tumors with age include accumulation of DNA damage, disregulation of growth control, decreased apoptosis and postmitotic damage induced by free radicals as well as decreased DNA repair [19]. Whether some of these changes relate specifically to an effect of age is unclear. Furthermore, there is little evidence that the clinical course of cancer in older individuals is different from that in the young. More important potential factors in the age-associated increased mortality in patients with cancer may be that patterns of care and treatment decisions differ from those in younger patients. Most of the data that are available indicate that the well elderly individual tolerates usual regimens of chemotherapy as well as younger patients. Frequently, it is the physician's fear of side effects of the therapy in the elderly that limits effective treatment.

In addition to epithelial cell tumors, small and large bowel lymphomas and carcinoid tumors also occur mainly in the elderly, usually in the distal small intestine, and present with intestinal obstruction and/or acute gastrointestinal bleeding. About 10% of non-Hodgkin's lymphomas involve the gastrointestinal tract, and in some of these patients, several segments of the digestive tract may be involved simultaneously.

Vascular Disease of the Bowel

Vascular diseases induce varying degrees of ischemia depending upon the degree of vascular occlusion and the adequacy of an anastomotic blood supply.

Acute ischemic syndromes resulting in tissue infarction and gangrene occur most commonly in the elderly. Since older patients often have concomitant cardiovascular, renal or other systemic disorders, the mortality rates for acute intestinal ischemia are much higher than in younger patients.

The existence of chronic ischemic syndromes of the small bowel is controversial [20]. Classical symptoms of postprandial abdominal pain akin to exercise-induced angina are rarely seen. Some of these patients may complain of weight loss and nonspecific gastrointestinal complaints. The diagnosis of chronic mesenteric ischemia is very difficult since abdominal symptoms are common in the elderly, biochemical findings do not help and angiographic examinations also may not be definitive because obstruction of 2 or even 3 major mesenteric arteries is found commonly without any abdominal symptoms. The message is that arteriosclerotic occlusions are common in the elderly population but intestinal angina is quite rare [21]. If localized arteriosclerotic changes in major mesentery vessels are seen in a patient with appropriate clinical symptoms, intravascular balloon angioplasty may help to determine whether the syndrome of intestinal angina really is present.

Inflammatory Bowel Disease

Although IBD occurs predominately in the young, increasing numbers of cases are being diagnosed after 60 years of age and there is evidence for a second peak of IBD during the life span [22], although this concept has been challenged in part by the suggestion that IBD-like disease in most elderly patients is due to ischemic vascular disease [23]. New-onset ulcerative colitis is relatively uncommon in the elderly but colonic Crohn's disease appears to be occurring with increasing frequency. Furthermore, the better results of medical and surgical therapy in younger patients are allowing many more patients with existing IBD to reach 'senior citizenship'. These issues and others that concern IBD in the elderly have been discussed in an excellent recent review [24].

What are the clinical features that distinguish the initial diagnosis and that reflect changes in manifestations and in therapy when dealing with IBD in the elderly? Most older studies suggested that it took longer to recognize the diagnosis in elderly IBD patients perhaps because the differential diagnosis was complex. Whereas the differential diagnosis of IBD is relatively easy in younger patients, it represents a major challenge in the old. Ulcerative and particularly Crohn's disease of the colon may mimic ischemic disease of the bowel, cancer [25] or diverticulitis, or may even be geographically associated with diverticula [26]. Crohn's disease in older patients is characterized by more distal colonic and less small bowel involvement. Patients also may have more inflammatory and fewer stricturing patterns of Crohn's disease, and late-onset Crohn's disease is less often familial than early-onset disease [25, 27].

Older patients have more comorbidities than the young, so that surgery for IBD in this age group is often more complicated and accompanied by increased mortality. Early studies suggested that older patients required earlier surgery, but this clearly is not the case when adequate medical treatment is provided. There are data that suggest that postoperative recurrences of Crohn's disease in the elderly may be less common than in the young and, surprisingly, most poly-poid masses that are found in patients with ulcerative colitis represent sporadic adenomas and not dysplastic masses [28].

It is important to emphasize that the management of IBD does not differ in any major way between older and younger patients. Of course, the most important exception in terms of pharmacologic therapy is that systemic cortico-steroids may be especially deleterious to older patients. On the other hand, there is no evidence that older patients tolerate either 5-aminosalicylic acid compounds or, more importantly, the immunosuppressive drugs that are used in treatment less well than the young. If there is an increased mortality in elderly IBD patients compared to the general population, this does not appear to result from more deaths with colorectal cancer. Recent studies have clearly demonstrated that osteopenia occurs commonly in patients with IBD. In some patients, this loss of bone mass reflects small bowel malabsorption of vitamin D and calcium, while in others, it reflects the deleterious effect of corticosteroids [29]. However, bone loss that is independent of these well-known etiologic factors is seen and is particularly harmful in the elderly patient who may already have underlying osteopenia. Repeated documentation and intensive treatment of osteopenia with calcium 1,200 mg and vitamin D 800 IU daily, often together with biphosphonates, is mandatory in these elderly patients. Treatment of the inflammation will also lower the pathogenic effect of inflammatory cytokines upon bone health [30].

Age does not influence the appearance of carcinoma of the large and small intestine in patients with chronic IBD, but cancer usually develops after prolonged duration of the underlying disorder. Extraintestinal malignancies are more common in the elderly and include esophageal tumors and reticuloendothelial neoplasms.

Differential Diagnosis

The diagnosis and differential diagnosis of IBD in the elderly is challenging. Older individuals are more likely to have diverticulosis, vascular disease or lymphomas and physicians have a low index of suspicion for ulcerative colitis and Crohn's disease in such patients. The differential diagnosis of ischemic bowel disease from IBD in older patients presenting with abdominal pain and rectal bleeding is particularly difficult. Ischemic disease usually remits after an acute attack and is far less likely if the clinical and colonic endoscopic features in the patient are prolonged. Diverticulosis is very common in the elderly, so that the differential diagnosis between localized Crohn's disease and diverticular inflammation may also be very difficult. Indeed, segmental Crohn's disease-like lesions have been described as occurring in areas of diverticulosis. Histologically, these lesions closely resemble the microscopic picture of Crohn's disease [31]. If the inflammation in these areas does not respond to IBD therapy (usually used with concomitant antibiotics), then segmental colonic resection is curative even in the presence of small bowel disease, and the inflammation usually does not recur in the colon.

Morbidity and mortality from surgical management of IBD mainly reflect the extent of coexisting medical conditions and the potential need for emergency surgery. The standard operation when colectomy for IBD is mandatory is ileal pouch-anal anastomosis. This author is unaware of evaluation of the functional outcome of this operation for elderly patients. One might be concerned that age-related anal sphincter dysfunction could lead to increased fecal incontinence.

In summary, small bowel disorders in the elderly present clinical challenges. It is clear that the barrier to successful management of these disorders in older individuals is the failure to consider causes that occur as commonly or present more frequently than in the young. Overall, once a clinical syndrome is recognized and investigated in an older patient and an appropriate diagnostic evaluation is followed, most patients respond to specific treatments almost as well as younger patients. It is the failure to consider a diagnosis or to approach the evaluation of the patient less completely than in the young that leads to increased morbidity and mortality in small bowel diseases in the elderly.

References

1   Thompson WG, Heaton KW: Functional bowel disorders in apparently healthy people. Gastroenterology 1980;79:283–288.
2   Koruda MJ, Sheldon GF: Surgery in the aged. Adv Surg 1991;24:293–331.
3   Ratnaike RN: Diarrhoea in the elderly: Epidemiological and aetiological factors. J Gastroenterol Hepatol 1990;5:449–458.
4   Mounts AW, Holman RC, Clarke MJ, Bresee JS, Glass RI: Trends in hospitalization associated with gastroenteritis among adults in the United States, 1979–1995. Epidemiol Infect 1999;123:1–8.
5   Abbas AM, Denton MD: An outbreak of rotavirus infection in a geriatric hospital. J Hosp Infect 1987;9:76–80.
6   Holt PR: Diarrhea and malabsorption in the elderly. Gastroenterol Clin North Am 2001;30:427–444.
7   Lewis SJ, Potts LF, Barry RE: The lack of therapeutic effect of *Saccharomyces boulardii* in the prevention of antibiotic-related diarrhoea in elderly patients. J Infect 1998;36:171–174.
8   Kyne L, Warny M, Qamar A, Kelly CP: Asymptomatic carriage of *Clostridium difficile* and serum levels of IgG antibody against toxin A. N Engl J Med 2000;342:390–397.
9   Schiller LR, Santa Ana CA, Morawski SG, Fordtran JS: Studies of the antidiarrheal action of clonidine. Effects on motility and intestinal absorption. Gastroenterology 1985;89:982–988.
10 Schiller LR, Santa Ana CA, Schmulen AC, Hendler RS, Harford WV, Fordtran JS: Pathogenesis of fecal incontinence in diabetes mellitus: Evidence for internal-anal-sphincter dysfunction. N Engl J Med 1982;307:1666–1671.
11 Price HL, Gazzard BG, Dawson AM: Steatorrhoea in the elderly. Br Med J 1977;i:1582–1584.
12 Swinson CM, Levi AJ: Is coeliac disease underdiagnosed? Br Med J 1980;281:1258–1260.
13 Isaacson PG: Intestinal lymphoma and enteropathy. J Pathol 1995;177:111–113.
14 Roberts SH, James OFW, Jarvis EH: Bacterial overgrowth syndrome without 'blind loop': A cause for malnutrition in the elderly. Lancet 1977;ii:1193–1195.
15 Riordan SM, McIver CJ, Wakefield D, Bolin TD, Duncombe VM, Thomas MC: Small intestinal bacterial overgrowth in the symptomatic elderly. Am J Gastroenterol 1997;92:47–51.
16 Haboubi NY, Montgomery RD: Small bowel bacterial overgrowth in elderly people: Clinical significance and response to treatment. Age Ageing 1992;21:13–19.
17 Lipski PS, Kelly PJ, James OFW: Bacterial contamination of the small bowel in elderly people. Is it necessarily pathological? Age Ageing 1992;21:5–12.
18 Pearce VR: The importance of duodenal diverticula in the elderly. Postgrad Med J 1980;56:777–780.
19 Newcomb PA, Carbone PP: Cancer treatment and age: Patient perspectives. J Natl Cancer Inst 1993;85:1580–1584.
20 Shaw RS, Maynard EP III: Acute and chronic thrombosis of the mesenteric arteries associated with malabsorption: A report of 2 cases successfully treated by thromboendarterectomy. N Engl J Med 1958;258:874–878.
21 Marston A, Clarke JMF, Garcia JG, Miller AL: Intestinal function and intestinal blood supply: A 20 year surgical study. Gut 1985;26:656–666.
22 Lapidus A, Bernell O, Hellers G, Persson PG, Lofberg R: Incidence of Crohn's disease in Stockholm county 1955–1989. Gut 1997;41:480–486.
23 Brandt L, Boley S, Goldberg L, Mitsudo S, Berman A: Colitis in the elderly: A reappraisal. Am J Gastroenterol 1981;76:239–245.
24 Robertson DJ, Grimm IS: Inflammatory bowel disease in the elderly. Gastroenterol Clin North Am 2001;30:409–426.

25 Wagtmans MJ, Verspaget HW, Lamers CBHW, van Hogezand RA: Crohn's disease in the elderly: A comparison with young adults. J Clin Gastroenterol 1998;27:129–133.

26 Gledhill A, Dixon MF: Crohn's-like reaction in diverticular disease. Gut 1998;42:392–395.

27 Polito JM 2nd, Childs B, Mellits ED, Tokayer AZ, Harris ML, Bayless TM: Crohn's disease: Influence of age at diagnosis on site and clinical type of disease. Gastroenterology 1996;111: 580–586.

28 Wolff BG: Factors determining recurrence following surgery for Crohn's disease. World J Surg 1998;22:364–369.

29 Ljunghall S, Ljunggren O: Inflammatory bowel disease and osteoporosis. Ital J Gastroenterol Hepatol 1999;31:103–109.

30 Fries W, Martin A: IBD-associated bone loss: Is inflammation the explanation? (letter). Gastroenterology 1997;112:2161.

Peter R. Holt
St. Luke's Hospital Center,
1111 Amsterdam Avenue, New York, NY 10025 (USA)
Tel. +1 212 523 3679, Fax +1 212 523 3683, E-Mail pholt@chpnet.org

Pilotto A, Malfertheiner P, Holt PR (eds): Aging and the Gastrointestinal Tract.
Interdiscipl Top Gerontol. Basel, Karger, 2003, vol 32, pp 187–199

....

Diarrhea in Old Age

Ranjit N. Ratnaike

Department of Medicine, The University of Adelaide,
The Queen Elizabeth Hospital, Adelaide, Australia

Introduction

Diarrhea, whether acute or chronic, seriously affects the quality of life of both the older person and his/her carer. Diarrhea may not be regarded as a serious problem due to its wide prevalence among all age groups and most importantly because the illness usually resolves spontaneously. Older persons are predisposed to and at a greater risk of acquiring diarrhea. They are also vulnerable to life-threatening fluid loss and electrolyte abnormalities, with increased morbidity and mortality [1, 2]. A rapid decline in nutritional status may occur from even a single episode of diarrhea [3].

Terminology and Definitions

The World Health Organization defines diarrhea as three or more unformed bowel actions in 24 h, acute diarrhea as an episode of diarrhea that lasts less than 2 weeks and persistent diarrhea as an episode that lasts for 2 weeks or longer [4]. Chronic diarrhea is defined as diarrhea for at least 3–6 weeks [5].

Predisposing and Risk Factors

Diarrhea is more prevalent in the aged due to numerous predisposing and risk factors, often against a background of ill health, undernutrition or malnutrition, and diminished physiological reserves. Aging itself does not significantly affect the gastrointestinal tract structurally or functionally to predispose to diarrhea [6], but a decrease in immune and nonimmune gastrointestinal defenses occurs, as subsequently discussed. Iatrogenic factors are prominent in predisposing to diarrhea. Inmates in long-term aged care facilities risk diarrhea from nosocomial infections, common source outbreaks and person-to-person spread of infection, especially from infected patients with fecal incontinence. Cognitive or physical handicaps increase the risk of infective diarrhea due to suboptimal personal and domestic hygiene affecting food preparation and preservation.

Aging and Immune Defenses

Secretory IgA produced in the small intestine prevents viral, bacterial and parasitic colonization by inhibiting viral replication, binding to bacteria, neutralizing bacterial toxins and preventing pathogen adherence to enterocytes. Secretory IgA is highly T cell (particularly T_4) dependent, and both the quality and proportion of T helper and T suppressor subpopulations decrease with age [7]. The secretory antibody response may also be affected due to aging by a loss of follicles in Peyer's patches, where antigen sampling, the generation of tolerance and immunization occurs. Importantly, the treatment of many malignancies weakens the immune response.

Aging and Nonimmune Defenses

Gastric Acid and Gastric Motility

The usual gastric acid pH is below 4, and at a pH of 3.0, the stomach is virtually sterile. At a pH of 4–5, bacteria in saliva are present in the stomach, and at a pH greater than 5, bacteria, viruses and protozoa survive. Gastric acid production decreases with age [8]. Hypochlorhydria is associated with gastric carcinoma, chronic atrophic gastritis, pernicious anemia, the watery diarrhea, hypokalemia and achlorhydria (WDHA) syndrome, and with therapeutic agents used to decrease gastric acidity in peptic ulcer, gastroesophageal reflux disease and the Zollinger-Ellison syndrome.

In the stomach, gastric motility increases contact between pathogens and acid. This activity decreases when increased gastric emptying occurs due to gastric surgery, pancreatic exocrine deficiency and prokinetic agents, for example metoclopramide, domperidone, cisapride, erythromycin and diazepam.

Small Bowel Motility

This powerful defense mechanism cleanses the lumen of pathogens, preventing mucosal adherence and mucosal invasion. Decreased intestinal motility may lead to bacterial overgrowth (see below) and bacterial deconjugation of bile salts that leads to a secretory diarrhea. Bile salt deconjugation may also cause fat malabsorption due to a decrease in the critical micellar concentration.

Intestinal Flora of the Colon

Commensal bacteria prevent pathogenic bacterial overgrowth in the colon. This is achieved by elaboration of antibiotic-like substances, stimulation of peristalsis, induction of immunologic responses, depletion of essential substrates from the environment, competition for adhesion sites and the creation of restrictive metabolic environments [9]. Antibiotics often breach this colonic line of defense and this is of particular relevance in older persons, who consume more antibiotics than younger persons.

Mechanisms of Diarrhea

Diarrhea occurs when there is a disruption in the balance between intestinal absorption and secretion. Each day, the small intestine converts about 10 liters of fluid and digested food into approximately 1.5–2 liters of ileal content that the colon then transforms to about 200 g of solid stool. The essential mechanisms that cause diarrhea are few, despite the numerous etiological factors.

Secretory Diarrhea

Secretory diarrhea occurs due to biochemical intracellular changes induced by a secretagogue (e.g. cholera toxin) which binds to surface receptors on intestinal epithelial cells. Secretory diarrhea is voluminous and unaffected by fasting. The intestinal mucosa is normal. Stool osmolality parallels the plasma osmolality with no osmotic gap.

Osmotic Diarrhea

Osmotic diarrhea occurs when a compound with a high osmolality within the intestinal lumen causes fluid retention and secretion into the lumen, thus altering the normal intestinal function of initiating and maintaining a water gradient. An essential diagnostic feature is that diarrhea ceases when the osmotic agent is not ingested.

Mucosal Damage

In the small intestine, mucosal damage leads to villous atrophy of varying severity and malabsorption may ensue. In the colon, in addition to diarrhea, blood and mucus may be present, depending on the severity of inflammation.

Na^+-K^+ Exchange Pump

In the intestine, the Na^+-K^+ exchange pump regulates water and electrolyte transport using energy derived from the breakdown of ATP by ATPase.

Iatrogenic causes	***Table 1.*** Common causes of diarrhea in the elderly
Fecal incontinence	
Infections	
Irritable bowel syndrome	
Malabsorption	
Inflammatory bowel disease	
Neoplasms	
Metabolic causes	

Inhibition of ATPase by therapeutic agents discussed below can lead to fluid secretion and diarrhea.

Etiology of Diarrhea

The etiology of diarrhea is extensive. Diarrhea may be a consequence of disorders intrinsic to the gastrointestinal tract, a manifestation of a systemic illness or an iatrogenic consequence (table 1).

Iatrogenic Causes
Drug Therapy
The many therapeutic agents that cause diarrhea by a variety of mechanisms [10] are shown in table 2. Diarrhea has been reported to occur with cimetidine [11] and omeprazole [12] through an alteration of normal gastric flora and small bowel bacterial overgrowth. Recently, lansoprazole-associated microscopic colitis has been documented in the elderly [13]. Prokinetic agents which increase gastric emptying may contribute to the survival of enteropathogens. Drug-induced small bowel hypomotility and hypermotility can also cause diarrhea. Hypomotility due to anticholinergic drugs may result in bacterial overgrowth, deconjugation of bile salts and diarrhea, although constipation is the most frequent side effect. Anticholinergic drugs in common use are propantheline for urinary incontinence and benztropine for Parkinson's disease. Nursing home patients on drugs with strong anticholinergic effects are reported to require long-term laxative usage. Spurious diarrhea may be a consequence of constipation. Drugs that have a cholinergic activity lead to increased gastrointestinal tract motility and diarrhea, as with tacrine hydrochloride [14] and donepezil [15], used in Alzheimer disease, and irinotecan hydrochloride, an agent used to treat primary and refractory colorectal, ovarian and lung malignancy [16]. Cisapride, used in gastroesophageal reflux disease, induces mild diarrhea by increasing interdigestive and postprandial

Table 2. Drugs associated with diarrhea

Cardiovascular system
Methyldopa, digitalis, quinidine, propranolol, hydralazine, ACE inhibitors, procainamide

Gastrointestinal system
Laxatives, lactulose, antacids (Mg salts), H_2-receptor antagonists, proton pump inhibitors (particularly lansoprazole), cholestyramine, chenodeoxycholic acid, olsalazine, misoprostol, enprostil

Musculoskeletal system
Colchicine, indomethacin, auranofin, naproxen, phenylbutazone, mefenamic acid

Central nervous system
Anticholinergic agents, levodopa, alprazolam, lithium, fluoxetine (Prozac), tetrahydroaminoacridine (Tacrine)

Endocrine system
Oral hypoglycemic agents: clofibrate, thyroxine

Miscellaneous
Antibiotics: clindamycin, amoxicillin, ampicillin, cephalosporins, neomycin
Antimetabolites: 5-fluorouracil, methotrexate
Osmotic cathartics: magnesium-containing antacids, lactulose, sorbitol, acarbose, propranol

ACE = Angiotensin-converting enzyme.

small bowel motor activity. The host-protective commensal bacteria in the colon are significantly depleted by antibiotic therapy and may lead to suprainfection with organisms such as *Clostridium difficile*. Examples of other agents associated with diarrhea are neomycin and colchicine, which cause small bowel villous atrophy and malabsorption, and auranofin, which may lead to colitis.

Antibiotic-Associated Colitis
Many antibiotics may cause mild, self-limiting diarrhea. Although uncommon, superinfections may occur with *Clostridium perfringens*, *Salmonella* and *Shigella*. The best-known and most serious consequence of antibiotic-associated diarrhea is colitis due to *C. difficile*. The severity of the illness ranges from mild almost inconsequential diarrhea to pseudomembranous colitis, a serious toxic illness with severe diarrhea, abdominal pain and pyrexia. Colitis may be present with or without a pseudomembrane, which is the result of tissue necrosis. Almost all antibiotics are implicated, including vancomycin and metronidazole, used in treating *C. difficile* infection. Lincomycin, clindamycin, cephalosporins, amoxicillin and ampicillin are best known due to their frequent use. Antibiotic-associated colitis may occur at the onset of treatment or within the next 6–8 weeks. Immediate withdrawal of therapy is often remedial. Severe cases should

be treated with metronidazole or oral vancomycin. Metronidazole is the preferred antibiotic due to vancomycin-resistant enterococci, its equivalent efficacy and relapse rates and lower cost. Vancomycin is used in patients unresponsive to metronidazole, if relapses occur and in immunocompromised patients. Antidiarrheal agents should not be used, due to the potential danger of toxic megacolon. If relapses occur in institutionalized patients, hygiene practices must be urgently reviewed. Spores of *C. difficile* survive for up to 5 months and have been isolated from bedding and bedpans.

Surgical Intervention

Diarrhea is a prominent feature of small bowel resection. Bowel adaptation can occur in adults with more than 60 cm of small bowel, or 30 cm of small bowel *and* an intact ileocecal valve.

Radiation Enteropathy

Radiotherapy is often used to treat those patients who are the oldest and most unwell in order to avoid major surgery; in addition, treatment may be ceased temporarily if necessary. Older persons have an increased incidence of malignancies such as carcinoma of the cervix, uterus, rectum and prostate that are treated with radiation therapy. Diarrhea is a frequent consequence due to several factors. A recent advance in radiotherapy, supravoltage radiation, causes minimal or no skin lesions, thus allowing a higher dose of radiation to be delivered, but has the disadvantage of significant side effects such as diarrhea of small and large bowel origin [17]. Diarrhea may occur immediately after therapy, often with spontaneous recovery [18], although 10% of patients may present with diarrhea after 20–30 years [19].

Infectious Causes

An infection may involve the small or large intestine. Significant mucosal invasion of the colon and diarrheal stools with blood and mucus is termed dysentery. Other features are tenesmus, urgency, cramping and infraumbilical abdominal pain. Besides bacterial pathogens, other infectious causes of diarrhea are parasites. Protozoa such as *Giardia lamblia*, *Entamoeba histolytica* and *Cryptosporidia* are common causes. *Giardia lamblia* affects the small intestine and may cause acute or chronic diarrhea; malabsorption may also be a feature. Other causes are nematodes (round worms) such as *Strongyloides stercoralis*, and trematodes (flukes) such as *Schistosoma mansoni* and *Schistosoma japonicum*. Viruses such as rotavirus can cause diarrhea in all age groups. Norwalk virus infections are associated with vomiting, and outbreaks have occurred in nursing homes. As a result of immunosuppression, a chronic carrier state may be reactivated, for example with cytomegalovirus.

Whipple's Disease

Whipple's disease can occur in the elderly [20]. The disease is uncommon, though lethal if not treated. The causative organism, *Tropheryma whippelii*, targets the small intestine but frequently affects other systems. Due to small bowel involvement, malabsorption, weight loss and abdominal pain occur. Arthralgia or arthritis is a frequent complaint and may be the only presenting symptom, predating other manifestations by years. The diagnostic histopathological features occur in the small intestine and are variable villous atrophy and distension of villous architecture by an infiltrate of foamy macrophages with a coarsely granular cytoplasm that stains a brilliant magenta color with periodic acid-Schiff. A recent diagnostic test is the polymerase chain reaction of the 16S ribosomal RNA of *T. whippelii*. Treatment consists of an adequate regime of antibiotics. Relapses are common.

Tropical Sprue

Tropical sprue is a primary malabsorption syndrome in residents or visitors to certain areas of the tropics. An infective etiology is most likely. Unlike celiac disease, the entire small intestine is invariably involved and therefore both folate, and vitamin B_{12} malabsorption (due to terminal ileal involvement) occurs. The symptoms are malaise, weight loss, diarrhea and abdominal discomfort. The specific treatment is a combination of folic acid and tetracycline, usually for several months until histological improvement of small intestine morphology occurs.

Small Bowel Bacterial Overgrowth

Small bowel bacterial overgrowth (blind loop syndrome, stagnant loop syndrome) is associated with diarrhea and even malabsorption. In older subjects, the etiology is often unknown. Recognized etiological factors are diverticula, strictures, fistulas, blind loops and conditions that decrease motility. Diarrhea is due to bacterial deconjugation of primary bile salts to dihydroxy bile acids (predominantly deoxycholic acid), which affect net fluid and electrolyte secretion in the colon. Bile salt deconjugation also impairs micelle formation and may lead to steatorrhea. Bacterial overgrowth can be diagnosed by the ^{14}C-xylose breath test. The many patients in whom a cause is not demonstrable are effectively treated with a course of antibiotics, in cycles to prevent antibiotic resistance and further bacterial overgrowth. Tetracycline and erythromycin are commonly used.

Malabsorption

Malabsorption occurs invariably due to a pancreatic or a small bowel cause. The common feature is steatorrhea producing bulky, foul-smelling stools that are difficult to flush away and often float due to air, not fat. In diagnosing steatorrhea, the ^{14}C-triolein breath test is the test of choice.

Pancreatic Causes of Malabsorption

In older persons, pancreatic insufficiency is an important cause of malabsorption [21], and the entity 'idiopathic pancreatitis' is a major cause of malabsorption [22]. Pancreatic insufficiency and steatorrhea are uncommon in carcinoma of the pancreas. Chronic pancreatitis as a cause of diarrhea should be suspected if there is a history of recurrent upper abdominal pain, weight loss and diabetes mellitus. Pancreatic calcification and a normal small bowel biopsy strongly suggest a pancreatic etiology. Pancreatic enzyme replacement therapy is the principal treatment for steatorrhea.

Small Intestine

The etiology of small bowel malabsorption is extensive. Celiac disease, a common and often unsuspected cause of diarrhea in the elderly, is discussed below. Other important causes are discussed in the section on infectious diarrhea. Due to malabsorption, vitamin, mineral and protein deficiency may manifest as anemia, a bleeding diathesis, peripheral neuropathy, osteomalacia or edema.

Celiac Disease

Celiac disease (gluten-sensitive enteropathy, celiac sprue) may occur for the first time in adult life but may not be considered as a cause of diarrhea in older persons. Gluten causes villous atrophy, more so in the proximal small intestine, resulting in fat malabsorption and a range of vitamin, mineral and protein deficiencies with a spectrum of clinical signs and symptoms. Celiac disease should be considered in a patient with diarrhea and folate deficiency, iron deficiency, or metabolic bone disease or hypoproteinemia and edema. The presentation may also be due to malignancies of the small intestine such as lymphoma and adenocarcinoma, or of the pharynx and esophagus from long-standing untreated celiac disease. Celiac disease is associated with a number of autoimmune disorders, especially type I diabetes mellitus [23]. Serological tests are now available to diagnose celiac disease. The most sensitive and specific serological tests for diagnosing celiac disease are anti-endomysial antibody and, more recently, antibody to tissue transglutaminase, the autoantigen for endomysial antibody [24]. These tests are negative in patients with serum IgA deficiency, which occurs in 1 in 50 patients with celiac disease. Histological evidence of villous atrophy on a normal diet with reversal on a gluten-free diet remains the best test.

Lactose Intolerance

Lactose intolerance is the commonest cause of carbohydrate malabsorption. Secondary lactose intolerance rather than the congenital primary form is more common, due to small intestinal mucosal damage from celiac disease, an infection or iatrogenic causes such as drugs or radiation therapy. The symptoms are explosive watery diarrhea, cramping abdominal pain and distension, and flatulence. Yogurt, a useful protein supplement, causes no ill effects, as bacterial lactase in yogurt is activated at body temperature [25]. The breath hydrogen test is an accurate, relatively simple and rapid diagnostic test.

Irritable Bowel Syndrome

Irritable bowel syndrome is not as common in the elderly compared to younger persons but is an important cause of diarrhea. Irritable bowel syndrome is defined as 'chronic or recurrent symptoms attributable to the intestines and occurring in varying but characteristic combinations of abdominal pain, bloating (distension) and symptoms of disordered defecation, especially urgency, straining, feeling of incomplete evacuation and altered stool form and frequency' [26]. The diagnostic criteria change cyclically, and the ROME II diagnostic criteria are now in vogue [27]. Four mechanisms suggested are: altered intestinal motility; increased visceral sensitivity; disturbed intestinal reflexes (intrinsic and extrinsic), and psychological disorders [28]. The nature and exhaustiveness of investigations required is debatable. A sensible approach is one that satisfies both the patient and physician. This includes allaying patient anxiety (within reason) and ruling out, especially in older persons, a malignancy or an easily treatable condition such as celiac disease. Indeed, recent studies point to the strong association with celiac disease [29]. The long-held belief of an association between irritable bowel syndrome and lactose intolerance continues to be espoused [30]. New therapeutic advances focus on serotonin (5-hydroxytryptamine; 5-HT) mediated processes, including 5-HT$_3$ antagonists, such as ondansetron and granisetron, as well as 5-HT$_4$ agonists, such as tegaserod and prucalopride. The side effects of many of these compounds preclude their use. Diarrhea, constipation and abdominal pain are treated symptomatically.

Carcinoma of the Colon

Carcinoma of the colon is the most common malignancy in old age after carcinoma of the prostate. The rectosigmoid is the site of tumor in two thirds of cases. A colonic malignancy should be suspected in patients with iron deficiency anemia with no obvious cause, sudden weight loss or a change in bowel habit. Pain is an uncommon symptom except in advanced disease.

Fecal Incontinence

Many patients may not admit to the embarrassing problem of fecal incontinence, which is especially prevalent in acute-care hospitals and in patients in long-term care. Fecal incontinence is a common sequel to constipation and fecal impaction (spurious diarrhea, overflow diarrhea). Other causes of 'true' fecal incontinence are impaired rectal sensation, reduced reservoir capacity or impaired puborectalis function [31]. Patients, carers and health professionals should be aware that fecal incontinence is treatable. Depending on the etiology, the options available include preventing constipation and fecal impaction, using a small dose of an antidiarrheal agent such as loperamide, undertaking sphincter exercises or surgical repair.

Diverticular Disease

In older persons, the incidence of diverticular disease is significantly increased. Diarrhea is associated with acute or chronic inflammation due to a mechanical obstruction within the diverticula. The presentation is a febrile illness with bloody diarrhea, lower abdominal pain, tenderness and a possible mass due to an abscess. This is an abdominal emergency requiring hospitalization, antibiotic therapy, restricted oral fluids and intravenous fluids. Three to four weeks after the acute episode has resolved, a colorectal malignancy needs to be excluded.

Ischemic Colitis

In older patients, ischemic colitis may mimic inflammatory bowel disease or diverticulitis. The presentation may be acute or chronic. Ischemic colitis occurs when the vascular supply to the gut is decreased due to primary or secondary atherosclerotic disease, diabetes mellitus or reduced perfusion from any cause of vasculitis or a hypercoagulable state such as polycythemia. Digitalis preparations increase the risk of ischemic colitis. The diagnosis is based on the typical barium enema findings of 'thumb printing' or 'saw tooth' indentations.

Ratnaike

Inflammatory Bowel Disease

Inflammatory bowel disease may present for the first time in the elderly and should be an 'exclusion priority' in patients with diarrhea and rectal bleeding. In ulcerative colitis, a peak of incidence occurs in the third and fourth decade and a second peak in the eighth decade. Comparison of elderly and younger patients with inflammatory bowel disease shows no significant differences in the course of the illness or response to treatment.

Collagenous Colitis and Lymphocytic ('Microscopic') Colitis

The clinical picture is one of chronic watery diarrhea. The pathological findings are a band of subepithelial collagen in collagenous colitis, and in microscopic colitis, the surface epithelium of the colon shows damage and infiltration by large numbers of lymphocytes. Colonoscopy and barium studies are normal.

Endocrine and Metabolic Causes

Diarrhea is frequently associated with both hyperthyroidism and hypothyroidism and also with diabetes mellitus. Alpha-2-adrenergic agonists, such as clonidine, are useful, but side effects limit their use. Diarrhea occurs with the Zollinger-Ellison syndrome, gastrinoma, carcinoid tumors, thyroid carcinoma, somatostatinoma, glucagonoma and vipomas such as ganglioneuroma, ganglioblastoma and pheochromocytoma.

Diagnosis, Management and Prevention

Valuable initial steps are to clarify what is meant by diarrhea, to establish the normal bowel pattern and determine if the problem is due to fecal incontinence. A diagnostic approach is to establish whether the diarrheal illness is acute or chronic. Is the small or large bowel likely to be involved? Is diarrhea a manifestation of a disease intrinsic to the gastrointestinal tract or secondary to a systemic illness? Is the diarrhea iatrogenic? It is essential to establish at the onset what medication the patient is on, including over-the-counter and 'natural' health products. A comprehensive drug history *and* the physician viewing all medication may often avoid unnecessary, inconvenient and expensive investigations.

If an infective etiology is suspected, and bacterial culture considered, consultation with laboratory staff helps in determining the most appropriate enrichment and isolation techniques. Stool examination for leukocytes is popular in North America to point to an infective etiology. Microscopic examination of feces with concentration on cysts and ova is an important preliminary screening test to detect protozoan and helminth pathogens.

The management priority is to prevent dehydration and electrolyte loss and maintain nutritional status. The conventional 'markers' of dehydration are unreliable in the elderly. Seven signs and symptoms that strongly correlate with dehydration, independent of age-related changes, are: dry tongue; longitudinal tongue furrows; dry mucous membranes of the nose and mouth; eyes that appear recessed; upper body muscle weakness; speech difficulty, and confusion [32]. Oral fluid intake is adequate if supervised. Older persons have a decreased perception of thirst and may also be unable to ask for or independently obtain fluids. Drinks with a large osmotic load should not be consumed, such as Coca-Cola (680 mOsm/kg), apple juice (870 mOsm/kg), orange juice (935 mOsm/kg) and grape juice (1,170 mOsm/kg); drinks with caffeine have a diuretic action.

In an institutional setting, if an outbreak of diarrhea occurs, public health authorities must be notified immediately to investigate the outbreak and help with control measures. Most mild episodes of diarrhea are self-limiting. Antibiotics are indicated in dysentery, especially if systemic symptoms occur. Trimethoprim-sulfamethoxazole, norfloxacin or, if systemic symptoms are prominent, ciprofloxacin may be used. Preventive measures include the use of drugs with minimal side effects and promoting optimal personal, domestic and institutional hygiene, including food preparation and storage.

References

1   Lew JF, Glass RI, Gangarosa RE, Cohen IP, Bern C, Moe CL: Diarrheal deaths in the United States, 1979 through 1987. A special problem for the elderly. JAMA 1991;265:3280–3284.
2   Bennett RG, Greenough WB III: Approach to acute diarrhea in the elderly. Gastroenterol Clin North Am 1993;22:517–533.
3   Giannella RA, Broitman SA, Zamcheck N: Influence of gastric acidity on bacterial and parasitic infections: A perspective. Ann Intern Med 1973;78:271–276.
4   World Health Organization: The Management and Prevention of Diarrhoea. Programme for Control of Diarrhoeal Diseases, ed 3. Geneva, World Health Organization, 1993.
5   Powell DW: Approach to the patient with diarrhea; in Yamada T (ed): Textbook of Gastroenterology. Philadelphia, JB Lippincott, 1991, pp 732–778.
6   Holt PR: The process of aging and small bowel diseases in the elderly; in Ratnaike RN (ed): Small Bowel Disorders. London, Arnold, 2000, pp 77–95.
7   Makinodan T, Kay MM: Age influence on the immune system. Adv Immunol 1980;29:287–330.
8   Husebye E, Skar V, Hoverstad T, Melby K: Fasting hypochlorhydria with Gram positive gastric flora is highly prevalent in healthy old people. Gut 1992;33:1331–1337.

9 Rolfe DR: Interactions among micro-organisms of the indigenous intestinal flora and their influence on the host. Rev Infect Dis 1984;6:S73–S79.

10 Ratnaike RN: Drug-induced diarrhea in older persons. Clin Geriatr 2000;8:67–88.

11 Donowitz LG, Page MC, Mileur BL, Guenthner SH: Alteration of normal gastric flora in critical care patients receiving antacid and cimetidine therapy. Infect Control 1986;7:23–26.

12 Thorens J, Froehlich F, Schwizer W, Saraga E, Bille J, Gyr K, Duroux P, Nicolet M, Pignatelli B, Blum AL, Gonvers JJ, Fried M: Bacterial overgrowth during treatment with omeprazole compared with cimetidine: A prospective randomised double blind study. Gut 1996;39:54–59.

13 Thomson RD, Lestina LS, Bensen SP, Toor A, Maheshwari Y, Ratcliffe NR: Lansoprazole-associated microscopic colitis: A case series. Am J Gastroenterol 2002;97:2908–2913.

14 Zemlan FP, Keys M, Richter RW, Strub RL: Double-blind placebo-controlled study of velnacrine in Alzheimer's disease. Life Sci 1996;58:1823–1832.

15 Shintani EY, Uchida KM: Donepezil: An anticholinesterase inhibitor for Alzheimer's disease. Am J Health Syst Pharm 1997;54:2805–2810.

16 Rivory LP: Irinotecan (CPT-11): A brief overview. Clin Exp Pharmacol Physiol 1996;23:1000–1004.

17 Berken CA: Nd:YAG laser therapy for gastrointestinal bleeding due to radiation colitis. Am J Gastroenterol 1985;80:730–731.

18 Radiation induced proctosigmoiditis (editorial). Lancet 1983;i:1082–1083.

19 Pia-de-la-Maza M, Gotteland M, Ramirez C, Araya M, Yudin T, Bunout D, Hirsch S: Acute nutritional and intestinal changes after pelvic radiation. J Am Coll Nutr 2001;20:637–642.

20 Ratnaike RN: Whipple's disease. Postgrad Med J 2000;76:760–766.

21 Montgomery RD, Haboubi NY, Mike NH, Chesner IM, Asquith P: Causes of malabsorption in the elderly. Age Ageing 1986;15:235–240.

22 Reber HA: Chronic pancreatitis; in Howard JM, Jordan GL, Reber HA (eds): Surgical Diseases of the Pancreas. Philadelphia, Lea and Febiger, 1987, pp 475–495.

23 Lunt H, Florkowski CM, Cook HB, Whitehead MR: Bone mineral density, type 1 diabetes, and celiac disease. Diabetes Care 2001;24:791–792.

24 Vitoria JC, Arrieta A, Arranz C, Ayesta A, Sojo A, Maruri N, Garcia-Masdevall MD: Antibodies to gliadin, endomysium, and tissue transglutaminase for the diagnosis of celiac disease. J Pediatr Gastroenterol Nutr 1999;29:571–574.

25 Kolars JC, Levitt MD, Aouji M, Savaiano DA: Yoghurt – an autodigesting source of lactose. N Engl J Med 1984;310:1–3.

26 Heaton KW: Functional bowel disease; in Pounder RE (ed): Recent Advances in Gastroenterology. Edinburgh, Churchill Livingstone, 1988, pp 291–312.

27 Thompson WG, Longstreth GF, Drossman DA, Heaton KW, Irvine EJ, Müller-Lissner SA: Functional bowel disorders and functional abdominal pain. Gut 1999;45(suppl 2):II43–II47.

28 Villanueva A, Dominguez-Munoz JE, Mearin F: Update in the therapeutic management of irritable bowel syndrome. Dig Dis 2001;19:244–250.

29 Sanders DS, Carter MJ, Hurlstone DP, Pearce A, Ward AM, McAlindon ME, Lobo AJ: Association of adult celiac disease with irritable bowel syndrome: A case-control study in patients fulfilling ROME II criteria referred to secondary care. Lancet 2001;358:1504–1508.

30 Vernia P, Di Camillo M, Marinaro V: Lactose malabsorption, irritable bowel syndrome and self-reported milk intolerance. Dig Liver Dis 2001;33:234–239.

31 Sun WM, Chung O: Faecal incontinence; in Ratnaike RN (ed): Practical Guide to Geriatric Medicine. Sydney, McGraw-Hill, 2002, pp 519–535.

32 Gross CR, Lindquist RD, Woolley AC, Granieri R, Allard K, Webster B: Clinical indicators of dehydration severity in elderly patients. J Emerg Med 1992;10:267–274.

Ranjit N. Ratnaike, MD, FRACP, FAFPHM
Associate Professor of Medicine, Department of Medicine,
The University of Adelaide, The Queen Elizabeth Hospital, Woodville South, SA 5011 (Australia)
Tel. +61 8 8222 6887, Fax +61 8 8222 6042, E-Mail ranjit.ratnaike@adelaide.edu.au

Pilotto A, Malfertheiner P, Holt PR (eds): Aging and the Gastrointestinal Tract.
Interdiscipl Top Gerontol. Basel, Karger, 2003, vol 32, pp 200–211

....

Colon Cancer in the Elderly

Suthat Liangpunsakul, Douglas K. Rex

Division of Gastroenterology and Hepatology, Department of Medicine,
Indiana University School of Medicine, Indianapolis, Ind., USA

Introduction

Gastrointestinal cancers collectively are the commonest malignancies worldwide. These cancers increase sharply in incidence in people in their sixties and seventies. There are several hypotheses of cancer causation in older people, including decreased immune surveillance and prolonged duration of exposure to carcinogens; however, no one theory has been accepted universally [1].

Incidence of Colorectal Cancer

Colorectal cancer is the second most common cancer and third most common cause of cancer-related death in the United States in both males and females [2]. In 2000, there were 130,000 new cases and 56,300 deaths from colorectal cancer. The use of colonoscopy to identify and remove polyps has been effective at reducing both the incidence and mortality of colorectal cancer [3]. Between 1990 and 1996, the incidence rates for colorectal cancer decreased in the United States at an annual rate of 2.1%. Mortality rates have followed a similar trend; between 1990 and 1996, the overall mortality rate decreased at an annual rate of 1.7% [1].

Age and Gender Differences in Colorectal Polyps and Cancer

Both age and gender have an impact upon the risk of colorectal cancer. Men have been found to have a greater age-adjusted risk of colonic polyps and tumors than women [4, 5]. The reason is that estrogen may have a protective role in prevention of polyp formation by mechanisms of estrogen receptor genes [6], decreased secondary bile acid production [7] and decreased serum levels of insulin-like growth factors [8]. Our previous study indicated that approximately 15% of asymptomatic males and 7% of females aged 60 years or older have colorectal cancer or an adenoma which is large (≥ 1 cm), has a villous component or has high-grade dysplasia. These persons with adenoma are at increased risk for the subsequent development of colorectal cancer [9, 10]. A similar result was reported by McCashland et al. [4], who found that men have a greater risk of colonic polyps and tumors than women, with odds ratios of 1.5 and 1.4, respectively.

Colorectal carcinoma is primarily a disease of the older population, with 93% of cases diagnosed after the age of 50 years and an average age at diagnosis of approximately 70 years [11]. Increasing age has been shown to be a powerful determinant of a higher prevalence of colonic neoplasia in asymptomatic persons [4]. A similar pattern of an increasing prevalence of colorectal neoplasia with increasing age has also been noted in symptomatic subjects [12] and those with occult blood in the stool and in autopsy studies [13, 14]. In patients in whom the disease develops at an earlier age, there is a trend toward different morphological and clinical features compared to those who develop the disease at the age of 50 years or older. Moreover, early age of onset may be an indication of hereditary nonpolyposis colorectal cancer syndrome (Lynch syndrome), an autosomal dominant disorder that is characterized by a preferential localization of tumors in the proximal colon and the frequent occurrence of multiple primaries. Early-onset colorectal cancer has a unique clinical presentation and requires a different approach for colorectal cancer surveillance. This specific topic is beyond the scope of this review.

As mentioned earlier, colon carcinoma is especially common in men and women aged ≥ 65 years. The National Cancer Institute Surveillance, Epidemiology and End Results data demonstrated that the overall age-adjusted cancer incidence rate for persons in this age group is 20 times greater than the rate for persons younger than 65 years (235.8 per 100,000 population compared with 12.0 per 100,000 population) [15]. It is worth pointing out that the age-adjusted mortality is higher in men than in women. However, the lifetime risks of diagnosis and death from colorectal cancer are similar in both genders (fig. 1, 2). The explanation for this is that women live longer than men, and therefore have a greater opportunity to develop colorectal cancer. Since colon carcinoma affects a large number of individuals who, because of advancing age, already may be coping with concomitant physical illnesses such as heart disease, chronic obstructive pulmonary disease, diabetes, hypertension and other major health problems, these preexisting diseases may provoke adverse

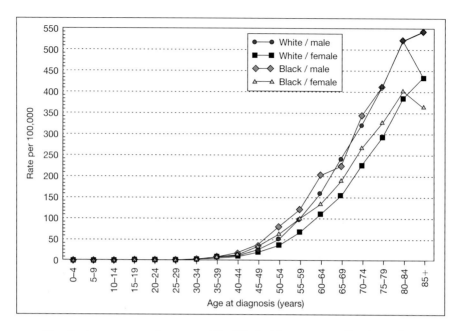

Fig. 1. Average annual age-specific US incidence rates of colorectal cancer, 1994–1998 (National Cancer Institute, Surveillance, Epidemiology and End Results Cancer Statistics Review 1994–1998, modified from http://seer.cancer.gov/FastStats/html/COLORECT.html). Colon carcinoma is especially common in men and women aged ≥65 years. The overall age-adjusted cancer incidence rate for persons in this age group is 20 times greater than the rate for persons younger than 65 years.

consequences and affect conventional approaches to the management of colorectal cancer. Thus, the management of colon cancer in these individuals is challenging.

Progressive Shift of Colorectal Cancer toward the Proximal Colon

In the past, the majority of colorectal carcinomas have been reported to arise in the distal colon in the rectosigmoid area. Recent experience, however, indicates that an increasing percentage of such lesions are located proximal to the sigmoid. No satisfactory explanation for this change in the natural history of colorectal cancer has yet been offered. However, increasing life expectancy was thought to be a determinant factor for such a change, since older patients are more likely to develop right-sided cancers. Comparisons of the odds ratios for different age categories for right- and left-sided polyps showed an increase

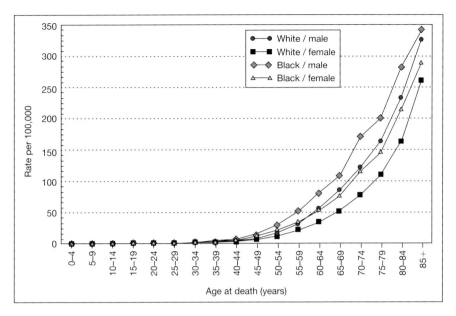

Fig. 2. Average annual age-specific US mortality rates of colorectal cancer, 1994–1998 (National Cancer Institute, Surveillance, Epidemiology and End Results Cancer Statistics Review 1994–1998, modified from http://seer.cancer.gov/FastStats/html/COLORECT.html). The age-adjusted mortality is higher in men than in women. However, the lifetime risks of diagnosis and death from colorectal cancer are similar in both genders.

with aging. Patients in the age group between 60 and 69 years have a 1.44-fold greater risk of right-sided polyps compared to those aged less than 50. As noted with polyps, right-sided colon cancers also increase with aging. A recent study demonstrated that with each decade of aging above 60, the risk of having right-sided colon cancer increases by a factor of 1.53–1.98 compared to those subjects less than 50 [4]. Currently, nearly 40% of colorectal cancers overall in the Unites States arise proximal to the splenic flexure [16]. In summary, most cancers still occur in the distal colon; however, in the elderly population, there is a progressive shift of the location of colorectal cancer toward the proximal colon. This finding has an impact on the method of colorectal cancer surveillance for patients in this age group.

Clinical Presentation of Colorectal Cancer in the Elderly

As in younger populations, symptoms of colorectal cancers in elderly patients vary depending on the anatomic location of the lesions. The prognosis is significantly worse in symptomatic than asymptomatic individuals. In people older than 50 years, persistent changes in the normal pattern of bowel habits should be viewed with suspicion. The commonest presenting symptom of colorectal cancer is rectal bleeding. Cancers arising from the left side of the colon generally cause hematochezia, or in their late stages may cause constipation, abdominal pain and obstructive symptoms. On the other hand, right-sided colon lesions produce vague abdominal aching, but are unlikely to present with obstruction or altered bowel habits. Constitutional symptoms, i.e. weakness, weight loss or anemia resulting from chronic blood loss, may accompany cancer of the right side of the colon. Because the elderly are more likely to have right-sided cancers, they are also more likely to present with otherwise asymptomatic iron deficiency anemia. Occult colonic bleeding is site but not stage dependent; cecal and ascending colon tumors cause a 4-fold higher mean daily blood loss (approximately 9 ml/day) than tumors at other colonic sites [17]. Even though colon cancer in the elderly tends to be located in the proximal colon, the physical examination of an elderly patient should still include a digital rectal examination [1]. In the presence of symptoms suggestive of a colon cancer, occult blood testing is not appropriate and may be misleading; regardless of the result, colonoscopy is strongly indicated.

Choices of Colorectal Cancer Screening Tests

An understanding of the biology of colorectal cancer is essential to guide the application of available screening tests. It is generally accepted that most colorectal cancers evolve from adenomatous polyps. Evidence supporting this belief includes the following: cancers rarely arise in the absence of adenomatous polyps; individuals with a history of adenomatous polyps are at increased risk of developing cancer, and removal of these premalignant lesions reduces the incidence of colorectal cancer.

A series of genetic alterations appears to be the impetus from which normal colonic mucosa develops into an adenomatous polyp and ultimately transforms into a cancer [18]. The time required for the transformation of a small adenomatous polyp into localized cancer and ultimately invasive cancer, the so-called 'polyp dwell time', is of great interest in colorectal cancer screening. Knowledge of the polyp dwell time can be utilized to determine the window of opportunity during which screening is effective in the prevention and early detection of colorectal cancer. The average polyp dwell time is not precisely known. However, the low incidence of advanced adenomas in postpolypectomy surveillance studies and in the incidence studies performed in persons with initially negative flexible sigmoidoscopies and colonoscopies suggests that growth

Table 1. Options for screening of average-risk individuals beginning at the age of 50 in the Agency for Healthcare Policy and Research guidelines

Annual FOBT
Flexible sigmoidoscopy every 5 years
Annual FOBT plus flexible sigmoidoscopy every 5 years
DCBE every 5–10 years
Colonoscopy every 10 years

Reprinted with permission from Rex et al. [24].

rates for colon adenomas are slow. Data from the National Polyp Study indicated that the mean age of adenoma patients precedes the mean age of cancers by 7 years [3, 19]. Using available data on the growth rate of colon adenomas and carcinomas, a mathematical model suggested that it takes 2–3 years for a small adenoma (≤5 mm) to grow to 1 cm in size, and another 2–5 years for the 1-cm adenoma to progress to carcinoma [20–22]. It has been estimated that it takes approximately 11 years for an adenoma with low-grade dysplasia and approximately 4 years for an adenoma with high-grade dysplasia to progress to carcinoma [23]. Knowledge of this transformation time has been one factor by which the recommended frequency of accepted screening tests is determined.

There are 5 options recommended for the screening of average-risk individuals (aged 50 and older) without other risk factors for colorectal cancer (table 1) [24].

Though colonoscopy has not been studied in randomized controlled trials or case-control studies to demonstrate its effectiveness as a screening test on colorectal cancer mortality, several lines of evidence suggest that colonoscopy is the most effective colorectal cancer prevention test currently available. Retrospective [25, 26] and prospective [27] studies of colonoscopy findings in patients with colon cancer proximal to the splenic flexure have consistently found that at least two thirds of these patients have no neoplasm distal to the splenic flexure. Furthermore, two recent studies demonstrated that advanced proximal neoplasia was found in 1.5–2.7% of patients without any polyps in the distal colon. When compared to patients with no polyps in the distal colon, the relative risk of finding an advanced proximal neoplastic lesion increased 1.1- to 2.6-fold in those with a hyperplastic polyp in the distal colon [28, 29]. Asymptomatic persons 50 years of age or older who have adenomas in the distal colon are more likely to have an advanced proximal neoplastic lesion than are persons without distal adenomas. However, if only sigmoidoscopy screening is performed in persons with distal polyps, about half the cases of advanced proximal neoplasia will not be detected. Additional factors favoring colonoscopy as the screening test of choice, particularly in the elderly, are the overall greater prevalence of both right- and left-sided adenomas and the rightward shift of adenomas and cancers with advanced age. The preferred screening strategy in the elderly with average risk for colorectal cancer should be colonoscopy every 10 years as long as examinations are negative for adenomas and cancer, the patient has a reasonable life expectancy and there are adequate local resources and expertise to provide services.

Another alternative screening strategy is flexible sigmoidoscopy every 5 years plus an annual fecal occult blood test (FOBT). This screening method is recommended when resources, expertise or reimbursement for screening colonoscopy are not available [24]. FOBT is the only colorectal cancer prevention test that has been examined in randomized controlled trials [30, 31], and colonoscopy following positive FOBT has been shown to reduce the mortality rate from colorectal cancer [30]. However, sensitivity for the detection of cancer is only 33–50% for one-time testing, though the yield improves with repeated tests every 1–2 years. Furthermore, most patients with adenomas without cancers will have negative tests [5]. As such, patients undergoing FOBT and flexible sigmoidoscopy should be aware of the limitations of each test. As mentioned earlier, development of colorectal symptoms after one or both tests are negative should lead to colonoscopy to evaluate the entire colon.

Though it is the least expensive screening test available to examine the entire colon, double-contrast barium enema (DCBE) has poor sensitivity to detect polyps and cancers. In a recent trial, DCBE missed 26% of rectosigmoid adenomas >1 cm and 25% of rectosigmoid cancer in patients with positive FOBTs [32]. In the National Polyp Study, DCBE detected only 48% of polyps >1 cm in size [33]. Because of the absence of data on DCBE in screening populations, combined with significant deficits in sensitivity, DCBE is generally not used as a primary screening strategy in average-risk persons.

Because of the evolution in computer-assisted radiographic images, computerized tomographic (CT) colonography and magnetic resonance (MR) colonography have been introduced as alternative methods for colorectal cancer screening. Though a recent study demonstrated high sensitivity and specificity in detecting colonic polyps [34], very few data are currently available in screening populations. At this time, CT and MR colonography are not recommended for colorectal cancer screening.

What should be the upper age limit for colorectal cancer screening in the elderly? So far, none of the national guidelines have provided an upper age limit for colorectal cancer screening; however, screening for any condition should stop when the risk of screening outweighs any potential benefits. Comorbid conditions that limit a patient's longevity need to be weighed against the potential survival benefit gained by the proposed screening test [35]. Given the dwell time of approximately 7–12 years for normal mucosa to develop into a cancer, screening should be discontinued in patients with estimated survival of less than approximately 10 years. Based on individual life expectancy in the United States, this occurs at the age of approximately 80 years in the absence of comorbid conditions [35]. This age cutoff, of course, is arbitrary. On the other hand, if patients older than 80 years have never had colorectal cancer screening, particularly colonoscopy, then the yield of screening is particularly high because the incidence of colorectal cancer continues to rise with advancing age. In summary, primary care providers should utilize an individualized approach considering the patient's age, comorbid conditions, estimated life expectancy and whether prior screening has been performed when considering colorectal cancer screening in each elderly patient.

Treatment of Colorectal Cancer in the Elderly

Staging and Prognostic Factors
The most widely used clinical and pathological staging for colorectal cancer is the Astler-Coller modification of the Dukes classification [36]. This system is based on the depth of tumor invasion into and through the intestinal wall, the number of regional lymph nodes involved and the presence or absence of distant metastasis. The TNM staging classification is also well accepted. This later classification has been modified to correlate with the Dukes system for staging colorectal cancers [36]. Pathological staging is the most important prognostic factor after surgical resection of colorectal cancers. The 5-year survival rates for surgically resected disease are stage dependent, being 100%, 90–97%, 63–78% and 26–56% for stages 0, I, II and III, respectively [37, 38]. On the other hand, the survival rates classified by the Astler-Coller modification of the Dukes system are 97%, 78%, 48–74% and 4% for stages A, B, C and D, respectively [37, 39]. Other factors associated with poor prognosis are bowel obstruction or perforation, an elevated preoperative serum carcinoembryonic antigen level and deletion in chromosome 18 [1].

Treatment
Surgical resection is the initial treatment of choice in elderly as in younger patients. The operative risk may be substantial in elderly patients because of comorbid conditions, such as cardiopulmonary disorders. In one study, the postoperative mortality in patients who had been operated on for colorectal cancer was 3.7% in patients 70–79 years old, 9.8% in those 80–89 years old and 12.9% in those >90 years [35, 40]. However, a recent study demonstrated that

the mortality rate for elderly patients undergoing surgical resection for colorectal cancer did not differ from that of younger patients, provided that the overall medical status was optimized [41]. A similar result was reported by a German group, who found that age per se is not a contraindication to colorectal surgery, especially during an elective tumor resection and when there is enough time to optimize other comorbid conditions [42]. However, there was a definite increase in mortality with age during emergency operations, especially in those patients with coexisting cardiopulmonary diseases [42].

In colon cancer, the need for postsurgical treatment is dictated primarily by the stage of the cancer. For patients with node-positive (stage III) disease, adjuvant treatment with fluorouracil and levamisole reduces the risk of death by 33% as compared to surgery alone [43]. Later studies demonstrated similar benefits from adjuvant chemotherapy with fluorouracil and leucovorin [44, 45]. Currently, fluorouracil plus leucovorin for 6–8 months is standard adjuvant treatment for stage III colon cancer after surgery. A recent pooled-analysis study demonstrated that patients with stage II colon cancer also received the same benefit from fluorouracil-based adjuvant therapy [46]. The 5-year overall survival rate was 71% for those who received adjuvant therapy, as compared with 64% for those not treated [46].

Though adjuvant chemotherapy is effective, elderly patients may not be offered chemotherapy or may choose not to be treated with chemotherapy because of a perception that they will have greater toxic effects or tolerate the treatment poorly. However, one randomized trial demonstrated no significant difference in the side effects of fluorouracil-based chemotherapy among all age groups [47]. A recent study also found that elderly patients did not have higher rates of nausea or vomiting, stomatitis or diarrhea than younger patients when treated with fluorouracil plus either leucovorin or levamisole. On the other hand, the incidence of leukopenia was significantly higher among elderly patients who received fluorouracil plus levamisole, but among those who received fluorouracil plus leucovorin, the increase was of borderline significance [46]. In summary, there is no important increase in side effects in healthy elderly patients treated with chemotherapeutic regimens compared to those experienced by younger patients.

Palliative therapy is an important consideration in elderly patients with colon cancer because 30% are not candidates for surgery [1]. Palliative resection can be helpful in providing control of bleeding and obstructive symptoms. Other nonsurgical palliative therapies include cryotherapy, electrocoagulation and radiotherapy, but their use is limited by frequent complications [1, 48]. Stent placement is an effective therapy for obstruction in the patient who is not a surgical candidate. Stent placement can also allow a one-stage surgical approach in the obstructed patient. The choice of treatment modality should be individualized to each patient.

Summary

Colorectal cancer is the second leading cause of cancer death in the United States. Age is a powerful risk factor for the development of colorectal cancer. The prevalence of adenomas increases with advancing age. Most cancers still occur in the distal colon; however, in the elderly population, there is a shift of the location of colorectal cancer toward the proximal colon. Thus, colonoscopy every 10 years is a particularly appropriate colorectal cancer screening strategy in the elderly. Surgical resection is the initial treatment of choice for colorectal cancer in elderly as in younger patients. Adjuvant chemotherapy should be considered in patients with stage III disease and in some patients with stage II disease. There is no significant increase in side effects in healthy elderly patients treated with chemotherapeutic regimens compared to those in younger patients. Management decisions in the elderly should follow the same principles as those in younger patients. A thorough medical evaluation of elderly patients is necessary to evaluate the patient's risk and to optimize surgical and therapeutic regimens.

References

1   Sial SH, Catalano MF: Gastrointestinal tract cancer in the elderly. Gastroenterol Clin North Am 2001;30:565–590.
2   Greenlee RT, Murray T, Bolden S, Wingo PA: Cancer statistics, 2000. CA Cancer J Clin 2000; 50:7–33.
3   Winawer SJ, Zauber AG, Ho MN, et al: Prevention of colorectal cancer by colonoscopic polypectomy. N Engl J Med 1993;329:1977–1981.
4   McCashland TM, Brand R, Lyden E, de Garmo P: Gender differences in colorectal polyps and tumors. Am J Gastroenterol 2001;96:882–886.
5   Rex DK, Lehman GA, Ulbright TM, Smith JJ, Pound DC, Hawes RH, Helper DJ, Wiersema MJ, Langefeld CD, Li W: Colonic neoplasia in asymptomatic persons with negative fecal occult blood tests: Influence of age, gender, and family history. Am J Gastroenterol 1993;88:825–831.
6   Issa JPJ, Ottaviano YL, Celano P, Hamilton SR, Davidson NE, Baylin SB: Methylation of the oestrogen receptor CpG island links aging and neoplasia in human colon. Nat Genet 1994;7:536–540.
7   Everson GT, McKinley C, Kern F Jr: Mechanisms of gallstone formation in women. Effect of exogenous estrogen (Premarin) and dietary cholesterol on hepatic lipid metabolism. J Clin Invest 1991;87:237–246.
8   Campagnoli C, Biglia N, Altare F, Lanza MG, Lesca L, Cantamessa C, Peris C, Fiorucci GC, Sismondi P: Differential effects of oral conjugated estrogens and transdermal estradiol on insulin-like growth factor I, growth hormone and sex hormone binding globulin serum levels. Gynecol Endocrinol 1993;7:251–258.
9   Atkin WS, Morson BC, Cuzick J: Long term risk of colorectal cancer after excision of rectosigmoid adenomas. N Engl J Med 1992;326:658–662.
10 Spencer RJ, Melton LJ III, Ready RL, Ilstrup DM: Treatment of small colorectal polyps: A population-based study of the risk of subsequent carcinoma. Mayo Clin Proc 1984;59:305–310.
11 Fante R, Benatti P, di Gregorio C, De Pietri S, Pedroni M, Tamassia MG, Percesepe A, Rossi G, Losi L, Roncucci L, Ponz de Leon M: Colorectal carcinoma in different age groups: A population-based investigation. Am J Gastroenterol 1997;92:1505–1509.

12   Rex DK, Weddle RA, Lehman GA, Pound DC, O'Connor KW, Hawes RH, Dittus RS, Lappas JC, Lumeng L: Flexible sigmoidoscopy plus air contrast barium enema versus colonoscopy for suspected lower gastrointestinal bleeding. Gastroenterology 1990;98:855–861.

13   Arminski TC, McLean DW: Incidence and distribution of adenomatous polyps of the colon and rectum based on 1000 autopsy examinations. Dis Colon Rectum 1964;7:249–261.

14   Vatn MH, Stalsberg H: The prevalence of polyps of the large intestine in Oslo: An autopsy study. Cancer 1982;49:819–825.

15   Kosary CL, Ries LAG, Miller BA, Hankey BF, Harras A, Edwards BK (eds): SEER Cancer Statistics Review, 1973–1992: Tables and Graphs; NIH Pub. No. 96-2789. Bethesda, National Cancer Institute, National Institute of Health, 1995.

16   Rex DK, Rahmani EY, Haseman JH, Lemmel GT, Kaster S, Buckley JS: Relative sensitivity of colonoscopy and barium enema for detection of colorectal cancer in clinical practice. Gastroenterology 1997;12:17–23.

17   Macrae FA, St John DJ: Relationship between patterns of bleeding and Hemoccult sensitivity in patients with colorectal cancers or adenomas. Gastroenterology 1982;82:891–898.

18   Vogelstein B, Fearson ER, Hamilton SR, Kern SE, Preisinger AC, Leppert M, Nakamura Y, White R, Smits AM, Bos JL: Genetic alterations during colorectal tumor development. N Engl J Med 1988;319:525–532.

19   Villavicencio RT, Rex DK: Colonic adenomas: Prevalence and incidence rates, growth rates, and miss rates at colonoscopy. Semin Gastrointest Dis 2000;11:185–193.

20   Carroll RLA, Klein M: How often should patients be sigmoidoscoped? A mathematical perspective. Prev Med 1980;9:741–746.

21   Figiel LS, Figiel SJ, Wieterson FK: Roentgenologic observation of growth rates of colonic polyps and carcinoma. Acta Radiol Diagn 1965;3:417–429.

22   Luk GD: Colonic polyps. Benign and premalignant neoplasms of the colon; in Yamada T, Alpers DH, Powell DW, Owyang C, Silverstein FE (eds): Textbook of Gastroenterology. Philadelphia, Lippincott, 1995, pp 1911–1943.

23   Kozuka S, Nogaki M, Ozeki T, Masumori S: Premalignancy of the mucosal polyp in the large intestine. 2. Estimation of the periods required for malignant transformation of mucosal polyps. Dis Colon Rectum 1975;18:494–500.

24   Rex DK, Johnson DA, Lieberman DA, Burt RW, Sonnenberg A: Colorectal cancer prevention 2000: Screening recommendations of the American College of Gastroenterology. Am J Gastroenterol 2000;95:868–877.

25   Lemmel GT, Haseman JH, Rex DK, Rahmani E: Neoplasia distal to the splenic flexure in patients with proximal colon cancer. Gastrointest Endosc 1996;44:109–111.

26   Dinning JP, Hixon LJ, Clark LC: Prevalence of distal colonic neoplasia associated with proximal colon cancer. Ann Intern Med 1994;154:854–856.

27   Rex DK, Chak A, Vasudeva R, Gross T, Lieberman D, Bhattacharya I, Sack E, Wiersema M, Farraye F, Wallace M, Barrido D, Cravens E, Zeabart L, Bjorkman D, Lemmel T, Buckley S: Prospective determination of distal colon findings in average-risk patients with proximal colon cancer. Gastrointest Endosc 1999;49:727–730.

28   Lieberman DA, Weiss DG, Bond JH, Ahnen DJ, Garewal H, Chejfec G: Use of colonoscopy to screen asymptomatic adults for colorectal cancer. Veterans Affairs Cooperative Study Group 380. N Engl J Med 2000;343:162–168.

29   Imperiale TF, Eagner DR, Lin CY, Larkin GN, Rogge JD, Ransohoff DF: Risk of advanced proximal neoplasms in asymptomatic adults according to the distal colorectal findings. N Engl J Med 2000;343:169–174.

30   Mandel JS, Bond JH, Church TR, Snover DC, Bradley GM, Schuman LM, Ederer F: Reducing mortality from colorectal cancer by screening for fecal occult blood. Minnesota Colon Cancer Control Study. N Engl J Med 1993;328:1365–1371.

31   Kronborg O, Fenger C, Olsen J, Jorgensen OD, Sondergaard O: Randomised study of screening for colorectal cancer with faecal-occult-blood test. Lancet 1996;348:1467–1471.

32   Kewenter J, Brevinge H, Engaras B, Haglind E: The yield of flexible sigmoidoscopy and double-contrast barium enema in the diagnosis of neoplasms in the large bowel in patients with a positive Hemoccult test. Endoscopy 1995;27:159–163.

33   Winawer SJ, Stewart ET, Zauber AG, Bond JH, Ansel H, Waye JD, Hall D, Hamlin JA, Schapiro M, O'Brien MJ, Sternberg SS, Gottlieb LS: A comparison of colonoscopy and double-contrast barium enema for surveillance after polypectomy. National Polyp Study Work Group. N Engl J Med 2000; 342:1766–1772.

34   Fenlon HM, Nunes DP, Schroy PC 3rd, Barish MA, Clarke PD, Ferrucci JT: A comparison of virtual and conventional colonoscopy for the detection of colorectal polyps. N Engl J Med 1999; 341:1496–1503.

35   Miller KM, Waye JD: Approach to colon polyps in the elderly. Am J Gastroenterol 2000;95: 1147–1151.

36   The National Cancer Institute (NCI) Surveillance, Epidemiology, and End Results (SEER): http://seer.cancer.gov/Publications/SummaryStage/.

37   Cohen AM, Tremiterra S, Candela F, Thaler HT, Sigurdson ER: Prognosis of node-positive colon cancer. Cancer 1991;67:1859–1861.

38   Cohen AM, Minsky BD, Schilsky RL: Cancer of the colon; in Devita VT Jr, Hellman S, Rosenberg SA (eds): Principles and Practice of Oncology. Philadelphia, Lippincott-Raven, 1997, p 166.

39   Willett CG, Tepper JE, Cohen AM, Orlow E, Welch CE: Failure patterns following curative resection of colonic carcinoma. Ann Surg 1984;200:685–690.

40   Damhuis RAM, Wereldsma JC, Wiggers T: The influences of age on resection rates and postoperative mortality in 6457 patients with colorectal cancer. Int J Colorectal Dis 1996;1:45–48.

41   Cohen AM, Shank B, Freidman MA: Colorectal cancer; in Devita VT, Hellman S, Rosenberg SA (eds): Cancer: Principles and Practice of Oncology. Philadelphia, Lippincott, 1989, pp 895–964.

42   Wolters U, Isenberg J, Stutzer H: Colorectal carcinoma – aspects of surgery in the elderly. Anticancer Res 1997;17:1273–1276.

43   Laurie JA, Moertel CG, Fleming TR, et al: Surgical adjuvant therapy of large-bowel carcinoma: An evaluation of levamisole and the combination of levamisole and fluorouracil. J Clin Oncol 1989;7:1447–1456.

44   O'Connell MJ, Laurie JA, Kahn M, Fitzgibbons RJ Jr, Erlichman C, Shepherd L, Moertel CG, Kocha WI, Pazdur R, Wieand HS, Rubin J, Vukov AM, Donohue JH, Krook JE, Figueredo A: Prospectively randomized trial of postoperative adjuvant chemotherapy in patients with high-risk colon cancer. J Clin Oncol 1998;16:295–300.

45   Francini G, Petrioli R, Lorenzini L, et al: Folinic acid and 5-fluorouracil as adjuvant chemotherapy in colon cancer. Gastroenterology 1994;106:899–906.

46   Sargent D, Goldberg RM, Jacobson SD, Macdonald JS, Labianca R, Haller DG, Shepherd LE, Seitz JF, Francini G: A pooled analysis of adjuvant chemotherapy for resected colon cancer in elderly patients. N Engl J Med 2001;345:1091–1097.

47   Aschele C, Guglielmi A, Tixi LM, Bolli E, Mori AM, Lionetto R, Rosso R, Sobrero A: Adjuvant treatment of colorectal cancer in the elderly. Cancer Control 1995;2(2 suppl 1):36–38.

48   Catalano M, Levin B: Cancer of the colon and rectum. Clin Geriatr Med 1991;7:331–346.

Douglas K. Rex, MD, FACG
Professor of Medicine, Division of Gastroenterology and Hepatology,
Department of Medicine, 550 N. University Boulevard, UH 2300, Indianapolis, IN 46202 (USA)
Tel. +1 317 274 0912, Fax +1 317 274 0975, E-Mail drex@iupui.edu

Author Index

Subject Index

Epidermal growth factor receptor,
    expression in gastrointestinal cancers
    50, 51
Esophageal body, aging changes 41, 75
Esophageal cancer
    adenocarcinoma 91
    epidemiology 3, 89, 91
    esophageal dysphagia 89–91
    squamous cell cancer
        clinical features 89
        lesion detection 89
        treatment 90, 91
Esophageal webs, dysphagia association
    89
Esophagitis, epidemiology 3, 4

Fecal incontinence
    causes 196
    epidemiology 8
    treatment 196

Gallbladder cancer, epidemiology 7
Gallstone, epidemiology 7
Gastric cancer
    classification 146
    clinical presentation 146, 147, 155
    computed tomography 150, 151
    diagnosis
        barium meal 150
        endoscopy 148–151
        laboratory tests 148
    epidemiology 5, 50, 51, 145, 146
    epidermal growth factor receptor
        expression 50
    etiology 147, 148
    Helicobacter pylori infection 147, 148
    management
        chemotherapy 153, 154
        palliative therapy 154, 155
        surgery 151–153, 155
    metastasis 155
Gastric mucosa
    acid secretion 46
    aging changes 43, 44, 46
    non-steroidal antiinflammatory drug
        susceptibility, see Non-steroidal
        antiinflammatory drug gastropathy

proliferative activity
    cell cycle regulation 48
    gastrectomy effects 46
    growth factors and receptors 48–50
    nutrition effects 49
    rat studies 47, 48
protective function classification 119,
    120
Gastroesophageal reflux disease
    consequences 74, 84
    diagnosis
        barium radiography 104
        endoscopy 104
        manometry 105
        pH testing 104, 105
        proton pump inhibitor trial 105
    epidemiology 2, 3, 84, 100
    esophageal dysphagia 84–86
    Helicobacter pylori infection 132, 133
    pathophysiology 100, 101
    risk factors 101, 102
    swallowing anatomy and physiology
        40–42
    symptoms 84, 85, 100–104
    treatment
        cost analysis 113
        H$_2$ blockers 85, 107, 109
        lifestyle and diet modification 85, 106
        long-term medical treatment 108–113
        prokinetic agents 85, 86, 106, 107, 109
        proton pump inhibitors 86, 107–112
        quality of life impact 111
        safety 111, 112
        short-term medical treatment 106–108
        surgery 86, 112, 113
Gastrointestinal bleeding, epidemiology 5
Geriatric assessment
    effectiveness of assessment programs
        20–23
    health status screening scales 16, 17
    historical perspective 13, 14
    inpatient setting 17
    multidimensional assessment 19
    office practice setting 17–19
    overview 12, 13
    prospects 23, 24
    structure and process 14–17